BETWEEN BENCH AND BEDSIDE

Between Bench and Bedside

Science, Healing, and Interleukin-2 in a Cancer Ward

ILANA LÖWY

HARVARD UNIVERSITY PRESS
Cambridge, Massachusetts
London, England   1996

Library of Congress Cataloging-in-Publication Data

Löwy, Ilana, 1948–
   Between bench and bedside : science, healing, and interleukin-2 in
   a cancer ward / Ilana Löwy.
      p.   cm.
   Includes index.
   ISBN 0-674-06809-2 (alk. paper)
   1. Interleukin 2—Therapeutic use.   2. Cancer—Immunotherapy.   3. Oncologists—
   Attitudes.   4. Clinical trials—Philosophy.
   I. Title.
   [DNLM: 1. Neoplasms—therapy.   2. Interleukin-2—therapeutic use.   3. Clinical Trials—
   personal narratives.   QZ   266 L922b 1996]
RC271.I47L68   1996
616.99'4061—dc20
DNLM/DLC
for Library of Congress
96–25407
      CIP

Contents

Prologue   *1*

Introduction: Observing a Clinical Experiment
in Context   *7*

1 The Culture of Clinical Experimentation in Oncology   *36*

2 Cancer Immunotherapy, 1894–1979   *84*

3 Cancer Immunotherapy and Mass Production of
Biological Agents, 1980–1990   *118*

4 The IL-2 Trial at the Cancer Foundation:
A Personal View   *164*

5 Making the IL-2 Trial Work: Professional Cultures,
Jurisdictions, and Practices   *219*

6 A Science-Laden Pathology between Bench
and Bedside   *279*

Notes   *289*

Acknowledgments   *363*

Index   *365*

BETWEEN BENCH AND BEDSIDE

Prologue

September 1989. I run up the stairs of the research building at the Cancer Foundation, peeling off my wet coat on the way. The rain has delayed the city buses, so I am already five minutes late for the group meeting scheduled to start at 1:30 sharp. This is the third year I have been observing the clinical trial of a new molecule, interleukin-2 (IL-2), in cancer therapy at the Cancer Foundation, a major French cancer treatment center. (In fact the term "trial" embraces several small trials, conducted and evaluated together.) As an external observer with uncertain status, I don't like to attract attention to myself by being late. Fortunately, the meeting has not started yet, although the small conference room is nearly full. Ten people are gathered around a big wooden table, chatting in small groups and trying to ignore the construction noise in the background. Several nod briefly when I enter the room, but as usual my presence doesn't attract much attention. I have become a permanent element of the background decor, like the outdated oncology textbooks in the bookcases and the yellowing, dusty photos of the Foundation's "greats" on the walls.

I am here to follow a highly publicized clinical trial: the application of interleukin-2 to cancer therapy. IL-2, a protein secreted by the white blood cells, is considered to be an important nonspecific stimulator of the immune system—the mechanisms that monitor the body's response to substances that are perceived to be "foreign," such as pathogenic bacteria, viruses, and possibly malignant cells.

I open a thick notebook, then glance around. Madeleine, a hematologist, is sitting almost, but not quite, at the head of the table, shifting her chair to situate herself in the most appropriate spot. While rearranging a thick bundle of computer printouts she occasionally looks toward the open door. François, an immunologist, and Georges, a medical oncologist, still haven't arrived, and the meeting can't start without them: the group is formally led by the trio François, Georges, and Madeleine, but François, the head of the immunology department at the Cancer Foundation Hospital, is the initiator of the trial and informally the incontestable leader of the group. Georges is responsible for the clinical tests and has all the data on the patients being treated with IL-2.

Madeleine is glancing at her watch again: it is 1:39. Just as she clears her throat to make an announcement, François rushes in. He apologizes briefly for his lateness, mentioning an important meeting, and takes his usual place at the head of the table. Madeleine swiftly moves her chair a little farther away to make their relative positions clear. She and François confer briefly in hushed voices and decide to start the meeting. Because Georges hasn't arrived yet, the usual order of discussion—first the patients, then the experimental results—will be reversed. Hoang, a Chinese postdoctoral student, opens her notebook to start presenting her results. At this point Georges arrives and seats himself behind Madeleine, away from the table. After a brief additional exchange, François, Georges, and Madeleine decide to follow the usual order of presentation.

Madeleine opens her thick folder containing the results of the blood samples of patients treated with IL-2 this week. Patients who participate in the trial receive intravenously several consecutive "induction" cycles of IL-2, separated by rest periods of five to seven days; then, if the clinical results seem encouraging and the patients are able to tolerate the therapy, after an interval of several weeks (generally three to four) they receive additional "maintenance" or "consolidation" treatment typically lasting five days. During a treatment cycle the patient receives continuous infusions of a solution of IL-2. The treatment induces severe reactions, including high fever, gastrointestinal troubles, irregular heartbeat, circulation problems, edema (swelling), and even psychiatric complications. Because these effects typically worsen over time, many patients are unable to complete the five-day treatment cycles. The blood samples, taken at the beginning and end of each treatment cycle, measure the influence of the IL-2 on their white blood cells (leukocytes). Three effects are observed: the increase in the number of white blood cells following the injection of IL-2, the increase of specific subgroups of leukocytes credited with the ability to kill cancer cells (identifiable by specific proteins—"markers"—on their surface), and the cytotoxic activity of the white blood cells—that is, their ability to destroy (to "lyse") cancer cells in the test tube under standardized conditions.

Madeleine first shows her graphics to François, who comments on them partly to himself and partly to the group. Periodically he asks Georges about the clinical status of the patients. His monologue is punctuated by Madeleine's interventions and, occasionally, Georges's brief, sometimes barely audible answers.

F.: Mr. K. Ah. I see . . . He's having a good rebound [increase in the total number of leukocytes at the beginning of a new cycle of treatment] . . . And how is his cytotoxicity? . . . Well, not bad. It might have been better.

M.: All the cytotoxicity tests seem to be low this week. Maybe there is some kind of problem with the targets [tumor cells cultivated in the laboratory, which are employed in standardized cytotoxicity tests]. They didn't look very good to me Monday. We'll have to check it.

F.: Mr K.—what is it?

G.: Mela [melanoma—a highly malignant skin cancer]. Skin and lung metastases.

F.: And his clinical status?

G.: He isn't reacting too badly to the treatment. So far. It's his third week.

F.: I see . . . It's too early for a clinical evaluation. He looks all right to me. It's promising. And this is Ms. N. A melanoma too. Well, she seems to be doing rather poorly. Low OKT-19 [a cell marker] . . . her CD-3 [another cell marker] is also not very high . . . Where is her cytotoxicity?

M.: Here.

F.: Yes. I see. It's not very good either. What about the clinics [the clinical findings]?

G.: It's her second week. Can't tolerate the treatment. Crazy as a bat. Went completely nuts after two days. Her platelet count is very low. [Platelets are responsible for blood clotting.] We stopped the treatment on the third day.

F.: Are you going to drop her from the program?

G.: We haven't decided yet. Maybe we'll try again next week.

F.: Mr. F. . . . Mr. F. . . . Who is Mr. F.? Oh, he's a new patient. It's his first week. What is it?

G.: A kidney [renal cell carcinoma—a kidney tumor].

F.: An "American?" [There are two ongoing clinical trials of IL-2 at the

Cancer Foundation. Most of the patients are in the "French" trial and are treated with IL-2 produced by a French pharmaceutical company, but some of the kidney cancer patients are participating in the "American" trial and are injected with IL-2 produced by a California-based biotechnology firm. The two products—and the two trials—are similar but not identical.]

G.: Yes. With interferon [some of the kidney cancer patients are treated with a combination of IL-2 and a second regulatory substance produced by the white blood cells, alpha interferon].

F.: He seems to be doing fine. It's too early to know, of course. And here are the data on Mr. M. . . . I see . . . It's his first week too. Also a kidney?

G.: Yes. French.

F.: O.K. We'll look at it later. Looks like a good start. The cytotoxicity results finally are not so bad this week.

M.: They were much better last week. We're going to retest all the cell lines Friday. I do feel that we have some kind of problem there. In addition I again had difficulty obtaining the eighth-day blood of some of the patients [blood samples drawn from the patients three days after the last intravenous infusion of IL-2]. I am fed up with explaining to the nurses again and again how important it is.

G.: (to whom the last comment was clearly addressed) Mmm.

F.: And here is our friend Ms. N. It's her second consolidation cure [a second stage of treatment, which follows the "inductive" stage]. She seems to be reacting well. Nice rebound. What about the clinics?

G.: She seems to be stable.

F.: Good. Mmm, I see that Mr. D. had a very good cytotoxicity this week. It's his first consolidation cure, isn't it?

M.: Yes. He's on the old French protocol.

F.: And his rebound is nice too. With high CD-3. Well, he continues to have the R. profile. [Ms. R. is the exemplary success of the earlier part of the program. The R. profile is the rather unusual pattern of blood-sample response to IL-2 that, it is hoped, will turn out to indicate a good clinical outcome.] How he is doing?

G.: (almost inaudibly) Regrowing [the tumor is growing back].

F.: But . . . his cutaneous metastases were all melting away just two weeks ago?

G.: He is regrowing now.

F.: That's surprising. His biological results look really good. Well . . . perhaps they have gone down a little bit. Yes . . . I see . . . maybe. We'll have to look at it more carefully. Are there more patients?

M.: No. That's all for today.

F.: What are the plans?

G.: A new melanoma is scheduled for next week. And two more kid-
  neys for the week after.
F.: French?
G.: One French, one American.
F.: Well, if there are no more patients, we can start looking at the lab
  results. Hoang, you may go ahead now.

I sit at the other end of the table, tucked between the "mouse technician," Marie, and the intern from Georges's ward, Sandra. I try to
follow the discussion carefully while taking detailed notes. It isn't easy,
and although I concentrate on my task I will probably miss some parts
of the verbal exchange. My observer status is apparent not only from
my note-taking but also from the fact that I am the only person besides
François who is not wearing a white laboratory coat. François's street
clothes, however, indicate his managerial standing. From time to time
Sandra glances at my feverish scribbling, as if to make sure that I don't
omit some important piece of information. She seems to be favorably
impressed by my ability to decode the sometimes cryptic exchanges
around the meeting table. But at the same time she and other participants seem to wonder why I continue to spend so much time observing trivial and routine meetings. Three years ago, at its inception, the
Cancer Foundation IL-2 trial held the excitement and the promise of
the unknown, and its organizers were not surprised that an external
observer wished to study it. Now, however, it has become increasingly
evident that this trial is not very different from other attempts to improve the (low) efficacy of drug therapies in advanced cancer in adults.
This book is an attempt to answer Sandra's silent question: What can
be learned from the study of a semiroutine clinical experiment in a
cancer treatment center?

Introduction: Observing a Clinical Experiment in Context

Interleukin-2 was advanced in the mid-1980s as a highly promising experimental therapy for cancer in adults in the wake of interest in interferon, another molecule belonging to the family of cytokins (substances produced in the body that regulate cell activation). Interferon was presented in the late 1970s as a revolutionary biological therapy of cancer, a therapy that stimulates—or is believed to stimulate—the body's antitumor mechanisms. High hopes for its putative antitumor properties prompted efforts to produce large quantities of interferon through genetic engineering techniques, and in the early 1980s industrialists were able to manufacture enough to permit large-scale clinical trials. The trials revealed that although interferon indeed has therapeutic effects in selected cancers, it is far from being a "miracle cure" for common human malignancies.[1]

In the late 1970s and early 1980s intensive studies by immunologists revealed that the molecule interleukin-2, secreted by white blood cells, stimulated the proliferation of cells active in immune responses, and thus permitted the culture of these cells in the test tube. This property made IL-2 an important research tool for biologists: a molecule able to stimulate immune mechanisms and thus potentially to improve the body's ability to fight infections may have numerous clinical applications. Its first clinical trials, however, focused not on IL-2's ability to improve immune responses, but on its possible anticancer properties. In the test tube IL-2 stimulated the proliferation of specific subgroups of lymphocytes (one of the main categories of white blood cells) known as killer T cells or natural killer cells, which are able to destroy tumor cells, and high doses of the substance were found to eliminate tumors in laboratory animals. In 1984 interleukin-2 was advanced as the next promising biotherapy of cancer, and oncologists joined immunologists in laboratory studies of the molecule. A 1985 article announced that treatment with industrially produced IL-2 and interleukin-activated white blood cells led to the regression of disseminated, incurable cancers in nearly half of the treated patients. The therapy was very expensive, highly unpleasant, and occasionally dangerous, but it did produce spectacular results.[2]

Although the study involved a very small number of patients, publication of its results led immediately to more clinical trials of the new therapy, and the price of shares of the biotechnology company that produced interleukin soared.[3] But clinical trials conducted from 1985 through 1990 on a larger number of patients yielded less cause for optimism. In the early 1990s most specialists agreed that interleukin-2 has a definite but limited therapeutic effect in a few human malignancies such as melanoma and renal cell carcinoma. This restricted but real clinical efficacy should be carefully balanced in each case, the experts proposed, against the costs and severe side effects of interleukin therapy.[4]

I observed the Cancer Foundation's IL-2 trial (comprising several small clinical trials) from its inception in November 1986 until July 1990. During that time IL-2 did not become an accepted method of treating advanced cancer, but neither was it dismissed as ineffective. Short-term and even a few long-term remissions were obtained in selected patients. The Foundation's oncologists conducted new clinical experiments to test the possibilities of combining IL-2 with other anticancer drugs or of developing new uses for the molecule. In addition, the IL-2 trial stimulated new areas of immunological research and helped promote close collaboration between immunologists and oncologists. It also played a role in the administrative reorganization of the Cancer Foundation and strengthened the links between the Foundation and industrialists.

Two diametrically opposed accounts of this trial are possible: a "white" one and a "black" one. A "white" account would faithfully adopt the analytic categories and point of view of the organizers. It would hail the trial's contribution to cancer therapy, to biological and medical knowledge, and to the more efficient organization of research and therapy at the Cancer Foundation. The IL-2 trial would be presented as a significant contribution to the cure for human cancer. Although IL-2 therapy is not (yet?) an efficient cure for "responsive" cancers (melanoma and renal cell carcinoma, both rare) or for common cancers in the adult, it did lead to remissions of otherwise incurable tumors in selected patients. From the perspective of those patients and their families, this achievement was very considerable. Other patients were perhaps not helped directly, but they gained access to the best available medical care and could continue to hope for a cure. In addition, they helped to advance medical knowledge. The trial contributed to a better understanding of the physiological and therapeutic effects of IL-2 in cancer patients, and this contribution was reflected in the publication of the results of the Cancer Foundation trial in well-known medical journals.

Another important achievement of the Cancer Foundation's IL-2 trial, the "white" account would maintain, was its success in breaking the pattern of mutual distrust between clinicians and scientists there. Before the trial, these two professional groups had had only limited contact. Thanks to the IL-2 trial, clinicians became aware of the scientists' concerns and discovered which clinical problems could be answered through collaboration with a research laboratory, while scientists gained access to patient-derived biological materials (such as blood or tumor fragments) and a better understanding of what was bothering the clinicians. This mutual awareness fostered the expansion of preclinical and clinical research at the Cancer Foundation. In addition the IL-2 trial facilitated the development of institutional arrangements modeled on interactions between laboratory and clinic in leading cancer treatment centers in other Western countries (in particular the United States). The professional benefits accruing to its organizers, the "white" account would assert, were no more than normal and just rewards for their hard work, their scientific and organizational talents, and their concrete achievements in promoting research and therapy at the Cancer Foundation.

A "black" account of the Cancer Foundation's IL-2 trial would reject the organizers' analytic categories and viewpoints. The "exemplary collaboration among clinicians, scientists, and industrialists" claimed by the organizers would be framed instead in terms of self-interest and self-promotion that increased the profits of industrialists and the glory and power of selected physicians and scientists; the Cancer Foundation IL-2 trial was objectively shaped by personal ambitions, however sincerely the major actors may have believed that they were motivated solely by scientific curiosity and the desire to improve the lot of cancer patients. A talent for self-deception, the "black" account would propose, is not necessarily a virtue. One should always ask who benefits and who loses in a given clinical experiment. More-over, a dispassionate look at the results of the IL-2 trial in the years 1987–1992 reveals a striking gap between the significant professional gains enjoyed by some of the organizers and the limited or nonexistent benefits to the great majority of patients. The existence of a such gap should make us wary of accepting the actors' statements and declared beliefs at face value.

In addition, the "black" account would maintain, during the time funds were dedicated to the IL-2 trial, the standard treatment for can-cer in France was far from being satisfactory.[5] In the 1970s and 1980s French oncologists (including those at the Cancer Foundation) had complained about a shortage of nurses, a lack of adequate psycholog-ical follow-up of patients and attention to the specific needs of older persons, and even a dearth of parking spaces for ambulatory patients and their families. In theory, decisions concerning the allocation of resources to experimental therapies of malignant tumors and to rou-tine management of cancer patients are made independently, but the fact remains that the amount of money available for cancer treatment is limited and that all choices are made within this larger context. A shift in public opinion in favor of, say, assigning a high priority to palliative care or the psychological needs of patients suffering from advanced, incurable cancer would probably affect not only the distri-bution of government funds but also the policies of cancer charities. There are more efficient ways to spend public money than in funding clinical trials of dubious efficacy.[6] Finally, a "black" account would note that the IL-2 trial revealed, and then rewarded, the political and managerial talents of some of its organizers while the French health system as a whole was threatened in the 1980s by such developments as the massive HIV contamination of the blood supply and blood products. Such events should serve as a warning against privileging entrepreneurial talents at the expense of ensuring responsibility and competence in a nation's entire health care system.[7]

My study seeks to avoid oversimplified, one-dimensional black-or-white accounts through a "contextualized" (that is, "historicized" and "sociologized") study of experimentation in the clinic. Scientific and clinical experimentation is a complicated, multilayered phenomenon involving the activities of a multitude of individual and collective ac-tors, which in turn are attached to specific practices and to concrete institutions, to local events and to long-term historical developments.[8] To paraphrase the historian of science Robert Kohler, a contextualized account of a clinical trial is not interested in medical science, that is, in finished intellectual products, but in scientists and physicians who introduce medical innovations, that is, in clinical experimentation as a social process.[9] Such an account investigates how that experiment was shaped by material constraints and institutional frameworks, sociocultural variables and political considerations, local events and larger developments in science, industry, and health care. It strives to achieve a "thick description" of a given event.[10] The goal of displaying complexity should not be equated with the tendency—particularly apparent in certain brands of journalism—to present the multiple aspects of a given question merely in order to imply the desirability of a middle ground. A careful examination of all the aspects of a complicated question may indeed lead to a conclusion that the best solution is to adopt one of the existing options or to reach a middle ground, but it may also open new ways of looking at familiar problems and indicate that the initial questions were not the right ones. Thick descriptions make such shifts in perception possible.

Contextualized studies of experimentation in the clinic may become even more important in the future. The IL-2 clinical trial was completed within a traditional—that is, pre-AIDS—framework for testing new therapies, in which decisions were made exclusively by professionals: scientists, clinicians, representatives of the pharmaceutical industry, and government agencies. In the 1980s, however, the pattern of testing new therapies for potentially lethal diseases underwent radical changes. Militant activism by AIDS patients has changed not only the process of testing and approval of new anti-AIDS drugs, but also the ways of testing therapies for other life-threatening diseases. In the United States patients suffering from such diseases now have rapid access to experimental drugs through innovative programs developed by the Food and Drug Administration (FDA) as a result of pressure by AIDS activists. Several European countries have recently developed similar approaches; France, for example, now has a fast track for approval of selected new drugs.[11] These new programs, some critics have warned, may lead to the exploitation of desperate patients by profit-oriented drug manufacturers.[12] However, in the late 1980s and early 1990s many AIDS activists viewed them as an important victory for their grassroots movements.[13] In the United States, cancer patients inspired by the AIDS activists' success have created their own advocacy group, CAN-ACT. In 1989 that group asked the FDA and other government organizations to expedite the release and testing of drugs able to stimulate the immune mechanisms of the body, such as interleukin-2 and interferon. Moreover, patients' influence is not limited to indirect pressure on government agencies. In a radical change in the traditional power structure of the process of new drug approval, representatives of people with AIDS have been invited to participate in the debates of the government-sponsored AIDS Clinical Trial Group.[14] This approach, if generalized, will give patients power over decisions that were previously considered the exclusive domain of the experts, such as decisions concerning the efficacy and safety of certain medical treatments. Users of health services will be able to contribute directly to the "genesis and development of medical facts."[15]

How do patients view clinical testing for new therapies? While AIDS activists tend to be imaginative and efficient when dealing with the concrete problems of people with AIDS (food, shelter, health insurance, discrimination), when discussing science they seem to rely mainly on simplified black-and-white images, in which good scientists and physicians, wholly dedicated to rapidly producing the miracle drug that will cure AIDS, are opposed to bad scientists, physicians, and federal bureaucrats, who defend their personal and professional interests and block the efforts of the good scientists.[16] In the words of John James, a key activist in the struggle to increase the influence of persons with AIDS/HIV infection on the process of drug approval in the United States, "officially sanctioned drug development responded to commercial and institutional *interests,* not scientific, medical or humanitarian *concerns.*"[17]

Stereotyped black-or-white images of physicians and scientists are shared not only by the lay public but also by biomedical scientists and medical practitioners. The persistence of these images may be rooted in the specificity of medical research. Patients—the subjects and objects of medical intervention—are at the same time distinct and conscious individuals and "medicalized bodies" subjected to the general laws of biology. Medicine manages this contradiction rather well, and one of the sources of modern medicine's success, according to one student of medical narratives, may be its steadfast ignorance of this epistemological paradox.[18] Such unawareness is, however, not always easy to sustain. It is nearly impossible for individuals to view themselves or a loved one as a "medicalized body," and it is difficult to study the emotionally loaded activities of physicians, such as attempts to find a cure for a life-threatening disease, in the same way one studies, say, efforts to develop a more efficient dishwasher. My own investigations were affected by irrational feelings toward medical research. Having been trained as a biomedical researcher, I was familiar with the problematic aspects of that activity. Even so, I caught myself feeling angry because the investigators at the Cancer Foundation were not always as perfect as I unconsciously wished them to be. On the other hand, a nagging internal voice often whispered: "Your attempts at a sociological analysis are a meaningless academic exercise. Only one thing counts: this therapy may save the lives of numerous cancer patients. And if not this therapy, certainly the next one." Thus the "black" and "white" accounts of the IL-2 trial presented above may be seen as mirroring my own contradictory feelings about it.

The persistence of stereotypic representations of experimentation in the clinic may also reflect their usefulness in coping with severe illness. It is perhaps easier—especially for patients suffering from life-threatening diseases and for their families and friends—to subscribe to schematic images that promote faith in medical miracle-workers and attribute blame for failures to self-centered and greedy professionals. Such "decontextualized" images may, however, be a serious liability in an era in which medical interventions are increasingly complex, medical certitudes are weakening, the scope of clinical experimentation is broadening, economic considerations are given more weight in the assessment of new therapies, and patients are playing a greater role in the design and evaluation of clinical trials.[19] A better understanding of the multiple factors that shape real-life clinical experiments and a better appreciation of the institutional tangle and the emotional muddle that surround such trials may help current and future patients to attain a closer approximation of the ideal of informed consent for individuals enrolled in clinical experiments. The contextualization of clinical trials may also help to guide action. It may help researchers and observers alike to identify intentional and contingent events that shape the trajectory of a given trial, bifurcations that lead to a change in direction, points beyond which radical modifications of the trial become very difficult.[20] It may thus contribute to more effective lay intervention in the approval and release of new treatments.

Clinicians and Scientists: Two Cultures or One?

Interleukin-2 was introduced to cancer therapy following an encounter between two distinct professional groups: biologists and physicians. The existence of differences between laboratory scientists and clinicians, "mice doctors" and "people doctors," is rarely contested. Yet the development of clinical experimentation in oncology is based on the assumption that, in principle at least, cooperation between these two professional groups is unproblematic because both recognize that the combination of their efforts is a precondition for the development of a "cure for cancer." To question this assumption is to look for trouble. In negotiating access to the Cancer Foundation IL-2 trial, I explained that the aim of my study was to observe the interaction between immunologists and oncologists during the transfer of an innovation from the laboratory to the clinic. My explanation was often met with puzzlement, sometimes with suspicion. The organizers of the IL-2 trial assumed that if the interaction between clinical oncologists and biologists at the Cancer Foundation was uneasy or problematic, the reason would necessarily reside in local, contingent problems. Consequently, a researcher who proposed to focus on the relationship between the laboratory and the clinics either might be viewed as wasting time on observing trivial work-related conflicts and frictions or, worse, might be suspected of secretly aiming to uncover professional mistakes, psychological difficulties, personality clashes, struggles over small parcels of power, and other unsavory events that hamper cooperation between scientists and clinicians in any given site.

My study is written from a different point of view: the view of science studies. It proposes that the collaboration between scientists and clinicians—that is, between persons who make experimental studies in the laboratory and those directly involved in the treatment of patients, and responsible for its consequences—is far from being self-evident. The view of the physician as a professional whose task is radically distinct from that of the biomedical scientist is actively endorsed by certain categories of physicians such as family practitioners. It is propagated by philosophers of medicine who explain that because medicine, unlike science, has a strong normative dimension, a practical goal, and is involved in specific, cure-oriented manipulations, it is therefore above all a form of practical understanding and cannot be reduced to purely scientific considerations.[21] Finally, sociologists of medicine have noted that the concrete tasks of producing knowledge and of healing remain distinct and are usually accomplished by non-overlapping professional groups. Physicians and scientists differ in the training that qualifies them for their respective roles, their patterns of organization, community structures, and professional objectives.[22]

In contrast, physicians who work in "high-tech," research-oriented medical specialties such as oncology tend to develop the self-image of scientific researchers and to blur the distinction between tasks of therapy and healing. Such blurring, I would claim, does not accurately reflect daily practices in the oncology ward. Usually it is not too difficult to distinguish between routine management of cancer patients and clinical research. Thus, counting the platelets in patients' blood during the IL-2 treatment was a therapeutic activity because the relationship between a low platelet count and the possibility of serious medical complications such as internal bleeding is a largely accepted, noncontroversial notion in the management of cancer patients. In contrast, counting specific subclasses of T leukocytes in the same patients was perceived as a research activity as long as the linkage between such a count and the clinical results of IL-2 therapy was not viewed as proven and its results were not automatically translated into routine patient management. The confusion of the tasks of healing and investigation in a cancer ward does not, I propose, reflect a growing fusion of the practical aspects of these tasks, but rather the growing convergence of their representations. Such convergence is rooted in the evolution of "scientific medicine."

Laboratory and Clinics in Historical Perspective

Since the beginnings of "scientific medicine" in the second half of the nineteenth century, biomedical research and clinical practice have provided legitimacy for one another. While physicians base their claim of effectiveness upon scientific knowledge, biomedical scientists justify their research in terms of its potential contribution to the solution of major health problems. The close association between the progress of scientific knowledge, the development of a scientifically grounded, sophisticated medical technology, and the improvement of health care is a relatively recent phenomenon. It originated in the transformation of medicine into a science-based discipline.[23] Following the development of anatomically based pathology in the early nineteenth century, diseases that had previously been viewed as aggregate symptoms (fever, drowsiness) and been accessible to the physician mainly through analysis of the patient's complaints and a few external symptoms were redefined as pathological changes in organs and tissues.[24] This redefinition cast doubt on the efficacy of existing—and supposedly time-proven—traditional therapies. It became increasingly difficult to accept that emetics, tonics, or bloodletting could cure fatty degeneration of the liver or heal tubercular changes in the lungs.

At the same time, the first attempts at statistical evaluation of the effectiveness of some of these therapies (such as Pierre Louis's "numerical method") revealed that untreated patients often fared better than those receiving traditional therapies. As a consequence, some physicians advocated restraint in the use of drugs and other therapies such as enemas and bloodletting. The extreme expression of this tendency was the "therapeutic nihilism" advocated by the Vienna clinical school, active in the mid-nineteenth century and led by Karl Rokitanski and Joseph Skoda. Physicians affiliated with this school asserted that because nearly all the existing therapies were based on ignorance, it was better to abstain from using them. The rationale for this approach was the assumption—which also underlies mainstream medical thinking today—that the only truly efficient way to improve therapy is to increase the amount of fundamental medical knowledge. A logical conclusion was that the doctor's main task is not to alleviate human suffering but to study disease. As one of the leading doctors of this school put it:

> Physicians should be judged according to their knowledge, not according to the results of their therapy. One should appreciate the physician as nature's investigator, not as an individual dedicated to the act of healing . . . Our strength lies in our knowledge, not in our actions. Therapy will result from our knowledge like a fruit growing from a flower. If the natural sciences blossom, practical medicine, their fruit, will also be established.[25]

The early debates on the importance of science in medicine were confined to the medical profession, and indeed to the small fraction of physicians associated with leading medical schools and hospitals. The laboratories in which medical science first flowered—those dedicated to anatomically based pathology, histology, and physiology—were not visible, let alone accessible, to the general public. With the advent of bacteriology, however, the status of laboratories underwent dramatic change. Thanks to the political skills of the pioneers of this discipline, for the first time the public became aware of the importance of medical laboratories.[26] Newspapers, magazines, and popular books transmitted the message that laboratory science and the application of laboratory-originated technology (serotherapy, vaccines) were efficient in preventing and fighting disease. Both the self-image of physicians and the public perception of medicine were deeply affected by this transformation. The progress of medicine became increasingly identified with scientific achievements.

Not all physicians were happy with this identification. Although validation by the laboratory served the specific interest of some groups, it hampered the interests of others.[27] But the process was essentially irreversible. From the late nineteenth century on, scientific, laboratory-based medicine became indissolubly associated with leading medical institutions, while the public was educated through the press and popular books such as Paul De Kruif's *The Microbe Hunters* to expect a steady stream of science-derived "miracle drugs."[28] This expectation was reinforced by codified and dramatized stories of medical discoveries such as insulin, sulfonates, and finally penicillin and other antibiotics, which helped establish a firm linkage between medical achievements and progress in science and technology. The tendency today to criticize some of the excesses of high-tech medicine and occasionally to turn to "alternative medicines" has not undermined the basic faith of the great majority of consumers in the life-saving potential of medical technology or the widely shared belief that the prevention and cure of major health problems such as cancer and AIDS will be achieved through scientific and technological progress.

The development of "scientific medicine" has culminated in the current identification of medicine with science-based technology. Medicine, however, is seldom studied in the same way as other technologies. Among the many studies of technology transfer, only a few deal with medicine, and these usually focus on issues such as the technical aspects of the diffusion of innovations, their cost-efficiency ratio, and the obstacles (bureaucratic red tape, the conservatism of certain groups of physicians) to the smooth transition of an innovation from the laboratory to the clinic, then to its diffusion among physicians. There has been little or no attention to the influence of medical innovations on the careers of their promoters, to institutional changes produced by these innovations, or to the impact of pressures by specific interest groups within or outside the hospital on the introduction and diffusion of new medical technology. Moreover—perhaps because it is difficult to question in depth a technology that deals with human suffering and death—investigations of technology transfer in medicine have ignored the development and consolidation of medical knowledge and clinical practices.[29]

Innovative approaches to the interaction between laboratory and clinics have, however, been developed by historians of medicine and historically oriented sociologists. Recent historical studies have pointed to the role played by laboratory-originated innovations in the structure of modern medicine.[30] These studies have shown that innovations destined to improve the understanding of pathological states (for example, the thermometer, the stethoscope, laboratory analyses of urine and blood, bacteriological tests, X rays) simultaneously induced cognitive and institutional changes. They changed perceptions of pathological phenomena and of the way medicine is organized. They also played an important role in the development of medical specialties and subspecialties. Such historical and sociological studies have undermined the idealized, linear view of the progress of medical knowledge and of simple, unidirectional relationships between the laboratory and the clinics,[31] and indicated the existence of a gap between the formal rationalization of medical decisions and the actual basis on which such decisions are made.[32] In doing so they have opened the way to a critical observation of the introduction of innovations into clinical practice today.

Observing Current Medicine

Observation of "medicine in action" is one of the established occupations of sociologists of medicine. Some sociologists observe the behavior of patients and health professionals, the division of tasks in hospitals and other health care institutions, patient-doctor relationships, and the professional roles of physicians, nurses, and paramedics. However, although sociologists of medicine emphasize the role of societal factors and cultural beliefs in defining what illness is and how one should deal with it, they are reluctant to deal with the problem of the social genesis of medical knowledge. The influential work of Eliot Freidson exemplifies this trend. Freidson was eager to show the social roots of physicians' professional activities, and he dedicated a segment of his 1970 book, *Profession of Medicine,* to the "social construction of illness." At the same time Freidson distinguished between illness as a purely biophysical state and illness as a human, social state, created and shaped by human knowledge and evaluation. Physicians, being human, are bound to show bias in their judgment. However, Freidson insisted, this bias can be reduced through the progress of medical research: "The increased sophistication of medical investigations and procedures begins to remove some of the practice of subjectivity from the frail hands of the physicians."[33]

Before the 1980s, medical sociologists interested in the production of medical knowledge focused on problems labeled as social and steered away from the technical and scientific aspects of medicine. Thus, whereas the effects of obvious and hidden variations in patient populations, the influence of lay knowledge on medical behavior, and bias in medical research were acknowledged as legitimate interests, the validity of, say, the biochemical or genetic knowledge underlying diagnosis was not. Medical sociologists who did study medical knowledge were usually investigating alcoholism, hypochondria, or psychiatric disorders rather than pneumonia or cancer.[34] They were not particularly attracted by the study of experimental therapies.

The notable exceptions to this lack of interest in clinical innovations were studies by Renée Fox and Judith Swazey on the introduction of new science-based therapies—corticosteroids, hemodialysis, kidney transplantation, the artificial heart.[35] These detailed and sensitive firsthand accounts of the sociocultural background of clinical experiments in the United States presented patients' and health professionals' reactions to clinical innovations. Fox's pioneering 1959 book, *Experiment Perilous,* is based on long-term participant observation in a hospital ward specialized in experimental treatments. This highly innovative investigation focuses on the ways physicians and patients cope with stress linked to medical experimentation and gives a subtle account of the daily dilemmas of medical experimentation. However, it stops short of probing the origins and the validity of the scientific knowledge underlying medical experiments, and of examining the professional interests of the physicians who direct it. Medical science and the interactions between biological research and clinical practice are seen as self-evident and unproblematic.[36] Although many of the decisions concerning the clinical management of individual patients are shown to be difficult, decisions concerning the conduct and outcome of clinical trials appear to flow "naturally" from scientific knowledge and clinical observation. My project, in contrast, aims precisely at analyzing this seemingly natural process of the "genesis and development of medical facts."

Recent trends in the history and sociology of science have led to the emergence of "social constructionism" in the sociology of medicine.[37] According to this perspective, medical knowledge—and indeed all scientific knowledge—is constructed by scientists. This conviction is based on two assumptions. One is that all observation is theory-laden: no observations are completely free from the observer's theoretical notions and preconceived ideas. The second is that scientific theories are underdetermined by evidence: however great and varied the empirical evidence is, there will be always more than one theory able to account for it. Thus, experiments do not confront a single, clear-cut hypothesis, but rather a network of interrelated beliefs and auxiliary hypotheses.[38] The belief that scientific knowledge is constructed has stimulated the search for social conditions underlying its development. Investigators associated with this approach have enlarged their inquiry to the more technical aspects of medical knowledge and to the conditions in which this knowledge is produced and disseminated. Most of the social constructionists' studies in medicine, however, have been based on published materials and have involved only limited direct observation of the activities of physicians and medical investigators. In addition, many of these studies have been based on *a posteriori* investigations and have suffered from the difficulties inherent in such reconstructions. Only recently have students of medicine become interested in direct observation of the production of new knowledge and new practices in the clinics.[39] My previous research on the transfer of an innovation from the laboratory to the clinics—a study of the introduction of tissue typing into the clinical practice of kidney transplantation—illustrates the difficulties of constructing accurate retrospective accounts. Although that study dealt with a very recent innovation, it was carried out after the innovation had become universally accepted and after it had induced important institutional changes in the organization of kidney grafts. But interviews with the participants, which were a central source of information in my research, proved to be problematic because the professional community had already adopted a reconstructed and standardized "discovery account" of the innovation, and this account shaped and distorted the actual participants' memories.[40] As a result of this experience, I vowed that my next research project would focus on medical sciences in the making and would entail direct observation of the sites in which new medical knowledge was being produced.

Observing Laboratories: The Advantages and Disadvantages of "Native Competence"

Sociologists started to observe hospitals in the 1950s, but the sociological observation of scientific laboratories is a much more recent phenomenon. In the 1950s and 1960s the sociology of knowledge was dominated by Robert K. Merton's approach, which excluded the sociology of knowledge from the preoccupations of sociologists of science.[41] Accordingly, the sociologists of science who did study scientific practice and scientific laboratories focused on issues such as social stratification, division of labor, and normative and reward structures.[42] New developments in the history and sociology of science, stimulated by debates on Thomas Kuhn's *Structure of Scientific Revolutions,* renewed interest in the sociology of scientific knowledge.[43] One result of this interest was the birth of a tradition of laboratory studies. Since the mid-1970s investigators have used anthropological and ethnomethodological approaches to observe the details of "laboratory life" and to learn *in situ* how knowledge is manufactured and how scientific facts emerge.[44] Several major studies of this kind had already been published when, in 1986, I began my observations of the introduction of IL-2 to cancer treatment, among them works by Harry M. Collins (1975), Bruno Latour and Steve Woolgar (1979), Karen Knorr-Cetina (1981), Andrew Pickering (1981), Michael Zenzen and Sal Restivo (1982), S. Leigh Star (1983), Michael Lynch (1985), and Trevor J. Pinch (1985).[45] Moreover, several of the "laboratory ethnologists" had observed biology and biochemistry laboratories: Latour and Woolgar had investigated a biochemistry laboratory, Lynch and Star (separately) neuroscience laboratories, and Knorr-Cetina a protein chemistry laboratory. I was therefore able to benefit from their experience.

Most laboratory ethnographies were the work of "naive" observers—sociologists, anthropologists, historians, philosophers—who ventured into the foreign land of a scientific laboratory to observe modern science. Their lack of familiarity with the setting they were investigating gave them a methodological advantage. As strangers to the culture under study, they were able to notice, and then to analyze, phenomena that both the "natives" (scientists, technicians) and observers familiar with the scientific culture usually took for granted. They were able to make visible and explicit tacit and unarticulated knowledge. Latour and Woolgar have strongly defended the advantages of being a naive observer in a laboratory: "The dangers of going native are particularly marked in the study of science, because as analysts we are inevitably caught up in the 'social science' tradition with explicit attempts to mimic natural science, and because of the currently widespread acceptance of the methods and achievements of science in the culture of which we are part."[46]

This approach to laboratory studies is not, however, the only possible one. Collins and Pinch advocate an alternative method for the observation of science: "participant comprehension" based on the acquisition of "native competence."[47] When Collins and Pinch observed the methods of investigation of paranormal phenomena, they were actively involved in these studies and finally became recognized specialists in testing these phenomena. Drawing on their experience, they affirmed that the disadvantages of "participant comprehension" were compensated by the advantage of directly experiencing the problems of the scientists they studied. Their insider status in studies of paranormal perception allowed them to observe phenomena such as the pressure of "official" science on "fringe" science, the experimenters' interactions with the media, with the subjects of their experiments, and with scientific colleagues, all of which, they affirmed, would be very difficult for less involved observers to perceive. Collins and Pinch acquired their unique inside knowledge during their study, attaining native competence only near the end of the project. The other possibility is to take "natives" and to train them as sociologists. For example, in the early days of the Chicago school of sociology, Robert Park trained members of specific social groups as sociologists. A probation officer later studied youthful delinquents, a social worker studied the ghetto, and an ex-hobo wrote a book on the hobo culture.[48] A similar approach has recently been used in medical sociology; nurses were trained as sociologists and returned to hospital wards as participant observers, usually working full-time or part-time in nursing.[49]

I was trained as an immunologist, and before turning to science studies I worked for ten years in immunological research. I did not, however, see my position as an inside observer of biomedical research as a handicap. Although naive observers are able to perceive some of the particularities of the observed culture invisible to "natives," familiarity with the language and the customs of the observed "tribe" may be an important asset, particularly if the goal is to provide a thick description of the phenomena being studied. My conviction that inside observers can be efficient students of science is rooted in, among other things, my previous studies of the historical and sociological work of Ludwik Fleck. Fleck is today viewed as a pioneer in the sociology of science.[50] In his articles, and especially in his 1935 book, *Genesis and Development of a Scientific Fact,* he developed his ideas on the social construction of scientific knowledge. He stressed the importance of

collective structures—"thought-collectives"—in the forn
entific ideas and observations. Fleck's ideas influenced Kui
of science and those of promoters of the sociology of sciei
edge. Fleck himself was not, however, a professional so
philosopher. He was a practicing bacteriologist and im
with no formal training in the humanities or social scienc
highly original thought has its roots in his scientific prac
theoretical outlook stemmed from his reflections on bacter
immunology in the 1920s and 1930s, while his critical perce
sharpened by his theoretical and institutional marginality
profession. Fleck's analyses of concrete examples of scientis
ior in the laboratory are among the best descriptions of ¡
practices in the sociological literature.[52] Fleck's example sh
native competence and total immersion in laboratory life are
essarily obstacles to perceptive historical reflection and soc
observation.

Fleck developed his theoretical thought in nearly complete is
In contrast, during my observation of the IL-2 experiment
tained strong links with sociologists and historians of science a
efited from their collective experience and from the generous
many colleagues. My concurrent immersion in studies of lat¡
teenth- and early twentieth-century medicine and philosophy o
icine also helped me to maintain some objective distance in r€
to the biomedical culture I was studying. Like Fleck, however,
observing a field in which I had a native competence. My profes¡
experience as a cellular immunologist was comparable to the pi
sional experience of most of the participants in the IL-2 study anc
acquired in a similar institutional setting. Ethnology has been de¡
by Clifford Geertz as "our own construction of other people's
struction of what they and their compatriots are up to."[53] In my st
I was one step closer to "other people's constructions" than an ave¡
anthropologist is. I was unable to know with certainty what the
vestigators I was observing were "up to," but it is reasonable to assu
that my educated guesses on this subject were as good as those of a
of their own colleagues. Latour and Woolgar's question "How do ¡
know that they know?"[54] could, in my case, be answered: probably
the same way they know that they know.

My experience as an immunologist greatly facilitated my entry int
the field during the IL-2 trial. I was familiar with the theoretical back

ground and technical details. I was already acquainted with some of the scientists I was to observe. In addition, while I had worked in immunology laboratories I had developed friendly relations with other immunologists at the Foundation. Those scientists were not directly involved in the IL-2 project, but their help was invaluable to my study. They supplied important information about the general policies of the institution, its internal conflicts and problems, and how the IL-2 trial was viewed by other scientists there.

My training in immunology was particularly important in the first part of my investigation. It is unlikely that a truly external observer would have been admitted to the very first stages of a new clinical experiment or would even have known that such an experiment was planned. My technical knowledge gave me easy access to numerous sources of information and facilitated my integration into the group. On the other hand, it was sometimes a hindrance. Several of the scientists in the project had difficulty understanding why a qualified immunologist with reasonably good career perspectives would abandon the bench for such an "exotic" occupation as science studies. They listened politely to my explanations but clearly did not really believe them. It took me a while to realize that some of them viewed my request to participate actively in the project—a very ordinary proposal from the point of view of a sociologist familiar with participant-observer techniques—as an expression of a wish to return to the laboratory, and an indirect admission that I had made a mistake in leaving experimental work. My professional identity and my place in the IL-2 trial were never entirely clarified. One consequence of this lingering ambiguity was frequent renegotiation and modification of my status as an observer. My specific position as an ex-immunologist-turned-sociologist probably also affected the scope of my observations. For example, it is possible—though difficult to prove—that things were hidden from me that would not have been concealed from a naive observer. It is also reasonable to assume that the unavoidable changes in the area observed that are induced by the presence of an external observer would have been different had I been a naive student of science.

As a trained biologist I was usually perceived by the researchers in the immunology laboratory as "one of us." But I was also viewed as a possibly dangerous or at least a disturbing presence, with latent potential to uncover the dark side of laboratory life. Any external

observer studying such a delicate subject as clinical experimentation in oncology would probably be viewed as a potential danger, but my technical knowledge and my insider/outsider status probably made my presence even more unsettling. I developed friendly relationships with many of the scientists and physicians in the IL-2 project, and my presence in the IL-2 group meetings was usually well-tolerated or politely ignored. However, each time a potentially disruptive incident happened—an obvious error made by the hospital's physicians, a violent verbal interaction between several persons in the group, an indiscreet remark concerning a colleague—heads automatically turned in my direction, and there was uneasiness in the air.

One way to limit the uneasiness linked to the presence of an external observer in the IL-2 group was to rename my role. When I first arrived at the Cancer Foundation I was called—in particular when introduced nonparticipants in the trial—our epistemologist" (that is, in the French context, a philosopher). Clearly, a philosopher was viewed as a less dangerous, and probably also more prestigious, person than a sociologist. I repeatedly protested, explaining that I was not a philosopher, and that my aim was not a general reflection on the nature of biomedical research but a detailed study of a specific clinical experiment in context. Finally a compromise was found. From "our epistemologist" I was transformed into "our historian"—a definition that was acceptable to me and less threatening to the group. The advantages of the new definition of my role were neatly captured by the group's leader, François, who later, each time he introduced me to newcomers to the IL-2 group, explained in a mockingly serious tone: "ours is indeed a very important study. Look, we even have our own historian. The person over there is present at all our meetings and writes down every single word we utter, so that nothing will be lost for future generations."

The ambiguity of my position at the Cancer Foundation—an insider, an ex-collaborator and still a colleague, and/or an external, potentially threatening observer—was mirrored not only in the way others viewed me but also in my own feelings. Back in the laboratory after an interval of several years, I wanted both to be accepted as a colleague by other participants and to be fully recognized in my singularity as a historian-sociologist of science and medicine. I constantly oscillated between two frames of reference—the old, "scientific" one and the new, "sociological" one. Sometimes I experienced a feeling of superiority because of my supposedly broader point of view, but at least as often I felt awkward and inadequate both as an immunologist and as a sociologist. My rather complicated *exercice de style* at the Cancer Foundation forced me to reevaluate both my past assumptions as an experimental scientist and my present assumptions as a historian and a sociologist.

The ambiguities pertaining to my status in the IL-2 trial operated only in my interactions with scientists (or with physicians who were working as scientific researchers). They did not extend to relationships with clinicians. I have no medical training and no experience in treating patients, and was therefore a true external observer of the physicians' work. My investigation of the medical aspects of the IL-2 trial was limited. It did not include direct contacts with patients or extended observations at an oncology ward. I justified the omission of the patients' point of view on the grounds that my research subject was already complicated and that I lacked familiarity with methods employed by medical sociologists in studying patients. My reluctance to have direct contacts with cancer patients was, however, far from being motivated by methodological considerations only. Undoubtedly I would have felt less resistance to extending my study to the users of a new technology if I had been observing, say, the production of fertilizers or computers. From a science studies point of view pharmacological manipulation of a cancer patient is not in principle very different from tinkering with electrodes during the construction of a laser.[55] But the emotional impact of observing terminal patients is obviously not the same as that of looking at pieces of wire. It is difficult to ignore the fact that sick persons, unlike instruments or chemical reagents, communicate their reactions to the way they are manipulated—they are not only objects but also subjects. In addition, researchers who observe patients cannot forget that at any moment they may themselves become the objects of the technological activity they are studying: every human being is a potential patient. The observation of a clinical experiment in an oncology ward was already a difficult experience. The inclusion of terminally ill patients as objects of study was, I felt, just too much.

Organization and Rationale

The choice of the Cancer Foundation IL-2 trial as the subject of my study was at least partly fortuitous: the trial started while I was looking for a "typical" example of the application of a new, science-based

technology to therapy, and I was acquainted with some of the participants. The trial also seemed particularly suitable for my research
purposes. It promised to be an important clinical experiment, and
moreover I was familiar with the scientific background of this trial
and had some knowledge of its institutional context. In addition, unlike most clinical trials dominated by clinicians, the IL-2 trial at the
Cancer Foundation was initiated and led by a laboratory-based immunologist. It therefore seemed particularly appropriate for a study
of the interactions between physicians and scientists.

At first I did not question the reasons for the study of the therapeutic
effects of IL-2 at the Cancer Foundation. This clinical trial was
grounded in what seemed to be uncontested immunological knowledge and had been preceded by extensive animal experimentation. The
IL-2 treatment was to be applied to cancer patients who could not be
helped by any existing therapy and who were therefore obvious candidates for an experimental treatment. Moreover, the Cancer Foundation IL-2 trial was not the first of its kind. It faithfully reproduced
similar experiments conducted in prestigious medical institutions in
the United States. Only gradually did I realize that clinical trials of IL-
2 were in fact more problematic. In preliminary experiments in humans, IL-2 had been found to be more toxic than previously thought,
the usefulness of the injection of IL-2-activated lymphocytes was contested, and the clinical results obtained in cancer patients were not
very impressive.[56] Early hopes of rapidly increasing the efficacy of the
IL-2 treatment or of reducing its toxicity were not fulfilled during the
first years of the introduction of the therapy. Nonetheless, in the years
1985–1990 more and more leading cancer centers conducted clinical
trials of IL-2. I gradually became interested not only in *how* the Cancer
Foundation trial was being conducted, but also in *why*. The two questions, I found, were closely related. The cognitive, social, and political
conditions that favored the initial spread of clinical trials of IL-2 also
shaped the form these trials took. This brought me to a larger interest
in clinical trials, in the history of cancer immunotherapy, in the culture
of clinical experimentation in oncology, and in the specific history of
IL-2 as an anticancer drug.

Chapters 1 through 3 analyze the historical and social background of
the Cancer Institute IL-2 trial: the development of a distinct culture of
clinical experimentation in the oncology clinics, the history of the application of immunological methods to cancer therapy, and the specific
story of IL-2 as cancer therapy.

Chapter 1 discusses the origins and current development of the culture of clinical experimentation in oncology. The treatment of advanced, inoperable cancer is closely associated in the West with the expansion of experimental therapies. From the 1970s on, oncologists have increasingly tended to view clinical trials of new anticancer therapies not as an exceptional, research-centered approach, but as a routine way to deal with advanced cancer. This unusual shift in the meaning of clinical trials has its roots in the history of cancer chemotherapy. The introduction of chemotherapy into cancer treatment after the Second World War was directly linked to the slightly earlier development of large-scale clinical trials of new drugs (such as antibiotics). In the 1960s and 1970s oncologists elaborated successful chemotherapies for several types of cancer, in particular for the majority of childhood cancers. This success led to the belief that efficient drug therapies would be found for other types of cancer too. Once this belief was adopted by numerous cancer specialists, the combined effect of the scarcity of treatments for disseminated cancer, the nearly infinite number of possible clinical trials with combinations of anticancer drugs, and the conviction that efficient therapies for cancer were close at hand favored the wide diffusion of clinical trials of cancer chemotherapies. The proliferation of these trials in the years 1970–1990 did not lead to the development of efficient cures for the cancers common in adults. It did lead, however, to the development of a distinct subspecialty— medical oncology—centered on the application of drugs to cancer treatment and organized (especially in the United States) as a trial-oriented professional segment. Although important national and local differences persist in the diffusion of clinical trials of chemotherapy, in Western countries these trials gradually became an accepted way of coping with otherwise hopeless clinical situations.

Chapter 2 discusses the history of tumor immunology and of the immunotherapy of human cancers between 1880 and 1980. Tumor immunology was developed in the 1960s and 1970s during an encounter between experimental oncology and cellular immunology. Both subspecialties were once low-prestige branches of pathology, and both became leading subspecialties in the biomedical sciences. The change in their status was made possible by a switch to well-defined animal models, quantifiable experimental approaches, and codified laboratory techniques that facilitated the integration of these subspecialties into mainstream biological research. The history of the immunotherapy of malignant tumors followed a somewhat more complicated path. Attempts to apply immunological methods to cancer therapy started in the late nineteenth century and continued up to the mid-twentieth, but at first they did not lead to significant advances either in cancer therapy or in the understanding of the mechanisms of "resistance" to malignant growths. The revival of immunology in the 1950s and 1960s, however, increased the interest in these attempts and led to the development of a therapeutic method based on the stimulation of immune mechanisms of cancer patients with bacterial vaccines. This method was described by its advocates as a fourth mode of cancer treatment—along with surgery, radiation therapy, and chemotherapy. But the initial enthusiasm for the new therapy waned in the late 1970s as results of larger, randomized clinical trials indicated that it had a negligible or nonexistent effect. These disappointing results were attributed to technical imperfections rather than to mistaken principles. In the late 1970s and 1980s substances credited with the ability to stimulate immune mechanisms—first interferon, then interleukin-2—were introduced into cancer therapy and presented as improvements on the imperfections of earlier immunotherapies.

Chapter 3 focuses on the history of interleukin-2 as an anticancer drug in the 1980s. IL-2 was introduced into the treatment of disseminated cancer by the laboratory of Dr. Steven Rosenberg at the U.S. National Institutes of Health in collaboration with the California biotechnology firm Cetus. In the first clinical trials of this molecule in humans, in 1985, patients received high doses of recombinant IL-2 together with interleukin-activated white blood cells. The new treatment was very expensive and labor-intensive and induced severe side effects, but Rosenberg and his collaborators affirmed that it had induced spectacular regressions of otherwise incurable tumors in nearly half of their patients. The results of later clinical trials of IL-2 did not confirm all the initial claims made for it. The new therapy was less effective than Rosenberg had alleged, the infusion of LAK cells (lymphokine-activated cells, white blood cells activated for three days with interleukin in a test tube) into patients was found to be of negligible clinical value, and no meaningful correlations were uncovered between the activation of subgroups of lymphocytes and the clinical results of interleukin therapy. On the other hand, IL-2's drawbacks—high toxicity and low efficacy—were no different from those of intensive chemotherapy regimens that became, from the 1970s on, an accepted treatment for disseminated cancer. Moreover, the new treatment had an advantage over the existing therapies: it linked the clinics to advanced research in experimental oncology, in immunology, and in molecular biology. These advantages facilitated the spread of clinical trials of IL-2 in the years 1985–1990.

Chapters 4 and 5 recount my field observations during the introduction of IL-2 to cancer therapy at the Cancer Foundation. They also follow changes in my trajectory as a participant-observer. My initial project was to study how physicians and scientists interacted during what I assumed would be an application of a laboratory-based method, adoptive immunotherapy: the activation of autologous (one's own) lymphocytes by IL-2 in the test tube and subsequent injection in the patient. Over time, however, the clinical experiment was modified so that IL-2 therapy came in many ways to resemble routine chemotherapies. In the later stages of my stay at the Foundation I realized that I was observing not direct collaboration between clinicians and immunologists, but rather different approaches employed by the participants to compensate for the fact that such collaboration did not become an indispensable feature of the IL-2 trial. The changes in the initial trial project may also account for some of my difficulties at the Cancer Foundation. I suspect that one of the main reasons I was allowed to observe this trial was to be a witness of a successful collaboration between immunologists and oncologists. The presence of an external witness may have become a liability for some of the participants when the predicted success became more problematic.[57] Finally, while writing this book I learned about the role played by the IL-2 trial in the subsequent reorganization of laboratory investigations at the Cancer Foundation. This newly acquired knowledge further modified my perceptions of the clinical trial.

Chapter 4 describes my experience at the Cancer Foundation, as well as my observations at several other hospitals (two in Israel, three in the United States) where IL-2 was applied to cancer therapy. These observations in different institutional settings seemed to me a useful tool for distinguishing the general characteristics of IL-2 clinical trials from the effects of national differences and of local conditions. The Cancer Foundation trial went through several successive phases: preclinical collaboration with a French producer of IL-2, initial collaboration with an American biotechnology firm in a pediatric clinical trial of lymphokine-activated white blood cells and IL-2, a switch to clinical trials of the American and the French IL-2 in adults, the introduction of lymphokine-activated white blood cells into these trials, and finally the development of (partially) routine, or standardized, uses of the new therapy. Each stage brought a different organizational pattern, modified relationships among actors, and influenced my perceptions of the trial and my status as an external observer.

Chapter 5 is an extended commentary. It discusses debates over jurisdiction and professional strategies during the Cancer Foundation IL-2 trial, and examines the mechanisms that facilitated cooperation among different professional groups. It focuses on interactions among scientists (immunologists), clinicians (oncologists), and industrialists (IL-2 producers) and on the shaping and reshaping of their jurisdictions during the trial.[58] These jurisdictions were outlined in a preliminary agreement among its senior organizers. Commonly elaborated therapeutic protocols served as links among the three groups and their heterogeneous domains of activity, delimiting areas of professional competence and defining specific skills. Agreement concerning the broad outlines of collaboration did not always prevent friction over issues such as the right to use space and equipment, to employ technicians, to recruit patients, to change protocols, to supervise students' work, to obtain biological materials from the clinics, to control patient-derived biological substances, and to present authorized accounts of the trial. Many of these conflicts occurred in the domain of semiroutine, trial-related laboratory tests (such as those measuring the antitumor activity of lymphocytes in IL-2-treated patients). This intermediary zone was where the preoccupations of the clinicians were articulated with those of the immunologists and industrial researchers.

The physicians and scientists were preoccupied with the potential of IL-2-activated white blood cells to selectively kill malignant cells. The Cancer Foundation IL-2 trial started with the assumption that interleukin-2 acts through the stimulation of specific immune mechanisms. The promoters of the trial believed that these mechanisms, then imprecisely understood, would become better defined through further investigations. A loosely defined entity—IL-2-activated killing lymphocytes—facilitated the creation of linkages between the professional cultures of scientists and physicians and the development of common research strategies. It also facilitated alliances with the biotechnology industry, government agencies, and cancer charities. Once the research results failed to confirm the initial assumption—no direct link was found to exist between the activation of one or more distinct subpopulations of lymphocytes by IL-2 (the laboratory domain) and a cancer cure (the clinical domain)—additional material, social, and discursive techniques were developed in order to maintain close ties among physicians, scientists, and providers of resources. Material techniques, such as preclinical investigations in which scientists employed biological materials derived from patients enrolled in the IL-2 trial, aimed at the construction and consolidation of exchange zones between the heterogenous domains of the laboratory and the clinic. Social techniques, such as regular meetings of a formal collaborative structure—the IL-2 group—stimulated contacts between physicians and scientists. Discursive techniques, such as joint writing of research projects, grant proposals, reports, and scientific papers, helped to elaborate shared vocabulary and shared criteria of evaluation of results. Together these techniques reduced the distance between the concerns of scientists and clinicians, limited trial-related tensions, and facilitated the presentation of interleukin therapy as an exemplary collaboration between immunologists and oncologists. Chapter 6 summarizes the results of the trial and my observations of it and reflects on the specificity of the disease known as cancer.

The book proceeds from the general to the particular: from the culture of clinical experimentation in oncology, to immunotherapies of cancer, to therapeutic uses of IL-2 in the oncology clinics, to a description of a single clinical experiment—the Cancer Foundation's IL-2 trial. My decision to follow one clinical experiment in detail was based on the assumption that a thick description of a single trial might provide more valid information about experimentation in the clinics than a "thinner" description of several trials. This assumption may be contested. Every clinical experiment is unique and may include atypical traits that make generalizations difficult. Moreover, the Foundation's trial may have had more than its share of unusual characteristics. It undoubtedly belonged to the international culture of clinical experimentation in oncology, but at the same time it was shaped by a unique combination of national and local factors. The central role of the immunology laboratory in the initiation and conduct of the IL-2 trial reflected the importance of immunologists in the organization of French biomedical research in the 1980s[59] and also its special status as the sole research laboratory affiliated with the Medical Division of the Cancer Foundation. Similarly, the presentation of the trial as an example of exceptionally successful collaboration between the laboratory and the clinics reflected both the dearth of collaborative efforts between clinical oncologists and scientists in France and the specific history of complex relationships between researchers and clinicians at the Cancer Foundation. The unique personalities and career patterns of individual physicians and scientists who organized the Foundation's IL-2 trial also affected the clinical experiment. As a result of these combined factors, the IL-2 trial played an important role in the reorganization of laboratory research at the Cancer Foundation Hospital and in changes in the power relationships within that institution.

Is such a potentially atypical clinical trial an adequate model for studying clinical experiments? My tentative answer is yes. Because there are few systematic studies of the conduct and effects of clinical trials, one cannot exclude the possibility that, if examined closely, other clinical trials would also show some of the supposedly unusual features of the Cancer Foundation IL-2 trial. And even if the Cancer Foundation trial was truly exceptional, this in-depth study may still increase our understanding of experimentation in the clinics, because it is reasonable to assume that some of the presumably atypical features of the Cancer Foundation IL-2 trial—such as its role in that institution's internal politics—can be found in less extreme form in more conventional clinical trials as well.

The Cancer Foundation IL-2 trial turned out to be a different enterprise from the one I had expected to follow. I planned to observe the implementation of a new, laboratory-based therapy in a medical oncology ward. I found myself also observing an effort to consolidate a fragile cooperation between clinicians and immunologists, and a complex strategic endeavor that played an important role in the administrative reorganization of a major cancer treatment center. My belated understanding of some of the central aspects of the trial hampered my research. Scientists often perform at the end of a given investigation experiments necessary to complete a logical sequence of inquiry. Such *a posteriori* reconstruction is viewed as legitimate because scientists assume that the laws of nature are invariable and that the sequence in which experiments are performed does not affect their outcome.[60] Researchers who deal with time-dependent variables are less lucky. It is not easy to obtain reliable *a posteriori* accounts of events that should have been observed several years ago, and it is impossible to find out what the participants would answer if they were asked the "right" questions, meaning the questions that would be asked if the end of the story were known in advance. In writing down my experience at the Cancer Foundation I became aware of the shortcomings of my research. I realized that the impossibility of moving backward in time, as well as the large scope of the subject, prevented me from making as well-rounded a study as I had aspired to. Even so, I believe that this has been a useful investigation. Subsequent expeditions into this uncharted territory may lead to a more finely shaded understanding of experimentation in the clinics.

A Note on Heterogeneous Perspectives

My research was initially focused on a single event: the clinical trial of IL-2 at the Cancer Foundation. I realized, however, that the IL-2 trial was embedded in a specific cognitive and material environment— the culture of clinical experimentation in oncology. An adequate contextualization of the IL-2 trial was not possible, I felt, without a study of the origins, development, and current status of this culture. To examine the trial within its larger context, I used approaches borrowed from the history of science, the history of medicine, the sociology of scientific knowledge, the ethnography of the laboratory, and the sociology of medicine. A combination of these methodological approaches in a single study is unusual. An attempt to combine the insights of distinct professional groups, some of which (for example, sociologists of medicine and ethnographers of laboratories) converse rarely if ever, may produce a patchy and heterogeneous story. But a patchwork narrative seems better than no narrative at all or one that is full of holes. My rather uncomfortable choice to combine several methodological approaches stemmed directly from the difficulty of finding a single theoretical framework that would permit the satisfactory investigation of a clinical experiment. The heterogeneity of my description matches some of the complexities of my subject.

In 1971 the English historian E. P. Thompson noted that historians, unlike anthropologists, have a tendency to attribute simplistic motives to their subjects: "we know all about the delicate tissue of social norms and reciprocities which regulate the life of Trobriand islanders and the psychic energies involved in the cargo cult of Melanesia, but at some point this infinitely complex social creature, Melanesian man, becomes (in our histories) the eighteenth-century English collier who clasps his hand spasmodically upon his stomach and responds to elementary economic stimuli."[61] Historians of early modern science— unlike the historians of the early modern English peasantry criticized by Thompson—cannot be blamed for oversimplification. Attentive to the multiple dimensions of scientists' activities, these historians have shown how the social identities and class reactions of court society, and then of the early urban gentry, became permanently embedded in the culture of the experimental sciences.[62] Their studies linked laboratories with royal courts, workhouses, arsenals, factories, city halls, academies, and markets and placed the experimental sciences in the midst of politics, social life, economy, culture. However, to paraphrase Thompson, this infinitely complex social creature, the seventeenth-century scientist, somehow became (in some historical accounts of present-day science) the twentieth-century research worker who is either developing a specific set of practices in the laboratory, or shaping institutional policies, or constructing networks that extend the influence of laboratories, but who seldom does all these things at the same time.[63] Thus the studies of "big science" carefully analyze scientific institutions and the politics of science but seldom trace the production and validation of scientific knowledge. Similarly, laboratory studies investigate experimental systems and laboratory cultures but rarely study scientists' interactions with the state, industrialists, or the military. This compartmentalized perspective is regrettable. Studies centered on a single aspect of scientists' activity have greatly increased our understanding of how science works today. However, if one is dealing with a complex, multilayered phenomenon, a single focus may sometimes become a handicap. The culture of clinical experimentation in oncology is just such a complex phenomenon and, I propose, should be studied through a combination of methodological approaches. The heterogeneity and patchwork aspect of the following chapters is perhaps not too high a price to pay for an attempt to develop a multifocus view on experimentation in the clinics.

The Culture of Clinical Experimentation in Oncology

Cancer Therapy: The Origins of a Science-Laden Medical Practice

Cancer research and cancer therapy are usually presented as complementary domains. Experimental cancer studies are viewed as synonymous with the search for efficient therapies for human malignancies. These studies are often inseparable from the practice of clinical oncology, itself often based on large-scale application of experimental and semiexperimental therapies.[1] Specialized institutions for cancer patients usually have large research departments. Most of the papers published in oncology journals deal with experimental and preclinical research. In the leading teaching and research institutions, bedside excellence and devotion to patients do not, as a rule, ensure access to power positions; professional rewards tend to be closely linked to research activity. Thus many leading oncologists have spent an important part of their career in the laboratory, and their clinical work is often related to experimentation with new anticancer therapies.

Government agencies and private fundraising organizations have repeatedly argued that increased funding for experimental cancer studies and for clinical experimentation will improve the lot of cancer patients.[2] In the 1980s, inspired by the success of AIDS activists, organized groups of cancer patients, their family members, and friends asked for more funding for cancer research, rapid approval of new cancer drugs, and increased access to experimental therapies for cancer patients. The rationale behind this demand is the expectation not only that research will solve the "cancer problem" sometime in the future but also that intensification of research and greater access to experimental therapies will help cancer patients here and now.[3] Organizations such as the American Cancer Society, though not necessarily agreeing with all aspects of patients' activism, supported their demands for more research funds.[4]

The consensus on the existence of a direct causal link between support for preclinical (laboratory-sited) and clinical research in oncology and the alleviation of the plight of cancer patients has two complementary aspects. One is the explicit claim that adequate funding for research will soon bring a cure for cancer and thus improve the situation of future cancer patients. The other is the implicit claim that such funding will also improve the lot of current cancer patients. The latter claim has also been used in publicity for hospitals. Thus a 1991 advertisement for the University of Southern California/Norris Cancer Hospital in Los Angeles explained that "because the Norris houses over 100 research scientists and clinical investigators, patients can benefit immediately from treatments not commonly available."[5] The culture of clinical experimentation in oncology was and is shaped by the combination of belief in a future science-based solution to the "cancer problem" and the pressure of the currently insoluble problems of numerous cancer patients suffering from incurable, fatal disease.

The links between "cutting-edge" research and cancer therapy first emerged at the beginning of this century, with the development of radiation therapy for malignant tumors. The diagnosis of cancer had long been viewed as a death sentence. The perception of cancer as incurable strongly colored the lay representations of its pathology and structured the organization of care for patients.[6] In the second half of the nineteenth century improvements in surgical techniques and the introduction of anesthesia and asepsis led to the first attempts to excise internal malignant growths.[7] In selected cases surgery indeed eliminated the tumor without killing the patient, but through the early twentieth century its long-term efficacy remained very low.[8]

The first serious challenge to the perception of cancer as incurable came from the development of radiation therapy. The observation that X rays induce skin burns led around 1896 to attempts to employ this technology in the treatment of skin cancers, and by 1904 special X-ray tubes were also being used to treat internal tumors. In 1905 Drs. Jean Bergonié and Louis Tribondeau demonstrated that X rays preferentially kill rapidly dividing cells; this finding provided a scientific rationale for the selective use of X rays on malignant growths.[9] The use of X rays was, however, dangerous: not only did they provoke burns, but it also became clear that in high doses they could induce cancer. At first physicians did not know how to measure and standardize X-ray radiation, and they lacked information on the biological effects of X rays. The therapy improved slowly, mainly through trial and error. Important technical advances such as the introduction of William D. Coolidge's hot cathode-ray tube in 1913 and J. T Case's development of a 200-kilovolt apparatus in 1921 allowed better control of radiation doses and favored the diffusion of X-ray equipment among hospitals specialized in the treatment of cancer.[10]

In 1904 doctors observed that radium produced burns similar to those induced by X rays. Because the radiation emitted by radium is directly proportional to the amount of pure compound present, it was easier to control than X rays. In selected cases the use of tubes and needles containing radium permitted direct delivery of radiation to the tumor ("curietherapy"). Radium was rapidly introduced for the treatment of skin cancer and other skin disorders, and its use was gradually extended to other tumors. In the 1920s radium therapy was improved through the development of radium collars and radium bombs, and in the 1930s external beam machines were used in the therapy of gynecological and head and neck tumors.[11]

The diffusion of X-ray and radium therapy led to the formation of a new professional group of radiotherapists—physicians specialized in the administration of radiation therapy or in clinical research on that subject. However, the high price of radium limited the diffusion of the new therapeutic approach and encouraged the centralization of cancer treatment. Private organizations such as the American Society for the Control of Cancer and the Ligue Franco-Américaine contre le Cancer collected funds to purchase radium and to finance basic and preclinical research in oncology. (Basic research investigates fundamental biological processes. Preclinical research is always related to human diseases and is therapy- or diagnosis-oriented.) They also strongly encouraged the development of specialized institutions that combined preclinical research with cancer therapy.[12] Cancer patients treated in these institutions were able to benefit from the latest technological advances: specialized surgery, new X-ray machines, and more efficient ways of delivering radium radiation. The existence of these centers favored in turn the diffusion of complex and expensive technologies such as radium beam machines. The cancer treatment centers developed between the two world wars were the forerunners of the "big medicine" era in industrialized countries. They also played an important role in the development and then consolidation of links between advanced physical and biological research, high-tech medicine, large budgets, and hopes for a cure for cancer.[13]

Besides their role in the institutionalization of cancer therapy and in research, cancer charities increasingly shaped professional and lay ideas about cancer. Their activity was guided by the belief that cancer, if recognized early enough, was curable. This idea, which acquired the status of official dogma, was first proposed in the eighteenth century by the French doctor Henri Dran. After observing the evolution of breast cancer in numerous patients, Dran concluded that cancer was always first a localized disease and only later spread to local lymph nodes, then to more distant targets.[14] The "incurability" of cancer was, according to this view, only a by-product of the failure to recognize the disease during its localized, curable stage. Cancer charities therefore encouraged early detection of cancer as an indispensable complement to research and therapeutic efforts. Health professionals and the lay public were trained to recognize the early, usually benign, manifestations of cancer.[15]

Between the two world wars both professionals and the general public showed growing interest in the "cancer problem." The activity of cancer charities enhanced public awareness of the need to seek professional help upon detection of early signs of cancer. Improved surgical techniques increased the rate of surgical cures for slowly spreading malignant growths, while radiation therapy allowed cures for selected cancers, in particular skin cancers and, in some cases, head and neck, breast, and uterine cancers. However, the percentage of cures for cancer remained low; skin cancers were the only significant exception. At the same time, the number of deaths from cancer in Western countries continued to rise. Cancer was increasingly identified as the main scourge of modern times and thus became an important political problem. The foundation of the National Cancer Institute (NCI) in 1937 was a response to these political preoccupations in the United States. During its first years the NCI was a small and modestly endowed institution, as were its counterparts in Europe.[16] The scale of funding for oncological research changed dramatically after the Second World War.

The Development of the Jurisdiction of Cancer Chemotherapy

The development of cancer chemotherapy in the 1940s and 1950s stemmed from the conjunction of several factors: growing faith in scientific medicine, boosted by the discovery of antibiotics; growing public—and hence political—impatience with the steadily rising level of cancer deaths, in contrast to a declining death rate from infectious diseases; a significant increase in allocations for biomedical research; and a belief in the virtues of "big science," boosted by the success of war research, exemplified by the Manhattan Project.

The first successful cancer chemotherapy was a by-product of war research. On December 2, 1943, the story goes, the Germans bombarded Allied ships in the Italian port of Bari, destroying ships that contained poisonous nitrogen mustard gas. Army doctors treating victims of this bombing observed that white blood cells disappeared from the blood of soldiers who had come into close contact with the gas, and they concluded that the substance selectively eliminating white blood cells might be of use in leukemia therapy.[17] This popular story aptly combines the elements of disaster with those of salvation. The historical account told to professionals is less dramatic. The capacity of certain chemical compounds to selectively kill white blood cells was already known around 1914, when Dr. James Murphy of the Rockefeller Institute attempted to demonstrate the key role of lymphocytes in graft rejection by irradiating the grafted animals or treating them with benzol in order to inhibit the activity of the lymphocytes.[18] During the First World War physicians noted that nitrogen mustard was selectively toxic to blood cells: autopsies of soldiers who had died of exposure to the gas showed that the white blood cells had disappeared from bone marrow and lymphatic tissue.[19] There was sporadic investigation of the topic in the 1930s,[20] but it did not become the subject of a systematic study until 1941, when a group of Yale University researchers, led by the pharmacologists Drs. Alfred Gilman and Louis S. Goodman, obtained funds from the U.S. Office of Scientific Research and Development (OSRD) (an organization that centralized U.S. war research efforts) for research on chemical warfare. Among other things, they studied the effects of nitrogen mustard on rapidly dividing tissue and found that injections of the gas induced remissions in mice with lymphoma; in December 1942 they found that the same drug induced transitory but complete remission in a patient with lymphoma. Though not officially published until 1946, these results were presented in a medical meeting in early 1943 and were rapidly confirmed by other groups.[21]

The partial success of nitrogen mustard therapy led to an organized effort to find less toxic and more efficient antitumor agents. In fact the nitrogen mustard study was not the first attempt to explore systematically the anticancer properties of chemical compounds. Ironically, official histories of chemotherapy usually start with studies of a substance viewed today as a precursor to immunotherapy (or biotherapy) of cancer—"Coley's toxins." Coley's toxins—a nonpurified mixture of bacterial toxins from streptococcus and *Serratia marcescens*—were introduced to cancer therapy in the late nineteenth century. The therapy had very unpleasant side effects (high fever, pain), and only a few patients responded to injections. Consequently, Coley's toxins were abandoned with the advent of radiation therapy.[22] In the mid-1930s Dr. Murray Shear, at the U.S. Public Service of Cancer Investigations at Harvard University (a service that merged in 1937 with the Pharmacology Laboratory of the old National Institutes of Health to form the National Cancer Institute), became interested in the effects of Coley's toxins on tumors and set up a research project to study this phenomenon in the laboratory. Shear assumed that Coley's toxins contained an unknown antitumor molecule, which was, however, seldom present in adequate concentration in preparations of the toxins; hence the rarity of cures in toxin-treated patients. Pursuing this lead, Shear and his collaborators isolated an active polysaccharide from the bacterium *Serratia marcescens*. They also developed a method to evaluate the polysaccharide's activity in a standardized experimental model—the necrosis of sarcoma (muscle cell tumor) S37 in mice—thus setting the pattern of testing the anticancer activity of chemical compounds in a single, well-defined animal model. However, the project met with limited practical success. Small-scale trials of bacterial polysaccharide in cancer patients revealed that this substance was not very effective: tumors regressed but were not totally destroyed, and they regenerated later, while patients rapidly developed polysaccharide immunity, so that prolonged therapy was difficult. Moreover, the polysaccharide induced severe side effects such as high fever and a sharp fall in blood pressure. *Serratia* polysaccharide was therefore declared unsuitable for clinical use.[23]

After the Second World War public and private funding for cancer research in the United States and, to a lesser degree, in other industrialized countries expanded rapidly. Part of this money was invested in the search for molecules that would cure cancer. Screening programs for anticancer drugs were developed in several Western countries. In Great Britain a program was developed by Dr. Alexander Haddow at the Chester Beatty Research Institute. Because this program was associated with the Royal Cancer Hospital, researchers were able to test promising compounds in the clinics. Haddow's studies were supported by the Medical Research Council and by a private fund, the British Empire Cancer Campaign. At the same time an important drug development initiative was launched by Imperial Chemical Industries.[24] In France small-scale essays of chemotherapy were introduced in anticancer centers in Orléans and Lyons, and beginning in 1946 the Institut National d'Hygiène (the precursor of the Institut National de la Santé et de la Recherche Médicale; INSERM) centralized all information on the application of drugs to cancer therapy.[25] There was also a Japanese research program on anticancer drugs led by Dr. Yoshida at the University of Tokyo.[26] Most of the cancer chemotherapy studies, however, were carried out in the United States, the only country capable at the time of investing large sums in such investigations.

The reorganization of cancer chemotherapy studies in the United States was deliberately modeled on industrial research.[27] The switch to "big science" in this domain was probably facilitated by the fact that the first successful studies on cancer chemotherapy were made within the framework of military research and were supported by the OSRD. Wartime research on poisonous gases led to the introduction of nitrogen mustard and other alkylating agents to cancer therapy. In addition, wartime studies on nutrition led to the introduction (by Dr. Sidney Farber) of antagonists of folic acid to leukemia therapy, while wartime research on antibiotics led to the finding that some antibiotics (such as actinomycin D) had antitumor properties. In 1945 Shear and his collaborators established a screening program at the NCI. This program, which lasted until 1953, lacked autonomous clinical facilities and collaborated with the Philadelphia Institute for Cancer Research for the clinical part of these studies.

At the same time an important screening program was initiated at the Sloan-Kettering Institute, in New York City. The Sloan-Kettering Institute was developed thanks to the efforts of Alfred P. Sloan, the president of General Motors and trustee of the Memorial Hospital in Manhattan, who in 1945 contributed $4 million to support a research institute associated with the hospital and directed by Dr. Cornelius Rhoads. The institute was also named after Charles Kettering, director of research at General Motors, because Sloan felt that Kettering, an eminent industrial engineer, would be a worthy example for cancer researchers. Sloan's choice of the institute's director reflected this belief. During the war Rhoads had been the head of the Medical Division of the Chemical Warfare Service, and he became an enthusiastic supporter of the transfer of industrial research methods to cancer studies. This conviction led him to develop a large-scale screening program for potential anticancer drugs at the Sloan-Kettering Institute.[28] This program collaborated with the pharmaceutical firm Burroughs Wellcome and tested compounds prepared by Wellcome chemists. The screening was made with a single animal model—sarcoma S180 in mice. The Sloan-Kettering and NCI programs each screened several thousand synthetic and natural products.[29]

The most serious drawback to both the NCI and Sloan-Kettering programs, later observers noted, was the limited possibility of testing active compounds in patients.[30] This was a significant handicap: unlike the iconic model for the development of successful drug therapy—the testing, then the mass production of penicillin during the Second World War—drugs used in cancer chemotherapy were not very efficient. Because a malignant cell is similar to the normal cell from which it is derived, it is difficult to find compounds that will harm only malignant cells. The researchers hoped that the small initial therapeutic effects observed with antitumor drugs could be magnified through adequate calibration of doses, discovery of efficient ways to administer the drugs, and later the appropriate combination of several drugs. The search for the optimal posology, or combination of drugs, requires human subjects, and the initial low efficacy of a tested drug often makes the search particularly tedious. Early screening programs conducted by chemists and/or bench workers did not lead to the discovery of new anticancer drugs, and this failure was related to the absence of clinical experiments. Dissatisfaction with these programs increased the pressure for clinical testing of antitumor compounds.[31] From the mid-1950s on, efforts to improve the efficacy of cancer chemotherapy became indissolubly linked with the development of large-scale clinical trials.[32] In the years 1945–1954 the absence of adequate institutional structures made the coordination of such clinical trials difficult. However, when the Cancer Chemotherapy National Service Center (CCNSC)—founded in 1955—provided an efficient structure for clinical trials, the obligatory ties of chemotherapy to large-scale clinical trials became one of the strong points of the new domain. Cancer chemotherapy became one of the preferential sites for the interaction between basic, preclinical, and clinical research and allowed efficient articulation between several research domains (cell kinetics, pharmacology, toxicology) and the clinics. It therefore played a central role in the expansion of oncology, defined as a specialty that was based simultaneously in the clinics and in the laboratory.[33] The domain of cancer chemotherapy was able to draw upon resources destined for advanced biomedical research and to attract scientists and physicians interested in interdisciplinary research, in the solution of practical problems and in the control of a new domain of medical intervention.[34]

In the early 1950s chemotherapy was viewed by many cancer specialists as a new and promising approach to the treatment of cancer. Leading cancer centers increasingly employed nitrogen mustard therapy, while research on the antagonists of folic acid (led by Sidney Farber and his collaborators) produced, for the first time, temporary remission in acute leukemia.[35] Drug therapy was rapidly introduced to routine management of leukemia. Its diffusion illustrates the attraction of "desperate drugs," which allow doctors to "do something" in a hopeless situation. The first reports on drug therapies for leukemia were published in 1946. In 1947, 10 percent of leukemia patients treated in American hospitals received chemotherapy; in 1950 the proportion increased to 75 percent.[36] Chemotherapy for leukemia had a limited practical success: there were almost no cures, and remissions obtained with drugs were usually very short. Nevertheless, the spread of this treatment contributed to a growing conviction that an efficient anticancer drug would soon be found, if only enough resources were allocated toward this goal. For the first time in the history of cancer studies, a single project focused the interests of industrialists, academic researchers, and clinicians. The result was increased pressure on the sole remaining screening program in the United States (the NCI program ended in 1953 for lack of clinical facilities)—the one at the Sloan-Kettering Institute. The Sloan-Kettering program was relatively efficient—in the mid-1950s it screened about 75 percent of the approximately 20,000 substances submitted to such screening in the United States—but its capacity for further growth was limited, and it was unable to respond to increasing demands by physicians and industry. An additional problem was that the NCI Center for Clinical Research, finally opened in 1953, was able to accept only a limited number of patients.[37]

In the 1950s various special interest groups lobbied for cancer chemotherapy in the United States: leading cancer specialists such as Farber and Rhoads; American Cancer Society activists, led by Mary Lasker;[38] and the pharmaceutical industry. They transformed this therapy into an important political topic. In July 1953 the U.S. Congress asked

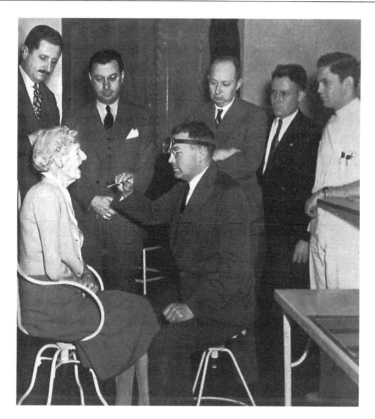

From *Cancer News,* March 1947: "Teamwork in Cancer Diagnosis: A group of physicians conducts a clinic with a patient at Memorial Hospital, Pawtucket, Rhode Island." (American Cancer Society. Photo courtesy The Countway Library of Medicine, Harvard University.)

the NCI to develop an extramural research program in chemotherapy for acute leukemia. It also allocated $1 million for leukemia research. In July 1954 growing congressional pressure led to the establishment of the Cancer Chemotherapy Committee (CCC), directed by Dr. Sidney Farber. The mission of the new committee was to improve collaboration through better circulation of information. The CCC started publishing a newsletter, *Current Research in Cancer Chemotherapy,* initiated a series of symposia on this topic, and began a compilation of relevant literature worldwide. At the same time the NCI increased funding for studies of cancer chemotherapy, allocating in 1954 $3 million to research on anticancer drugs.[39] The founding of the CCC did not, however, solve the problem of the organization of large-scale clinical trials. This problem was further complicated by the reluctance of NCI scientists and clinicians to share control of new chemotherapy clinical trials with outsiders.[40]

Continuous political pressure from Congress, together with growing pressure from some non-NCI cancer specialists and industry, led in April 1955 to the establishment of the Cancer Chemotherapy National Service Center, directed by Dr. Kenneth Endicott, to organize and coordinate clinical trials. The structure of the CCNSC was the result of a compromise: it was formally a part of the NCI, but the decisionmaking power was delegated to panels (a Chemistry Panel, a Clinical Studies Panel, a Pharmacology Panel, an Endocrinology Panel, and a Screening Panel) composed of extramural scientists and physicians. Also in June 1954 a central structure—the Cancer Chemotherapy National Committee—was established to coordinate industry, government agencies involved in the chemotherapy programs (the Atomic Energy Commission, the Veterans Administration, the Food and Drug Administration), and the charities (the American Cancer Society, the Damon Runyon Memorial Fund) that sponsored these programs. The fact that the chairman and the secretary of the new organization were also chairmen of the CCC ensured cooperation among the different institutions involved in chemotherapy studies.[41]

The search for cancer chemotherapies in the 1950s marked an unprecedented financial and organizational effort in the history of biomedical research.[42] Congress rapidly acknowledged the key role of clinical trials in cancer chemotherapy and allocated significant sums to the CCNSC: $5.6 million in 1956, $20 million in 1957, and $28 million in 1958.[43] The aim of the new program was, in the words of Dr. Gordon Zubrod, who headed the Acute Leukemia Task Force of the CCNSC, "to set up all the functions of a pharmaceutical house run by the NCI," while CCNSC chairman Endicott explained in 1957 that the problems of cancer chemotherapy would be resolved "when industry-government cooperation is as effective in the pharmaceutical area as it is in some of the defense areas."[44] In order to approach the ideal of industrial-type research on new drugs it was necessary to improve control over two variable components of the tests for new therapies: the tumor-bearing mice used in preliminary screenings of chemical compounds and the patients employed in clinical trials of new chemotherapies.

The control of mice became possible through the CCNSC inbred-mouse production program, financed, from 1956 on, by a special NCI grant. The goals of that program were explicitly formulated in industrial terms: its directors discussed the volume of input and output of the product, as well as the problems of standardization and of quality controls.[45] The mice-breeding program was at first conducted in the Jackson Laboratories, Bar Harbor, Maine, and was later extended to several commercial laboratories. At the same time the CCNSC, in collaboration with the Institute of Laboratory Animal Resources at the National Research Council, developed minimum standards for laboratory mice, while the screening panel of the CCNSC fixed the standards for transplantable tumors and for screening conditions. Three murine tumors (sarcoma 180, adenocarcinoma 755, and leukemia L1210) were employed in all screening tests, and there was strict codification of the evaluation of the levels of activity of the tested compounds on these tumors.[46] The control of patients was achieved

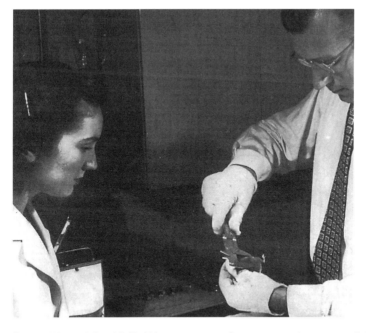

From *Cancer News*, May 1948: "A spontaneous breast tumor in a mouse is being measured with small calipers and recorded in the experiment notebook." (American Cancer Society. Photo courtesy The Countway Library of Medicine, Harvard University.)

through the centralization and standardization of clinical trials of new chemotherapies.

The organization of large-scale clinical trials of chemotherapy of cancer in the 1950s was a path-breaking enterprise: it established accepted patterns in cancer therapy and played an important role in shaping a distinct medical subspecialty, medical oncology. It was also a pioneering enterprise in the clinical testing of new therapies. In the 1950s and 1960s the CCNSC-coordinated cooperative groups for testing new anticancer drugs were the only permanent research groups doing clinical trials besides the cooperative groups of the Veterans Administration.[47] A brief history of controlled clinical trials may help us to understand why the culture of clinical experimentation in oncology—directly derived from clinical trials of chemotherapies—played an important role in the organization of the jurisdiction of cancer treatment after the Second World War.

Controlled Clinical Trials as an Organizational Innovation

Controlled clinical trials are usually presented as an important achievement of modern medicine: the development of an accurate way to measure the efficacy of a given therapy.[48] In the "dark ages" of medicine, the official story goes, there was no way to separate the objective effects of a given treatment from the subjective convictions of physicians and patients. Many positive results attributed to specific therapies were in fact placebo effects (that is, they reflected psychosocial effects of the treatment), while useless treatments—the classical example is bloodletting—survived for centuries because there was no way to evaluate their efficacy. The development of randomized, controlled clinical trials put an end to this anarchic situation. In such trials patients are randomly distributed between two groups: one receives the tested treatment and the other a control treatment (reference drug or placebo). In an optimal variant of the controlled trial, the experiment is "double-blind": neither the doctors who conduct the trial nor the patients who participate in it know who, among the enrolled patients, belongs to the tested group. On the other end of the scale, in selected cases such as tests of potentially life-saving therapies in invariably mortal diseases, carefully matched historical controls may replace randomization. Statistical tests are employed later to establish whether significant differences were obtained between the group that received the tested therapy and an appropriate control group. Therapy was perceived as the last stronghold of the nonscientific "art of heal-ing," and the elaboration of a method that made possible an objective, quantitative evaluation of results of a given treatment was usually viewed as a major medical innovation.

From the 1970s on, however, this emblematic achievement of sci-entific medicine has come under the close scrutiny of an active minor-ity of health professionals who have pointed to concrete problems with the design and implementation of controlled clinical trials and with the acceptance of their conclusions. Studies examining how clin-ical trials *were* or *are* conducted (in contrast to the majority of inves-tigations on this subject, which debate how they *should be* conducted) revealed that, official ideology notwithstanding, controlled clinical tri-als were far from being a universally accepted device for the evaluation of new therapies. Publications in the medical press and medical con-gresses in the years 1950–1980 pointed to the diminishing value of bedside observations: belief in efficacy often replaced proof of efficacy, and declarations in favor of clinical trials replaced actual trials.[49] From the mid-1940s to the mid-1970s the proportion of articles evaluating therapy steadily declined in prestigious medical journals, and more-over, researchers who evaluated these publications claimed that their quality declined too.[50] The overall decrease in the proportion of clin-ical studies may, according to some investigators, reflect the tendency to redefine medical research as basic biomedical research.[51] This re-definition induced in turn a tendency to substitute theoretically grounded belief in efficacy (it should work) for proof of efficacy (it works). For example, physicians were reluctant to accept the conclu-sion of studies indicating that the hospitalization of patients suffering from myocardial infarction in an intensive care unit did not bring significant survival advantage, because this conclusion did not fit their theoretical preconceptions.[52] Similarly, doctors did not accept the re-sults of randomized clinical trials which showed no benefit of extra-cranial/intracranial arterial bypass surgery for patients at risk for stroke, because they were convinced that this operation made sound physiological sense.[53]

Difficulties surrounding the introduction of controlled clinical trials were usually attributed to shortcomings in the scientific education of physicians and to their reluctance to adopt innovations. Some spe-cialists thought, however, that these difficulties also reflected a more fundamental problem: a contradiction between the principle of con-trolled trial and the clinical tradition, which emphasizes the uniqueness of each illness and the importance of individualized care for each patient.[54] Randomized clinical trials, some critics affirmed, are centered on disease and disease-related variables rather than on patient and patient-related variables; these trials had therefore contributed to the shift in focus in modern medical practice from the patient to the disease,[55] and to the mechanical transposition of techniques employed to study laboratory animals to the clinics.[56] This argument has been most eloquently developed by Dr. Alvin Feinstein. Feinstein points to the inability of randomized clinical trials modeled after artificially crafted experimental situations to answer complex questions of the kind most frequently found in the ordinary circumstances of clinical practice.[57] His criticism implies, however, that the current shortcomings of clinical trials have their roots in faulty investigation methods. A different method, directly derived from the clinician's knowledge, should allow an efficient and objective measurement of therapeutic effects.

Radical critics of controlled clinical trials share with advocates the perception of clinical trials as value-free measuring devices that allow (or should allow) the evaluation of efficacy of therapies. Controlled, randomized clinical trials are usually seen as a substitute for moral or political decisions, as a scientific (and thus neutral) method that, as the bioethicist Anne Fagot-Largeault puts it, "allows us to take moral decisions from the frail hands of humans, without burdening God with them."[58] Students of medicine have a different perception of clinical trials. "The demonstration of the collective benefits of individual clinical trials," sociologist of medicine Ian Robinson explains, "does not appear to occur spontaneously or effortlessly. It is a highly organized process with both professional and commercial reputations dependent not only on the proper running of trials, but also on the subsequent public management of findings stemming from them."[59] Clinical trials are seen not as value-free devices that objectively evaluate the efficacy of new therapies but as situated entities shaped by specific circumstances.[60] They should also be seen as a specific technology that, like the technologies associated with cars, bridges, or computers, incorporates the beliefs and values of the persons who developed it, and then is adapted locally to the conditions in which it is employed.[61] The history of the controlled clinical trial should thus shed light on its current structure and uses.

Since the eighteenth century physicians have tried to find ways to evaluate the effects of their therapeutic activity, but such evaluations have generally lain outside the mainstream practice of medicine.[62] The first attempt to coordinate clinical trials conducted in several medical centers and to create a cooperative group was made in the years 1928–1935 by the Cooperative Clinical Group for the Investigation of Syphilis Treatment. The clinical trials conducted by that group did not, however, contain some of the central characteristics of later efforts: randomization and double-blind tests. The organizers were reluctant to take collective responsibility and tended to rely on individual experience and expertise rather than on anonymous statistical evaluations. The centralization of scientific research during the Second World War made it possible to overcome some of the resistance to collaborative research on new therapies and to develop bigger and better-planned clinical trials, such as the research on the use of penicillin in treating syphilis sponsored by the U.S. National Research Committee in the years 1943–1945.[63]

After the Second World War large-scale cooperative research was maintained through the intervention of centralizing entities such as, in the United States, the Medical Research Committee of the OSRD, the Veterans Administration, and the Public Health Service; in England the Medical Research Council (MRC); and in France the Institut National d'Hygiène and, later, INSERM.[64] Large-scale studies sponsored by these organizations in the postwar period—in particular the MRC-sponsored study of the use of streptomycin in tuberculosis therapy (1946–48) and the MRC-sponsored trial of the whooping cough vaccine—later became the standard models of collaborative clinical trials.[65] They introduced such key innovations as centrally controlled randomization and objectively measured indicators. These innovations were presented later as the triumph of scientific rationality and the victory of (correct) statistical concepts. From the 1960s on, clinical trials became the icon of a rational, scientific approach to therapeutic practice.[66] As historian of medicine Harry Marks explains, however, the enthusiastic endorsement of statistical principles followed, rather than preceded, the establishment of randomized clinical trials. Statisticians offered physicians an elegant solution for the problems that beset their earlier attempts to establish an efficient collaborative framework, such as the neutralization of an individual researcher's biases and group interests. Randomization and the establishment of "objective indicators" became tools to facilitate the articulation of tasks and the neutralization of conflicts between professional segments involved in trials of new therapies.[67] At the same time clinical trials—

or, as Marks calls them, "the clinical trial enterprise"—offered an efficient way of dealing with organizational issues: as a 1980 National Institutes of Health publication on research with human subjects put it, "notwithstanding their prominent scientific and medical attributes large-scale clinical trials offer fertile ground for the successful application of modern management concepts and techniques."[68]

The main advantage of randomized clinical trials was, as advocates explained, that they replaced subjective estimations of therapy based on an individual physician's discretion with an objective, scientific evaluation.[69] Experience was, however, the traditional basis of specific expert knowledge—the "clinical tact" of the physician.[70] Early clinical trials such as the one conducted by the Cooperative Clinical Group before the Second World War integrated the expertise of participating physicians in the design and conclusions of the trial.[71] Why, after the Second World War, would the medical elite that had legitimated its status by its expertise readily surrender part of its power and actively propagate a method aimed at the elimination of individual doctors' clinical judgment? One possible answer may be linked to the structural changes in Western medicine during this period. The use of statistics to achieve objectivity, the historian of statistics Theodore Porter explains, is of particular importance for professional communities subjected to close scrutiny. They need to defend themselves against potential critics. Impersonal measurement and objectification through the use of statistics protect these communities against suspicion of personal bias and arbitrary decisions.[72] After the Second World War there was a shift toward public funding for health care and biomedical research. The majority of Western European countries developed centralized national health care systems, while in the United States biomedical research and health care delivery became increasingly dependent on various forms of government support. "Big medicine" became a powerful institution, but at the same time biomedical research institutions, teaching hospitals, and major health care facilities were increasingly subjected to scrutiny by science and health administrators, politicians, and the lay public, and occasionally had to protect themselves against potential accusations of misuse of government funds. The rapid adoption of the principle (if not always the practice) of controlled clinical trials was thus stimulated by the medical elite's increasing political vulnerability, itself a result of the development of state-dependent "big medicine" and biomedical science. Alternatively, the postwar success of clinical trials may be seen as another episode linked to the increase in the prestige and power of biomedical re-searchers in the struggle between academic elites and medical practi-tioners. Clinical trials, which involved alliances among medical re-searchers, the clinical elite, and drug companies, could be viewed as a means of consolidating this prestige and enhancing the control of academic physicians over practitioners.[73]

The specific circumstances of the introduction of large-scale con-trolled clinical trials also favored their diffusion. The first controlled and randomized clinical trials were those involving newly developed antibiotics such as penicillin and streptomycin. The results were de-void of ambiguity, and the trials became the model for evaluating the efficacy of therapies. Unambiguous results are, however, an exception rather than a rule in a clinical trial. Marks has shown that the general agreement on the value of many controlled clinical trials, especially those evaluating therapies for chronic diseases, was far from being free of controversies over goals and the interpretation of results.[74] In cases involving chronic illness, and in the absence of a treatment as effective as penicillin, definitions of therapeutic success cannot be sep-arated from debates over the pathophysiological nature of a given disease (what are the disease's essential traits and how they should be measured), the possible therapeutic responses to that disease (what is the treatment's main goal and how it should be evaluated), and indi-vidual and social perceptions of health and illness.[75] Doctors often have divergent opinions on these questions, and agreement may be difficult, especially in large-scale, multicenter trials.

One way to overcome these difficulties is to switch the focus of a clinical experiment from a search for technical innovations to a search for organizational ones. In complex organizations, sociologist Andrew Abbott explains, technical efficiency—the efficiency of isolated acts (in medicine, the development of efficient ways to prevent, detect, and cure disease)—is often subordinated to organizational efficiency—the ability to articulate tasks efficiently in a complex environment (in med-icine, to ensure efficient collaboration among professionals).[76] The pri-macy of organizational efficiency is not a result of deliberate choice but reflects the decisionmaking process in complex organizations. In such organizations innovations with high organizational efficiency have better chances to be selected for further testing; those with low organizational efficiency may be rapidly discarded and never be eval-uated for their technical efficiency. After the Second World War lead-ing cancer treatment centers became complex professional environments. Clinical trials of new cancer therapies increased the organizational efficiency of these centers by favoring the development and consolidation of links among distinct professional groups such as oncologists, biologists, pharmacologists, toxicologists, and cytologists. This function was not directly related to the technical efficiency of these trials, that is, to their success in developing an effective therapy for cancer. The history of clinical trials of chemotherapy in the United States in the 1950s is the history of an organizational innovation. This innovation promoted the development of networks that connected experts and sites, and then shaped a new domain of medical activity.

Clinical Trials of Cancer Chemotherapies in the United States

Early trials of chemotherapies conducted in the late 1940s—such as those at the Sloan-Kettering Institute and the Institute for Cancer Research in Philadelphia—were single-center assays involving a small number of patients (usually fewer than 50).[77] Two elements favored a radical change in the scale and methods of clinical trials of new cancer drugs after the Second World War: the development of multidisciplinary cancer treatment centers and the growing political importance of the "cancer problem," which led to the establishment of the CCNSC.

The trend to treat cancer patients in specialized centers began in the 1910s and 1920s and accelerated after the Second World War.[78] Centers and physicians gradually became more specialized. Although many cancer patients were still cared for by general practitioners and were treated in unspecialized hospital wards, cancer therapy was increasingly recognized as a distinct medical domain. The first stage of this recognition was linked with the high price of equipment used for radiation therapy, which favored the concentration of cancer patients in a small number of specialized centers. This concentration coincided during the interwar period with a general trend toward transforming hospitals into privileged sites of specialized medical treatments.[79] The second stage in the development of a specific jurisdiction of cancer therapy was linked with the development of clinical trials of chemotherapies after the Second World War. Nearly all new drug treatments were tested in leading cancer centers, which often combined therapeutic, diagnostic, and technical services, basic and preclinical research, and teaching activities. Clinical trials of new cancer therapies increased the organizational efficiency of leading cancer treatment centers. The centers facilitated the development of alliances among professional groups, and these alliances furthered the expansion of the specialized domain of cancer therapy.

The NCI screening program was a privileged site of development of such interprofessional alliances. The establishment of the CCNSC permitted the transformation of clinical trials of cancer therapies into an efficient organizational innovation. The Chemistry, Pharmacology, Endocrinology, and Screening Panels of the CCNSC were responsible for preclinical research, while the clinical trials themselves were co-ordinated by the Clinical Studies Panel. The CCNSC's guidelines, which aimed at the standardization of preclinical and clinical tests for new anticancer drugs, later established patterns for clinical trials in oncology. For example, according to Screening Panel guidelines, compounds were considered active in animals when minimum standards of activity were met at the maximum-tolerated dose. This approach was later transferred to the clinics. Cancer chemotherapy—and later the therapeutic application of biological substances such as interleu-kin-2—became synonymous with the use of maximum-tolerated (thus often highly toxic) doses of drugs.[80]

In the mid-1950s the Clinical Studies Panel promoted the establishment of 10 cooperative study groups, which were represented in about 100 hospitals. Many of these hospitals were controlled by the Veterans Administration, an official collaborator with the CCNSC. The organizers of these groups stressed the need to develop a highly organized domain of clinical activity. Members of panels reciprocally surveyed the application of protocols, the randomization procedures, and the quality of laboratory analyses of other members of the cooperative study group. These surveillance measures were justified by the need to raise the standards of cancer diagnosis and care, and by the low efficacy of anticancer treatments. As the head of the CCNSC, Kenneth Endicott, explained in 1957, "Specific measures are taken to secure uniformity, such as frequent meeting and inspection of individual laboratories by each member of the group. These restrictions would not be necessary if the treatment produced such dramatic effects as penicillin does in lobar pneumonia. Unfortunately such effects on cancer are the exception rather than the rule."[81] The low efficacy of tested treatments and the necessity to compare results obtained in different hospitals amplified the need to develop agreement on the staging of cancer (staging defines the severity of malignant disease on the basis of clinical and pathological findings) and on the quantifiable criteria

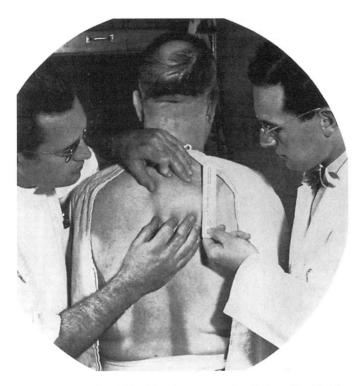

From *Cancer News,* July 1948: "The doctors on the clinic staff, aided by residents and interns, perform a complete examination, paying particular attention to any condition resembling cancer and reporting thereon." (American Cancer Society. Photo courtesy The Countway Library of Medicine, Harvard University.)

of response to drugs. The diffusion of cooperative clinical trials thus contributed to the standardization of diagnostic and therapeutic criteria in cancer treatment, reinforced the "quality control" of cancer therapies by leading specialists in the domain, and also increased the authority of the clinical researcher. The clinical studies panel recommended that "the patient's care should be under the complete control of the investigator."[82]

The organizational advantages of the cooperative study groups supervised by the CCNSC were immediately apparent. By contrast, the therapeutic advantages of the new drugs were at first less evident. In 1957 Endicott estimated that their main benefit was palliation: "although these drugs are not curative, they can temporarily relieve some of the manifestations of cancer, improve the patient's well-being and sometimes prolong life."[83] This relatively modest appreciation of chemotherapy was revised in the next decade following the development of curative therapies for acute lymphoblastic leukemia (ALL) in children. The proof that chemotherapy could actually cure cancer led to a radical modification of cancer therapy in the United States. Consequently, the structures that led to the elaboration of cure for ALL—Leukemia Group A (specialized in adult leukemia), Leukemia Group B (specialized in childhood leukemia), and, from 1962 on, the Acute Leukemia Task Force—became a universal model of clinical research in oncology.

Leukemia Group B was one of the 10 collaborative groups sponsored by the CCNSC, and it was clearly the most successful: in 1957 Endicott emphasized the advances in the treatment of childhood leukemia as the sole example of therapeutic progress brought about by the new approach to testing chemotherapies. At first this progress was limited to an important increase in the one-year survival rate.[84] From 1957 through 1961 Leukemia Group B organized numerous clinical trials and accumulated expertise in evaluating the performance of cytotoxic drugs. These trials afforded a better understanding of the effects of antileukemia drugs and led to their more efficient use in children. Greater experience with the use of cytotoxic drugs improved the management of their dangerous side effects. These improvements, however, did not lead to cures for childhood leukemia. The treated children survived longer, but they invariably relapsed.[85]

In the meantime cancer specialists obtained the first proof that a disseminated solid cancer (as distinct from a hematological, systemic cancer such as leukemia, which can be present anywhere in the body from onset and thus does not begin as a "localized tumor") can be cured with chemotherapy. This finding was not linked with screening programs or with the CCNSC-inspired cooperative studies. Like discoveries of the tumor-fighting properties of nitrogen mustard or folic acid antagonists, it stemmed from an unexpected observation followed by an investigation conducted by a single group of physicians and scientists. Clinicians who attempted to use methotrexate (a folic acid antagonist) to treat melanoma observed that this drug suppressed the secretion of gonadotropin (a sexual hormone). They thereupon used methotrexate in an attempt to cure the cancer of the cells that secrete gonadotropin—choriocarcinoma (a malignancy induced by embryonic cells, the trophoblasts). The study, conducted at the Endocrinology Department of the NCI in 1956, was greatly helped by the observation that there was a direct correlation between the measurable level of gonadotropin in the serum and urine of choriocarcinoma patients and the severity of their disease. The NCI endocrinologists could thus directly survey the therapeutic effects of methotrexate and rapidly determine the optimal therapeutic doses.[86] Other cytotoxic drugs (vinblastine, actinomycin-D) were later also found to be efficient against choriocarcinoma. In the early 1960s the NCI physicians reported apparent cures in nearly half their patients.[87] Although choriocarcinoma is a rare and atypical tumor, the discovery of a drug cure for a disseminated cancer had an important psychological effect. It also strengthened the links between endocrinology and chemotherapy. These links were later consolidated through closer integration of endocrinology studies into the chemotherapy program of the NCI.

The success of choriocarcinoma therapy helped convince specialists that other kinds of cancer would also respond to chemotherapy. Childhood leukemia was an obvious candidate for concentrated efforts to obtain a cure of major malignancy. In 1960 Kenneth Endicott left his position as director of the CCNSC to become director of the NCI. Dr. Gordon Zubrod, head of the CCNSC's Pharmacological Division, became the NCI's scientific director. These appointments probably reflected the political importance attached to the development of new chemotherapies. In 1961 Zubrod proposed the creation of a special task force "to engineer a cure" of acute lymphoblastic leukemia. Endicott liked the idea but thought that he and his colleagues should learn more about task forces. To do so they "visited friends at IBM, where such groups had been used with great effectiveness. The key elements in their success seemed to be selecting a single objective, identifying the best people in the company for the job, giving them time and resources to get it done, and disbanding the task force as soon as the objective was within reach."[88] The direct industrial inspiration, Zubrod and Endicott felt, was justified because the problem of the cure of ALL was seen as a technical one: five efficient drugs existed already, and researchers were convinced that it would be possible to find the right way to use them to kill all the residual malignant cells and to prevent relapses. This conviction was reinforced by early data from Leukemia Group A, which indicated that although less than 1 percent of ALL patients treated with chemotherapy became long-term survivors, there were no survivors among untreated patients.[89]

The Acute Leukemia Task Force, created in the spring of 1962, coordinated the activities of several professional groups: laboratory scientists, clinical investigators, pharmacologists, statisticians, industrial researchers, and members of the CCNSC staff. Its activity was not qualitatively different from that of the other CCNSC panels. It was, however, a much more intensive effort (in the participants' words, "an aggressive pursuit of new leads in the treatment of acute leukemia"), rendered concrete through numerous simultaneous studies and coordinated through monthly meetings of the principal investigators.[90] This effort rapidly led to several innovations. The screening of anti-ALL drugs was accelerated through the decision to use a single animal model, the L1210 (a leukemia of the mouse). Clinicians developed more effective methods to prevent the toxic effects of drugs. Infections were prevented by aseptic measures and energetic antibiotic therapy, while the danger of hemorrhage was limited through repeated platelet transfusions. The latter method became feasible thanks to the development (in collaboration with IBM) of a blood separator. The persistence of malignant cells in the meningeal fluid was treated by injecting methotrexate into the cerebrospinal fluid (and later by X rays to the head and spinal cord). Finally, probably the most important innovation was the introduction of multidrug regimens. Although drug combinations had been widely used in bacterial chemotherapy, they had not previously been employed in chemotherapy of cancer. Leukemia Groups A and B introduced the combination of two drugs and reported encouraging effects, while the Leukemia Task Force extended this experimentation and established fixed protocols that combined four or more drugs. The combination of all these methods led to therapeutic success. In the mid-1960s the first reports attested to the achievement of cures for ALL in children.[91] The success of the effort against ALL was closely followed by another therapeutic success directly inspired by ALL treatment—the cure for Hodgkin's lymphoma by a combination chemotherapy.[92] Clinical trials of chemotherapy for ALL and Hodgkin's lymphoma were nonrandomized, single-arm trials (that is, they did not oppose treated patients to a control group but compared treated patients with historical controls), a pattern that was later adopted for other clinical trials of new anticancer drugs. This approach was unusual: in the 1960s clinical trials of new drugs usually included control groups. The quasi-monopoly of oncologists over their patients (other doctors were seldom interested in the treatment of cancer patients) might have contributed to the persistence of historical controls in oncology. In the 1970s some doctors objected to this anomaly and contested the absence of randomization in clinical trials of new therapies of cancer.[93] However, the specialists who claimed that randomization of new cancer treatment trials was neither ethical nor necessary prevailed, and the NCI-sponsored clinical trials of new anticancer drugs continued to be nonrandomized.[94]

The success of the ALL task force and the promise of cures for adult cancers produced by the cure for Hodgkin's lymphoma had immediate political repercussions. Members of the National Advisory Cancer Council and of Congress insisted on creating task forces for virtually every type of cancer. Task forces were formed for lymphoma, solid tumors, chronic myelocytic leukemia, and brain tumors. The NCI also established the Breast Cancer Task Force, the Lung Cancer Working Party, the Brain Tumor Study Group, and the Polycythemia Vera Study Group. Although the CCNSC still faced some criticism, the principle of coordinated large-scale collaborative studies of cancer chemotherapy was widely accepted not only by oncologists but also by politicians and health administrators. The new approach was in agreement with politicians' and administrators' point of view on the proper management of resources. It was also in agreement with the belief that the "fight against cancer" should combine advanced scientific research and aggressive treatment. Moreover, it worked. It was thus strongly encouraged on the institutional level.[95]

In 1965 the CCNSC merged with the NCI Laboratory of Chemical Pathology and the Medicine Branch to form the National Chemotherapy Program, led by Zubrod. The new program was based on the principles that guided the Acute Leukemia Task Force and covered drug procurement, screening, pharmacology studies, and clinical trials. It obtained generous funding and enjoyed the support of a growing number of American cancer specialists, rapidly converted to faith in the therapeutic use of drugs in cancer therapy. The program's explicit goal was the extension of the early successes of the ALL and Hodgkin's lymphoma programs. New anticancer drugs were tested in an NCI-sponsored network. Drugs were made available first to a few selected anticancer treatment centers, then, if they proved promising, to a larger number of institutions and physicians sponsored by NCI grants or contracts. Drugs found to be efficient in the NCI network later went through the regular procedure of FDA approval, received a marketing permit, and became available for all medical practitioners.[96] Thus in the 1960s and 1970s the distribution of new, not yet approved, anti-cancer drugs remained under the near-exclusive control of NCI specialists. This pattern of testing new anticancer drugs was exceptional. As a rule drug companies, not government agencies, selected the initial investigators for new products. In contrast, the NCI specialists decided who among the numerous U.S. physicians treating cancer would be able to offer their patients access to experimental (and, for many desperate cancer patients, highly desirable) anticancer drugs. The 1982 NCI/FDA Joint Task Force report on anticancer drugs stressed that the aim of the NCI distribution system was to put the needs of the patient first. The drug distribution system was described as "an appropriate method for bringing important medication to patients who need them."[97]

The 1960s and 1970s witnessed the rapid expansion of multicenter clinical trials of solid tumor therapies. In the 1960s cancer specialists believed that the methods elaborated by the ALL task force would be successfully applied to the search for adequate chemotherapy for other cancers. The clinical results did not, however, confirm their expectations. Although oncologists developed efficient chemotherapies for several childhood cancers and a few rare cancers in adults, the National Chemotherapy Program and other task forces and study groups failed to find cures for common solid cancers in adults. The contrast between the high organizational efficiency of clinical trials of cancer therapies (that is, their ability to articulate the interests of numerous professional groups) and their low technical (that is, therapeutic) efficiency shaped the jurisdiction of cancer therapy in the United States and indirectly affected its development in other Western countries.[98] The high organizational efficiency directly favored the spread of clinical trials of anticancer drugs; the low technical efficiency stimulated experimentation with an ever-growing number of compounds and their combinations, and the routinization of the exceptional in the cancer clinics.

One of the central innovations induced by clinical trials of anticancer drugs was the standardization of criteria of therapeutic success in the treatment of solid tumors. The low therapeutic efficacy of the new anticancer drugs emphasized the need for agreement on the definition of success in a clinical trial of a cancer therapy. Such agreement was achieved through the development of the notion of "objective response." Only patients who had "measurable disease"—that is, patients with tumors whose size could be determined with reasonable accuracy in at least two dimensions—were (and are) seen as adequate candidates for enrollment in clinical trials. The definition of measurable disease was at first restricted to visible or palpable tumors and to tumors (such as lung and bone tumors) that could be seen on an X-ray film. But the development of new techniques of medical visualization such as magnetic resonance imaging and computerized axial tomography (CAT) scanners extended that notion and transformed an important fraction of patients suffering from advanced solid tumors into adequate candidates for enrollment in clinical trials.

In evaluations of the efficacy of new therapies for solid tumors, the importance attached to measures of reduction of cancer volume was based on two distinct assumptions. One was the belief—sustained by the ALL task force experience—that a therapy that initially produced only partial results had the potential to become a definitive cure. The second was the assumption—based on the cell-centered understanding of cancer that dominated both professional and lay perceptions of cancer from the 1930s on[99]—that a direct relation exists between a tumor's bulk and the severity of clinical manifestations of malignant disease. This assumption allowed an implicit equation between objective response to antitumor treatments, as measured by diminished tumor volume, and improvement in the clinical status of cancer patients. For example, the 1982 report of the NCI/FDA Joint Task Force on experimental therapies of cancer maintained that the 9.5 percent overall "response rate" of phase I (toxicity-testing) trials of anticancer drugs was reason enough for patients to choose an experimental therapy.[100]

It was easier to achieve agreement upon "hard" data, such as the measurable effects of a given therapy on a tumor's size, than on "soft" data, such as the effects of that therapy on patients' "quality of life."[101] "Quality of life" data were introduced into the evaluation of cancer therapies in the 1980s. The assessment of "quality of life" developed into a separate field aimed at the development of objective, quantifiable measurements of standardized indicators. These indicators, however, are usually measured by lower-status personnel such as nurses, psychologists, medical sociologists, or social workers, and are viewed as potentially more controversial than quantitative data.[102] Objective measures are presumably more efficient in facilitating collaboration among heterogeneous professional groups. They help to promote horizontal links among clinical researchers in different institutional settings and vertical connections between clinicians and research laboratories, the pharmaceutical industry, health administrators, and government agencies. They therefore became one of the cornerstones of the culture of clinical experimentation in oncology.[103]

Clinical Trials and the Development of Medical Oncology in the United States, Britain, and France

In the 1960s and 1970s cancer specialists in the United States mounted more and more efforts to treat a large variety of cancers with chemotherapy. The spread of chemotherapy created a need to train hematologists, gastroenterologists, gynecologists, and specialists in internal medicine in the management of highly toxic anticancer drugs. The increasing specialization of physicians who treated cancer with drugs led to the development of a distinct medical subspecialty, medical oncology. In 1971 the American Board of Internal Medicine decided to offer certification in this specialty. This decision was approved a year later by the American Board of Medical Specialists, and the first medical oncology certifying examinations were administered in 1973.[104] The number of board-certified oncologists grew rapidly, reaching 3,000 in 1984.[105] In the United States the medical oncologist was viewed not as a consulting specialist, but as the primary doctor caring for cancer patients, responsible (sometimes in collaboration with other specialists) for the entire management of cancer therapy.

The development of medical oncology as a distinct specialty may recall the development of radiation therapy as one in the 1910s and 1920s.[106] There was, however, an important difference between the two. Reactions to radiation are highly individualized. The radiosensitivity of specific human tumors cannot be studied in the animal, and even the extrapolation from one case of human cancer to another case of similar cancer is difficult. Early in the development of radiotherapy, its practitioners established its possibilities and limits, developed adequate equipment, determined effective radiation doses, and developed routine therapies for numerous human tumors. Radiation therapy, firmly grounded in medical practices and seldom closely associated with large-scale preclinical or clinical experimentation, rapidly diverged from radiobiological research. It became a technique-oriented medical subspecialty, relatively isolated from other biomedical specialties and from research in other disciplines. By contrast, chemotherapy immediately developed close connections with the research laboratory and with research in other specialties (pharmacology, toxicology, cell biology, biochemistry, endocrinology). These links were not affected by the difficulties of finding an effective drug therapy for the majority of adult cancers. Probably just the opposite was true. It is plausible to assume that the dearth of results with chemotherapy, combined with high expectations from the public (and politicians) of rapidly finding "the cure for cancer," promoted the conviction that even more intensive preclinical and clinical investigative efforts were needed, and contributed to the maintenance of a research-oriented ethos.

Support for clinical experiments in oncology was stimulated in the United States by local cultural traditions, derived from the frontier mentality. The frontier tradition valued an aggressive "fight against cancer," seen as the appropriate attitude for doctors and as a moral obligation for patients. Experimentation with new anticancer drugs was also stimulated by significantly increased funding for cancer research following passage of the Cancer Act in 1971.[107] Training in the administration of drugs in cancer therapy came to be closely associated with training in clinical experimentation, while the latter was modeled on the example of the ALL task force, that is, on large-scale cooperative studies. Medical oncology was organized as a trial-oriented professional segment. Specialists in cancer therapy were enrolled in a network of cooperative groups. These groups proposed a large number of clinical trials, a tendency encouraged by the trend in multidrug treatments and the nearly infinite number of combinations of drugs that might be proposed to patients. The collaborative groups favored the circulation of information and the development of professional contacts. They thus became an important site for the socialization of oncologists. The organization of cancer therapy around clinical experimentation reflected the strong pro-science tradition of American physicians and their close links with the laboratory.[108] It also reflected the history of chemotherapy trials in the United States and the key role of the NCI and of NCI-coordinated programs such as the CCNSC and, later, the National Chemotherapy Program and the Division of Cancer Treatment in the development of the new field. Around 1990, leading U.S. cancer treatment centers proudly announced that although clinical trials continued to have restrictive enrollment criteria, they were so numerous that nearly every patient suffering from advanced cancer could be eligible to participate in one.[109]

Enrollment in clinical trials of new therapies, once a fairly rare event, became part of the routine management of numerous cancer patients.

The central place of clinical trials in the development of medical oncology in the United States influenced other Western countries. The diffusion of the U.S. model was facilitated by North American supremacy in basic and preclinical oncological research. U.S. research institutions, and in particular the NCI, proposed programs to train postdoctoral students and physicians from abroad and offered resources that were not available elsewhere. Consequently, many European specialists in oncology were trained in the United States or have spent some time in one of the major American cancer research centers.[110] American institutions played an important role in the development of oncology as a research-oriented specialty in Europe from the 1950s on. Senior European researchers frequently visited leading U.S. research institutes and treatment centers, and their international and national reputations were influenced by the opinions of their North American colleagues. American dominance in cancer research also indirectly influenced the clinics. European specialists trained in U.S. hospitals were impressed by their dynamism and organizational efficiency and attempted to bring home some of their methods. Bedside medicine, however, continues to be shaped by local factors such as health policies, resources, the organization of the health care system, and local medical traditions and cultural differences. The distinct ways in which medical oncology developed in Britain and in France highlights the importance of such differences.

The British developed specialized training in oncology, but, unlike the Americans, they reserved this specialization for a small number of doctors. In 1981 there were only 40 to 50 consultants in oncology in Britain—per capita, less than one-tenth the number in the United States.[111] This trend became even more pronounced in the 1980s: in 1985 the number of certified American medical oncologists nearly doubled, while the number of British specialists remained unchanged.[112] British doctors complained about the dearth of certified oncologists and proposed various measures, such as merging the professional role of radiotherapy and chemotherapy specialists, training specialists such as hematologists or gastroenterologists in the use of anticancer drugs, or combining the roles of clinical researchers and oncologists.[113] They did not, however, show much enthusiasm for the U.S. model, which was seen as illustrating the harmful effects of overmedicalization. Moreover, not all British doctors recognized the need to train even a limited number of specialists in medical oncology. A 1981 editorial in *The Lancet* affirmed that "it seems unjustified to create a specialty around a few drugs, however toxic, although we must of course avoid the indiscriminate and unmonitored use of these drugs."[114] The British finally chose to develop a double training in medical oncology and radiation therapy. This shift led to a small increase in the number of consultant positions in oncology, but it did not modify the professional role of such consultants. They continued to offer principally advice and supervision, while the care of cancer patients was left mainly to general practitioners, specialists in internal medicine, or specialists in other disciplines (such as gastroenterology, hematology, pneumology, laryngology).[115]

For a long time France had no equivalent to the U.S. certification in medical oncology. As successors to regional anticancer centers created in 1921, in 1945 the government established a network of 20 regional, nonprofit, state-sponsored cancer treatment centers (Centres de Lutte contre le Cancer; CLCCs). From their inception the CLCCs were multidisciplinary institutions, employing surgeons, radiation therapists, anatomo-pathologists, and specialists in internal medicine. The physicians working in these centers had practical training in oncology but no formal certification in the field. Only one-fifth to one-quarter of cancer patients in France were treated in the CLCCs; most were treated by surgeons and radiation therapists working in general hospitals and private clinics.[116] The specialized teaching of oncology was organized according to a system of academic-style oncology chairs. After the Second World War such chairs were established in all the French medical schools, and most of the specialists occupying them became directors of the regional CLCCs. Their role—to coordinate the treatment of cancer on the regional level—was comparable to that of senior consultants in oncology in Britain. These specialists also trained medical students in selected aspects of oncology through the organization of teaching units ("certificates"). A national diploma in oncology was established only in 1989.[117] Yet the lack of such a diploma did not prevent a proliferation of doctors specialized in cancer treatment and awarded a "competence" (professional capacity certificate) in oncology by the French Medical Association (Ordre des Médecins). As of January 1, 1992, there were 1,103 doctors accredited with such "competence." These doctors had training in oncology (mainly in the use of cytotoxic drugs) and practical experience in the field but, unlike their American colleagues, were not exclusively specialized in cancer treatment. The establishment of a national diploma led to the emergence of a group of certified experts in oncology.[118] Thus French medical oncology in the early 1990s occupied a position between the American and the British approaches.

Several major anticancer centers played an important role in the development of cancer chemotherapy in France. This therapy became closely associated with the achievements of selected "great doctors." In the late 1950s and the 1960s the Institute for the Study of Blood Diseases (Institut de Recherches sur les Maladies du Sang) at the Saint Louis Hospital in Paris, directed by Dr. Jean Bernard, was one of the first centers in Europe to introduce chemotherapy to the treatment of childhood leukemia; similar projects concerning adult leukemia were conducted at the same time at the Institut Gustave Roussy, in the Paris suburb Villejuif, under Dr. Georges Mathé.[119] The French pioneers of cancer chemotherapy played an important role in the foundation, in 1963, of the European Organization for Research on the Treatment of Cancer, which has coordinated clinical trials of anticancer therapies.[120] This European collaborative network introduced mutual quality controls among nations and promoted standardization of diagnostic and therapeutic criteria.[121] Among other things, it played an important role in the introduction and standardization of hormone therapies for breast and prostate cancer. The rapid integration of selected leading French cancer treatment centers in an international network of clinical research in oncology contrasted with the paucity of research activity in other French institutions that treated cancer patients. To remedy this situation, in 1985 a government-sponsored commission proposed that CLCC research activities be better integrated with academic research programs and that oncology departments be created in teaching hospitals. Such departments, the commission recommended, should include a radiotherapy unit and a medical oncology unit specialized in chemotherapy, immunotherapy, and hormone therapy, and should have close links with a hematology unit.[122]

Although French researchers did not play a major role in the development of chemotherapies of cancer, new cancer treatments had high visibility in France. Leading oncologists who combined professional success, political power, and influence in the media presented their achievements in bestselling books combining popular science, personal memoirs, and philosophical reflections. These books praised the new therapies as an exemplary success of "scientific medicine" and proposed a variety of experimental approaches.[123] At the same time their narratives typically displayed awareness of the limits of current treatments and a sensitivity to the plight of patients. Thus Jean Bernard characterized randomized clinical trials as "necessarily immoral and morally necessary," and Claude Jasmin wrote of "the thin borderline that divides, in the country of the hopeless, the need to maintain hope and therapeutic excesses, the excitement and the glory of a discovery and the oblivion of the shared endeavor of two persons in which only one is risking his or her life."[124] From the 1960s on, these oncologists often secured their professional positions through preclinical and clinical research. The same specialists who wrote moving personalized accounts of the scientific and moral dilemmas of clinical trials in oncology often enthusiastically promoted these trials. In the 1980s the probability of a French cancer patient's being included in a clinical experiment to test a new anticancer therapy was lower than for an American patient. This difference probably does not reflect divergences in the therapeutic approaches of leading French and American oncologists, but rather the fact that in France a smaller percentage of patients suffering from cancer were treated in research-oriented institutions.

The Larger Context

Debates on the proper attitude toward patients suffering from untreatable malignancies usually oppose two points of view. Some specialists advocate, in the name of the patient's best interests, the continuation of active treatment and the enrollment of patients suffering from untreatable cancer in clinical trials of new therapies. They explain that, besides benefits for the collectivity, such trials bring direct benefits to patients by offering them a possibility of either a cure or an alleviation of suffering, and by allowing them to maintain hope in the last months of life.[125] Other specialists advocate, equally in the name of the patient's best interests, minimal intervention, palliative care, and the development of hospice networks. They stress the low efficacy and high toxicity of the great majority of experimental and semiexperimental treatments for advanced cancer. Such treatments, they claim, spoil the quality of the patients' remaining months or years of life and rob them of the opportunity for a dignified death.[126]

These debates on the ethics of clinical experimentation in oncology are usually cast in abstract terms.[127] Philosophers and medical experts alike often discuss decontextualized questions, such as the potential conflict between (abstract) "principles of sound science" and the (generally valid) "humanitarian impulses" of the doctors, or the unavoidable conflict between the physician's obligation as a healer to his or her patient and the physician's obligations as a scientist to all present and future patients.[128] Thus the 1982 NCI/FDA Joint Task Force report on anticancer drugs opposed "patients' needs" and the "scientific principles" of controlled clinical trials but did not mention the possible influence of professional structures, institutional frameworks, or career considerations on trial-linked decisions.[129] Debates on clinical trials of anticancer treatments describe physicians of unknown nationality, training, professional status, and institutional affiliation grappling with abstract moral dilemmas. Real-life patients participating in real-life trials of new anticancer drugs, however, face not abstract "caregivers" but well-defined groups of professionals with specific beliefs, interests, institutional constraints, and involvement in struggles for power and resources. The culture of clinical experimentation in oncology exists in all Western countries, but it takes a different shape in different sites. Debates on the ethics of experimentation in cancer clinics seldom consider these disparities. In the next few pages I attempt to give a concrete meaning to the general term "clinical trials of new cancer therapies" and to illuminate the links between the decision to enroll patients in a given clinical trial of a new cancer therapy and the national, institutional, and professional environments of that trial.

Let us examine the national context first. The different attitudes toward experimental or semiexperimental chemotherapies of advanced cancers of the adult in Britain and in the United States illustrate the ways in which the organization of the jurisdiction of cancer therapy may affect the therapeutic choices of cancer patients. In the early 1980s the per-capita expenditure on chemotherapy in Britain was one-fifth of the expenditure in the United States, and American patients with solid tumors were five to six times more likely to receive drug treatment than British patients with similar tumors.[130] This disparity was attributed to differences in the number of medical oncologists in each country and in their professional roles. Specialists tend to believe in the efficacy of their specialty. Research comparing the readiness of cancer specialists to enroll patients in clinical trials with the readiness of the same specialists to enter such trials themselves if they were in the patient's situation, found that medical oncologists favored to trials of new drugs more than radiation therapists or surgeons did, while radiation therapists favored radiotherapy and surgeons favored operations. In addition, cancer specialists were systematically more eager to enroll patients in a given clinical trial than to undergo that experimental treatment themselves.[131]

The high number of medical oncologists in the United States may thus stimulate drug consumption. Similarly, the low density of medical oncologists in Britain—and thus the lower number of potential "prescribers"—may favor a limited use of anticancer drugs. Indeed, the reluctance of British officials to increase the number of consultants in medical oncology was explained as a fear that such an increase would inevitably increase expenditures for cancer treatment.[132] Moreover, in the United States the fee-for-service system pressures doctors to "do something" for their patients, even if medical science is practically impotent.[133] American oncologists make their living by treating cancer and are interested in securing the loyalty of a large number of patients. They may therefore tend to develop a more optimistic view of chemotherapy. By contrast, in Britain there is no connection between the selection of therapy and a doctor's income. Physicians employed by the public health system are encouraged to make cost-effective choices and to incorporate such choices into their decisions. British doctors therefore tend to be more skeptical about the value of chemotherapy in extending the duration of "good quality" life.[134]

The spread of drug therapies for advanced cancer may also have affected how fully cancer patients are informed about their disease. American physicians, unlike their British colleagues, insisted in the 1980s on the importance of telling cancer patients the whole truth.[135] Thus American patients participating in clinical trials of interferons and interleukins signed a document stating that they knew they suffered from advanced cancer and that their disease could not be cured by any known therapeutic means. This was a relatively new policy; until the 1960s American doctors rarely announced the diagnosis to cancer patients.[136] This reversal in approach coincided with the diffusion of chemotherapies for cancer and the emergence of medical oncology as a distinct and populous medical specialty. The large-scale introduction of drugs to the treatment of advanced cancers made concealment of a cancer diagnosis difficult because chemotherapy typically induces side effects such as nausea, fatigue, and hair loss.[137]

American oncologists who try to convince their patients to accept harsh therapies may be more inclined to inform them about the severity of their disease, and more likely to view awareness of cancer diagnosis and prognosis as serving the patients' best interests.[138] By contrast, British doctors, obliged to ration resources, are more inclined to convince patients and families—and themselves—that a costly therapy such as chemotherapy for advanced, disseminated cancer will do more harm than good. This rule applies in particular to elderly patients or to those suffering from multiple health problems.[139] Accordingly, some experts propose that doctors who are more likely to withhold aggressive treatment may also be more inclined to believe that detailed knowledge of the diagnosis and prognosis may unnecessarily increase patients' plight.[140]

Differences in the public visibility of new therapies for cancer and in patients' freedom to select their treatment probably also affected the ways in which advanced cancer was treated in Britain and the United States in the 1980s. The diffusion of therapies not known to the lay public, such as total parenteral nutrition, depended in both countries only on the decisions of physicians and health administrators. In contrast, new treatments for cancer had much higher visibility, and physicians might come under public pressure to provide them. Desperate (and affluent) American patients who had heard about a new, experimental therapy were able to shop for a doctor who would conform to their wishes among the ample supply of medical oncologists. In Britain patients were reported to be less knowledgeable about new therapies and more inclined to trust their doctor, and thus rarely pressed for treatments that were not recommended. The regionalization of British public health services, which discouraged changing doctors and searching for different institutional settings for cancer therapies, also limited the possibilities of shopping around for experimental treatments.[141]

The enrollment of patients in clinical trials for new cancer therapies is affected not only by the structure of health services in a given country, but also by the institutional framework in which patients are treated. Differences among institutions within a (Western) country may be as great as, or greater than, differences between two countries. Leading research and teaching hospitals tend to develop strong "experimentalist" ethics. Such ethics may be encouraged by the size of a given institution and its need to compete with other, similar institutions. Big research and teaching hospitals are today complex, highly bureaucratized organizations. Specialists of organizational behavior have proposed that complex organizations, whatever their goals may be, tend to develop common features, a process called "institutional isomorphism."[142] One of the consequences of institutional isomorphism is that the adoption of innovation in complex organizations ceases to be a means of improving performance and instead becomes a means of achieving legitimacy in the organizational field.[143] The propagation of the culture of clinical experimentation in oncology may be seen as an example of institutional isomorphism. In complex organizations the success of diagnostic or therapeutic innovations may be judged not solely according to their contribution to improving the lot of patients but perhaps also according to their contribution to organizational goals such as maintaining a reputation and keeping up with state-of-the-art developments—a necessary condition for attracting funds, specialists, and patients in a highly competitive field.[144]

A cancer treatment center that aspires to maintain its image of being at the cutting edge of developments in oncology cannot afford not to test therapies characterized as "promising." In these research-oriented centers, professional rewards (recognition by peers, tenured positions, access to students, control of material resources) may depend to a large extent on a doctor's achievements as a basic or clinical investigator. The local value system often exerts strong pressures on its members to develop close relationships with the laboratory, to conduct preclinical and clinical research, and to enroll as many patients as possible in clinical trials. This trialist ethos is legitimated by the shared belief that enrollment in trials of experimental therapies not only contributes to the "general good" but also coincides with the best interests of individual cancer patients.[145] Adherence to a trialist ethos does not mean that every cancer therapy found to be moderately promising in preliminary tests reaches the stage of large-scale clinical experimentation and then clinical use. Institutional factors, professional structures, and industrial interests play large roles in shaping doctors' preferences for a given experimental therapy,[146] although those roles are seldom visible in debates over the therapies.

The culture of clinical experimentation is often less present in therapy-oriented cancer treatment centers than in those directly connected with academic medicine, and it is found even less frequently in general hospitals and in nonspecialized wards, in community practice, and in the private practices of doctors not affiliated with major teaching hospitals. Differences in the treatment of advanced cancer in distinct institutional frameworks may increase the range of choices open to well-informed or affluent patients. A patient who reaches the stage of "nothing more to be done" in a small or nonspecialized institution may be reclassified as a patient for whom "something more can be done" in a major research or teaching center. Patients who refuse the verdict of "nothing more to be done" may thus attempt to move to a big research hospital, while those who wish to avoid aggressive treatment may elect a peripheral institution.[147] The lower commitment to experimental therapy in nonspecialized institutions is not, however, an absolute rule. Oncologists trained in a leading teaching hospital may attempt to export the culture of clinical experimentation when they move to smaller and less specialized institutions, even more so if participation in multicenter clinical trials offers them access to other experts and reinforces their self-image as clinical scientists.[148] The tendency to promote clinical investigation may be encouraged by local health administrators interested in upgrading the visibility and prestige of their institution and enhancing its capacity to attract patients and resources.[149] It may also be stimulated by central political initiatives. Thus a French government commission strongly recommended the integration of the CLCCs into a national network of clinical experimentation, while the NCI initiated steps for greater diffusion of clinical trials in oncology.[150]

Clinical Experimentation as a Way of Coping with Cancer

The important disparities in the introduction of experimental therapies of cancer in different national and institutional settings should not mask the overall increase in experimental and semiexperimental treatments in the routine management of cancer patients in Western countries since the 1970s. This increase was affected by the structure of medical oncology as a trial-oriented occupational segment and by the development of "big science" and "big medicine" after the Second World War. It was also, I propose, influenced by the increase in the proportion of cancer patients treated in specialized institutions and followed by a single group of experts—the oncologists.

Working on specialized cancer wards is highly demanding and stressful. Oncologists have to face daily the suffering and the death of their patients, the frustration of being unable to help, and the anguish linked to the recognition of their own fragility.

Clinical trials may reduce the oncologists' work-related stress.[151]

They allow the clinician to "do something" for the patient, and thereby to alleviate frustration linked to lack of efficient therapies. The urge to "do something" is particularly strong when the patient is perceived as "too young to die." All other things being equal, such patients are more frequently enrolled in a "last-chance" trial of an experimental drug.[152] Clinical trials may also divide the long downhill trajectory of a cancer patient into a series of small, partial victories and may allow the physician to remain active even when little can be achieved.[153] They may also shift responsibility for the clinical outcome of a therapy of an individual patient from a single doctor to a more distant source.[154] Finally, a clinical trial may allow isolated failures to be interpreted as promises of future success ("the therapy did not save the patient, but we have learned a lot"). As one specialist put it, "there is so little that we have to offer so many of our patients that we tend to develop a sense of helplessness, unless we are regularly involved in a research project that at least seems to offer a hope for the future . . . Research is not just a luxury for the oncologist; it may be necessary to preserve our mental health."[155]

Enrollment in clinical trials of new therapies may also become one of the ways cancer patients cope with their "dread disease."[156] The number of cancer-related deaths has steadily risen in industrialized countries.[157] Today selected cancers (such as childhood leukemia and breast cancer) are no longer viewed as invariably fatal, but the high number of cancer-related deaths and the firsthand experiences of families and friends of cancer patients sustain the widespread fear of this pathology. The diagnosis of cancer is always a highly distressing event, and the cancer patient "is frequently ill-informed, misinformed, alienated, frightened, alone."[158] Patients and families often actively press for experimental treatment, in particular when they are unable to come to terms with an impending death (for example, when the patient is young or was in good health before diagnosis). They tend to maintain unrealistic hopes about the outcome of clinical trials.[159] If they are told that the result of a trial is not certain, they tend to interpret this information as lack of certainty about whether the new treatment will be better than standard therapy. They seldom consider the possibility that the new treatment may be worse than the standard one, because they are convinced that the "doctor wouldn't suggest it unless he thought it would help."[160]

In the late 1980s associations of cancer patients in the United States started to lobby in favor of access to clinical trials. Leading American oncologists joined them in arguing that a patient suffering from advanced cancer has nothing to lose (and much to gain) from enrollment in a clinical trial. In 1982 Dr. Vincent De Vita, then director of the NCI, testified before Congress that oncologists should not be afraid to test highly toxic drugs, because "the most serious toxicity of all is the unnecessary death from cancer."[161] During the same hearing one of the NCI experts, Dr. James Holland, explained that hesitation to use high, toxic doses of experimental anticancer drugs is against the patient's interests, because "underdosing, in an attempt to avoid toxicity, is much more deadly"; another NCI expert, Dr. Emil Freireich, warned that rigid regulation of clinical experimentation with cancer drugs may be very dangerous: "it is truly ironic that mechanisms designed for protection create serious harm to thousands of patients with cancer."[162] NCI doctors argued that patients suffering from fatal disease should be free to make their own evaluation of risks and benefits when faced with the decision to enroll in a clinical trial,[163] but the language they used (an excessively low dosage is "deadly," a limit on the testing of toxic drugs "creates serious harm" for "thousands of patients") strongly hinted that they perceived participation in clinical trials of new cancer therapies as a life-saving measure.

Even if a clinical trial does not lead to the discovery of an efficient anticancer treatment it does, some advocates of these trials affirm, fulfill an important function in bringing hope to desperate patients. Persons with advanced incurable cancer may became depressed and resentful when told that nothing more can be done to prolong life, and in such situations "an effective treatment for hopelessness is a legitimate scientific research."[164] Participation in a clinical experiment, the philosopher Andrew Feenberg proposed, may improve the participants' health independently of the physiological effects of the tested therapy.[165] Clinical trials are, it is true, designed above all to answer cognitive questions, but patients who enroll in a clinical trial with the hope of a personal advantage are not misled, because a clinical trial is in itself a form of treatment. Patients enrolled in such trials frequently benefit from the "symbolic efficacy" of medicine mediated by the placebo effect. Cultural and symbolic effects of medicine were and are a central component of healing, and the placebo effect should therefore be viewed as a perfectly legitimate consequence of medical activity.[166] From the "symbolic effectiveness" point of view too, patients have "nothing to lose" by participating in a clinical trial.[167]

Not all specialists agree, however. A patient suffering from an incurable, deadly disease, opponents of the trialist ethos claim, does have something to lose: quality of life and dignity.[168] The process of gradually accepting the inevitability of death may be disturbed by the unrealistic hopes evoked by a clinical trial. Physicians who conduct clinical trials have a tendency to be optimistic about the potential value of the trial, and their already overoptimistic evaluation is often further amplified by patients and families. Later, however, the return to a hopeless situation may induce more emotional distress than would be seen in the usual trajectory of a terminal disease.[169] Patients are obliged once again to go through the painful process of accepting the "nothing more to do" phase, and their depression is all the worse because of the loss of renewed hope.[170]

A crippling loss of hope may be linked to the failure of both orthodox and unorthodox experimental therapies. A comparative study of patients who received routine chemotherapy or unorthodox treatment for advanced cancer did not find a significant difference in the length of survival between the two groups, but revealed that in this particular sample, patients who were treated by orthodox (and inefficient) methods obtained higher scores on "quality of life" tests. The authors of the study attributed this result to the fact that patients in unorthodox treatment programs had higher expectations for improvement and were more disillusioned when the new treatment failed to bring the anticipated benefits.[171] Not surprisingly, this effect of unorthodox therapies is seldom evoked by advocates of these therapies. Evelleen Richards' innovative comparison between the different fates of an orthodox therapeutic innovation—interferon and 5-fluorouracil—and an unorthodox one—vitamin C—is oblivious to the fact that the great majority of cancer patients treated with vitamin C (often persons declared untreatable by orthodox medicine) were obliged at some point to face the fact that their disease would progress to a fatal conclusion, and to suffer the psychological effects of loss of hope. Her fine-grained sociological analysis does not discuss the consequences, for patients, of putting their faith in an unorthodox therapy that, its advocates agree, at best prolongs life. Consequently, Richards' reasonable plea for liberty of choice for cancer patients does not take into account the personal cost of such liberty for the sick person.[172]

The increasing importance of experimental trials of new cancer therapies in the trajectories of people suffering from advanced cancer and the personal costs of this development has been illustrated through stories of individual cancer patients.[173] Kenneth Shapiro's testimony about his life with cancer is centered on the ambiguous success of experimental cancer treatments. The author suffered from disseminated recurrent melanoma and was subjected to a large battery of semiconventional and experimental therapies. His reaction to these treatments was unusual: although he did not respond—or responded in an atypical way—to some routine or semiroutine therapies, he did respond well to several experimental treatments. Most remarkable was his response to a molecule credited with inducing interferon production; it rapidly eliminated all Shapiro's tumors. However, he was the only patient in the clinical trial who reacted to this therapy. The cancer eventually returned, and he agreed to additional semiconventional and experimental treatments. Shapiro's testimony—which usually avoids the uplifting tones of "my victory over cancer" type books—illustrates the difficult choices that oncologists and cancer patients face, the extent of ignorance about the natural history of cancer (although Shapiro affirms that he deeply respects his doctors, he also explains that they were almost always wrong), and the high physical and emotional costs, for the patient, of participation in clinical trials of new cancer therapies: "I sometimes wonder," Shapiro asks, "if the people who are recommending this drug or that drug would subject themselves to the therapy they are recommending."[174] On the other hand, although Shapiro claims that he accepted the inevitability of his death, he seldom refused to enter a new therapy trial.

The journalist Stewart Alsop narrowly escaped the dilemmas of experimental cancer therapy. He was tentatively diagnosed with acute myeloid leukemia and entered the NIH hospital, where he was offered the choice of several kinds of experimental therapies. All the patients admitted to that hospital had incurable cancer, were frankly informed of their health status, and were aggressively treated, up to their last breath. At some point Alsop's doctors proposed a bone marrow graft. At that time (1971), the success of bone marrow grafts as a cure for acute leukemia was very low. Alsop had found that of the twelve patients treated with this method at the NIH hospital, eleven had died either immediately or several months later, and the only one who survived suffered from recurrent infections. He wondered why doctors continued to propose treatment with such low chances of success, and he came up with two possible answers: the doctor's conviction that the patient would die soon and therefore the therapy was justified *in extremis,* and the fact that doctors, like other specialists, were eager to practice their specialty.[175] Alsop refused the bone marrow transplant but seriously considered experimental chemotherapy although he was aware that even when remission could be induced (half of the time), 95 percent of patients were dead within two years. Finally the decision was taken out of his hands. His doctors, baffled by some atypical aspects of his leukemia, decided to give him solely conservative treatment such as blood and platelet transfusion. Two years later he was still in reasonably good health (and wondered about the accuracy of the initial diagnosis).

A doctor similarly diagnosed with acute myelogenic leukemia did not escape the hard choices of a cancer patient. A sixty-five-year-old Los Angeles internist, Jack Lewis, was diagnosed as suffering from acute leukemia. His doctors at the UCLA hospital gave him the choice between aggressive, experimental therapy and no curative treatment. The chemotherapy, he was told, led to a remission in 35 to 45 percent of cases. After long hesitation, Lewis decided to try the experimental chemotherapy protocol. He suffered from extremely harsh side effects, including high fever, nausea, blisters and peeling of the skin, infection, and severe muscle pain. The therapy finally induced remission but left him in a very weakened state. "The day before I left the hospital," Lewis wrote,

> one of my doctors told me that he had never seen a patient do so well on this therapeutic regimen. I was aghast. When I questioned that if I did so well, what had the other patients on this regimen done, I was told that most had not survived the therapy. I asked my oncologist what was the definition of remission, which was the "joyous" state I was in. The answer was that the bone marrow showed no leukemic cells. How long might this last? Perhaps months, perhaps years. Maybe a cure? Who knows? Was it worthwhile? Who knows? . . . I have pondered many times whether I would have gone through this therapy knowing now what it is like. I can't honestly answer. It is easy to say now that I would not, but I am not sure this is the truth.[176]

Dr. Lewis died of a recurrent attack of leukemia after ten months of remission.

The writer and historian of women Gerda Lerner, who tells the story of the disease and death of her husband, Carl, describes the physical and psychological effects of experimental therapy in a hopeless situation. Carl Lerner was diagnosed with a malignant, inoperable brain tumor. The patient and his family were aware that there was no cure for that type of tumor, and that the disease would rapidly progress toward death. They were therefore interested when Carl Lerner's physician, Dr. Goldman, proposed that he enter a clinical trial of a new chemotherapy. On the other hand, Gerda Lerner was not sure whether Goldman's proposal was truly disinterested, whether he was able to distinguish clearly between his interest in research and his obligation to his patients.[177] She was partly reassured by the fact that her husband was not eligible for the official research protocol, and therefore would not be included in official statistics. On the other hand, she learned that the best one may expect from chemotherapy is short-lived remission and a temporary improvement of symptoms. Finally she put the case to her husband and brought him to see Goldman:

> then something extraordinary happened. Dr. Goldman, talking about the chemotherapy project, began to be transformed by real feeling and passion. Grant money, research designs, became a live force. "We will conquer this thing," he said, his eyes blazing with intensity. For a moment, even in my own misery, I perceived something noble and grand in his passionate hatred of the enemy sitting inside Carl's head and destroying his life. "Perhaps not in your lifetime," he continued, and this time his words were not cruel, simply honest, "but surely not too long from now we will learn how to arrest brain cancer with chemotherapy." Somehow, in the way he put it, there was some meaning in participating in this venture, that battle, which will go on when one's own life ceases. For a moment, with all his obvious frailties, he was at the same battleground with us, not because of Carl as a person, but because we shared a common enemy.[178]

Carl Lerner followed the experimental chemotherapy regimen, but his treatment was discontinued because of the severity of its side effects and the progressive deterioration in his health. The discontinuation of chemotherapy was, however, hidden from the patient, who might have viewed it as the loss of all hope.[179]

In advanced cancer, Gerda Lerner explained, "there was, as yet, no 'good way' to handle critical problems: there were only choices among 'lesser evils.' "[180] The same can often be said about clinical trials of new cancer therapies. In the absence of efficient therapies for the majority of advanced cancers of the adult, participation in a clinical experiment may indeed be viewed by numerous patients and doctors as a "lesser evil." Clinical trials increasingly became a part of the complex and sometimes chaotic trajectories of individual cancer patients. Such trajectories may include periods of intensive treatment and periods free from active medical intervention, the use of "parallel therapies" either alongside or alternating with "orthodox" medicine, contacts with numerous health professionals and with different health care institutions, and participation in one or several trials of experimental or semiexperimental therapies. The latter may be viewed as a part of the patient's duty to help himself and of the family's duty to make sure that every possible effort is made on behalf of the cancer victim. As an American oncologist put it, "a patient will never know what might have happened unless he is willing to try another therapy, assume the risks, and undergo assessment of the results. This is the practical approach to the treatment of cancer."[181] Practical, one may add, also in the sense that the culture of clinical experimentation allows patients and doctors to transform a "nothing more to be done" into a "something can be done" situation and to sustain the shared belief in the efficacy of scientific medicine.

Paradoxically, the role of clinical trials as a coping mechanism may have been expanded in the 1970s and 1980s by the persistent failure to develop efficient therapies for the majority of common cancers of the adult. This failure—combined with continuing faith in the possibility of developing new anticancer drugs or improving old ones—led to an impressive proliferation of trials of anticancer therapies. This proliferation had in turn an unexpected effect. Clinical trials had previously been criticized for subordinating the ideal of individual-oriented medicine to the necessity of applying a rigorously standardized therapy to all the enrolled patients in order to obtain statistically valid results. The dramatic increase in the number of experimental therapies turned this argument on its head. Clinical trials, some doctors have explained, facilitate the adaptation of therapies to the needs of individual patients. The existence of numerous experimental treatments for a given malignancy improves the patient's chances to find a therapy adjusted to the specific features of his or her disease.[182] The failure to develop efficient therapies had another consequence as well. Patients who participated in inefficient clinical trials often paid a high price in physiological side effects and in psychological strain related to loss of hope, while oncologists who invested their time, energy, professional reputation, and emotional resources in such trials faced the stress of repeated failures. The elevated personal cost of experimental cancer therapies for both patients and physicians might have increased the need to legitimate such trials through an optimistic evaluation of their results and through the reaffirmation of faith in the promise of future research.

The culture of clinical experimentation in oncology can be seen as an inseparable mixture of beliefs (such as the perception of cancer as a cellular disease, which can be cured through killing all "deviant" cancer cells, or the conviction that enrollment in a clinical trial is in the best interest of an individual cancer patient); practices (such as the administration of the highest tolerated dose of anticancer substances or the evaluation of progress as a measurable shrinking of tumors); and organizational devices (such as multicenter, nonrandomized trials, intertrial supervision of the quality of laboratory tests, or centralization of data). Together these beliefs and practices form a distinct entity, or, to paraphrase philosophers and historians of science, a "clinical form of life." The rapid diffusion of this "form of life" in the 1970s and 1980s was favored by institutional changes such as increased funding for clinical research in oncology, the centralization of cancer treatment in specialized, research-oriented institutions, and the development of a new professional segment—medical oncology. Its success is also related to the gradual transformation of clinical trials into a quasi-routine way of coping with advanced malignancies. The diffusion of clinical trials of anticancer drugs is also connected with general cultural attitudes. Modern society does not accept severe, potentially fatal illness as an unavoidable "fact of life," while modern medical science instrumentalizes sickness, suffering, and even death. Medicine analyzes the failings of the human body and translates them into a series of distinct medical or biological problems, then looks for a technical solution for each problem.[183] Malignant diseases have accordingly been conceptualized in this century as technical problems—as tissues, cells, chromosomes, enzymes, receptors, or genes that have gone astray. Biologists, oncologists, cancer charities, and politicians have repeatedly announced "breakthroughs" that would soon lead to a "victory over cancer," and this belief in a "scientific fix" has sustained the culture of clinical experimentation in oncology.[184]

The faith in a scientific solution to the "cancer problem" implicitly assumes the existence of direct relationships between developments in basic research laboratories and in cancer clinics. A closer look at the history of oncology, however, reveals a more complicated picture. The efficacy of cancer therapies has undoubtedly increased during the twentieth century. Surgical techniques have improved, antibiotics have increased the survival rates of surgery patients, radiation therapy has become more precise, and chemotherapy has become the treatment of choice for selected malignancies. But these improvements in cancer therapies have not been directly linked to developments in the basic biological sciences or to a better understanding of the mechanisms of malignant transformation of the cell. The two major therapeutic approaches developed in this century—radiation therapy and chemotherapy—were based on the observation, made in the second half of the nineteenth century, that tumors are made from cells that multiply with unusual speed.[185] Since that time, basic biological investigations have not made important contributions to the development of cures for cancer. Chemotherapy of cancer was presented in the 1950s and 1960s as a science-based treatment, but the development of efficient anticancer drugs did not stem from better understanding of fundamental biological mechanisms underlying malignancy. The capacities of chemical compounds to kill rapidly multiplying cells were discovered either by chance (nitrogen mustard) or in the course of another type of study (antagonists of folic acid, antibiotics) or—rarely—through mass screening of natural or artificial compounds. The development of drug therapies of cancer was grounded in trial-and-error approaches (critics called the NCI chemotherapy project a "nothing-is-too-stupid-to-test" program).[186] Laboratory investigations did contribute to the development of these therapies, but their role was often restricted to perfecting diagnostic tests and following up effects of treatments. The limited role of basic investigations in the development of new therapies for cancer contrasts with the widespread legitimation of fundamental cancer research by the promise to find a "cure for cancer" and with the self-image of cancer specialists as leading medical scientists.

The history of cancer immunotherapy told in the next chapter traces the attempt to develop a therapy based (in principle) on the application of fundamental immunological knowledge to the cure of malignant tumors. This attempt falls into two distinct periods: before and after the development of the culture of clinical experimentation in oncology. For a long time the main link between the research laboratory and the clinics was solely discursive—a shared use of immunological terms. Not until the 1960s, with the emergence of a new subspecialty—cellular immunology—and of a new clinical practice—large-scale tests of anticancer drugs—was immunological knowledge applied to the cure of malignant tumors, and the "fourth modality of cancer therapy" took its place alongside surgery, radiation therapy, and chemotherapy.

CHAPTER TWO

Cancer Immunotherapy, 1894–1979

The Invisible Past

In the 1980s "adoptive immunotherapy," a treatment based on the injection of interleukin-2 and interleukin-activated white blood cells, was presented as a highly innovative approach to curing cancer.[1] Most physicians like to present their endeavors as the culmination of a long history. The promoters of cancer immunotherapy, however, seldom mention that it is a century-old approach, because its past is problematic.

There have been three distinct waves of interest in cancer immunotherapy. This chapter describes the first and second. The first started in the late nineteenth century, peaked in the years 1910–1920, and ebbed in the following decade, with the subject remaining marginal until 1960. During the first wave researchers observed that tumors grafted into another animal were promptly rejected, concluded that immune mechanisms were responsible for the resistance, and established a research program to study the phenomenon in laboratory animals. At the same time physicians attempted to introduce immunological approaches (vaccination with cancer cells, inoculation with antitumor serum, or stimulation of the immune mechanisms with bacterial vaccines) into cancer clinics. The two areas of study remained separate, and in the late 1920s research efforts in both were discredited as nonreproducible, unreliable, poorly designed and executed, and lacking in therapeutic utility. Summing up in 1929 more than 600 articles on "resistance" to tumors, Dr. William Woglom of the Institute of Cancer Research at Columbia University concluded that "immunity to transplantable tumors . . . appears to be entirely unrelated to other forms of immunity . . . Resistance is effective during the first days following inoculation, but entirely powerless against an established tumor. Nothing may accordingly be hoped for at present in respect to successful therapy from this direction."[2]

Fifty years later the Australian immunologist Dr. Gustav Nossal assessed the effectiveness of immunological approaches to cancer therapy developed during the second wave of interest. In a 1979 lecture he concluded that "immunotherapy as presently practiced has fallen short of the hopes initially invested in it."[3] Interest in immunology and immunotherapy of malignant tumors had revived in the 1960s and early 1970s as a result of the conjunction of several events: the success of kidney transplantation in humans, which attracted attention to immune mechanisms involved in cell destruction; parallel basic research into mechanisms of destruction of foreign or malignant cells; and the emergence of clinical trials of anticancer drugs, which favored large-scale testing of immunotherapies in the oncology clinics. The second wave of cancer immunotherapy, unlike the first, was preceded by and related to investigations made in the test tube and in animal models of malignant tumors. But early, highly publicized reports of therapeutic success with immunotherapy for malignant tumors were not confirmed by multicenter clinical trials, and in the late 1970s the outlook for cancer immunotherapies again seemed poor.

In 1980 interferon, a molecule that, among its other physiological functions, is involved in the regulation of immune responses, received unprecedented publicity as the new hope for cancer cure, launching the third wave of interest in cancer immunotherapy. Because interferon was known mainly as an antiviral agent, its application to cancer therapy was at first promoted by virologists. But in 1985 the introduction of interleukin-2-based therapies promoted a strong revival of immunological approaches. Many of the senior investigators active in the introduction of interferon and IL-2 to oncology clinics had been involved in the second wave of cancer immunotherapy research. Having had their earlier high hopes dashed, it is not surprising that they attempted to stress the radical novelty of the current approaches.[4] But understanding the historical continuities in cancer immunotherapy is essential to comprehending these later developments.

The Parallel Trajectories of Cancer Immunology and Cancer Immunotherapy, 1900–1960

Lymphocytes between Laboratory and Clinics

In the 1970s researchers confirmed that certain subclasses of lymphocytes—the so-called cytotoxic, or cell-killing, lymphocytes—are able to destroy tumor cells in the test tube and seem to play a role in the destruction of tumors in laboratory animals. The assumption that certain subsets of lymphocytes play an important role in the destruction of malignant growths in the body was central to the development of interleukin-based cancer therapies. Interleukins, it was (and is) believed, stimulated subpopulations of lymphocytes with putative antitumor activity.[5] The description of cytotoxic lymphocytes is usually viewed as a direct consequence of increased understanding of the cellular mechanisms of immunity in the 1960s and 1970s. But in fact the idea that lymphocytes are involved in resistance to malignant tumors was successfully tested in the laboratory in the early twentieth century, only to be abandoned and then rediscovered fifty years later. The circumstances of the rise and subsequent neglect of the "lymphocyte hypothesis" illuminate the reasons for the separation, in the years 1920–1960, between experimental studies of tumor immunology and attempts to find immunotherapies for human cancers.

The observation that people who have had an infectious disease are often immune—that is, resistant—to subsequent exposures to the same disease was made in antiquity. It later became the basis of practices such as variolization (deliberate infection with smallpox, aiming at the induction of a light, localized form of the disease) and vaccination (deliberate infection with the less dangerous cowpox in order to protect against the more dangerous smallpox infection). The origins of modern immunology are, however, indissolubly linked with the development of bacteriology. The association between cancer and immune mechanisms also followed the rise of bacteriology. In the nineteenth century the definition of cancer as an abnormally growing tissue was based on anatomical and pathological observations, and cancer researchers at first explained malignancy as resulting from prolonged irritation or inflammation of the tissues or from the abnormal presence of embryonic tissue in an adult.[6] The discovery that infectious diseases are induced by specific microorganisms triggered the search for a putative "cancer germ(s)."[7] This search, together with the observation that tumors grafted into laboratory animals were usually rejected by the body's defense mechanisms, led researchers to connect cancer studies and resistance to infectious diseases.

Bacteriologists were interested in mechanisms that allowed the organism to get rid of pathogenic microorganisms. Two different theories explaining these mechanisms were proposed in the late nineteenth and early twentieth centuries. One—advanced by the "cellular school," led by Elie Metchnikoff, a Russian zoologist who worked at the Pasteur Institute in Paris—affirmed that pathogenic bacteria were eliminated by a particular subset of white blood cells—the macrophages or phagocytes—that is, cells that swallow particles and bacteria. The second, advanced by the "humoral school," led by the German investigator Paul Ehrlich, claimed that harmful microorganisms were destroyed by "humoral factors" (later called antibodies) in the blood serum.[8] Both schools, however, viewed immune mechanisms as specific manifestations of more basic physiological processes. Metchnikoff affirmed that phagocytic cells not only fought infection but, more generally, eliminated harmful and unnecessary substances from the organism; Ehrlich maintained that humoral antibodies were "lateral chains" found on all normal cells. The main physiological role of these lateral chains was to adsorb nutrition from the environment, and only secondarily did they participate in the defense of the organism against infectious disease.[9]

A physiological definition of resistance to infectious disease allowed a broad definition of immunity. Immunity was defined in a 1907 textbook as "a state of natural or acquired resistance of individuals, of races or of animal species facing harmful influences which, in the absence of a refractory state, can induce disease."[10] Early studies of immunity were divided into two chapters of equal importance: the studies of "natural immunity," that is, resistance to infectious disease without prior contact with the disease-inducing microorganisms (mechanisms of natural immunity explained, for example, why certain animal species are refractory to infections that affect other animal species); and "acquired immunity," subdivided into "natural acquired immunity," the consequence of an earlier encounter with the disease-inducing agent, and "artificial acquired immunity," resulting from vaccination. Cells were viewed as more active in natural immunity, humoral antibodies as more active in acquired immunity. This distinction was, however, far from being absolute. The initially nonspecific phagocytic cell, Metchnikoff affirmed, might become much more specific following interaction with an infectious agent. The phagocytes of an immunized animal destroyed the invading microorganisms more rapidly than did the phagocytes of a nonimmunized one.[11] On the other hand, no absolute distinction was made between specific "humoral factors" (antibodies) and nonspecific antibacterial substances found in blood serum.

The beginnings of immunology and of biochemistry were closely intertwined. Both were linked with the emergence of the concept of specific functional proteins. In the late nineteenth century this category included enzymes, alexine (complement) antibodies (lysins, precipitins, agglutinins), and bacterial toxins.[12] Thus Pasteur's collaborator Emile Duclaux explained that all antibacterial substances belonged to the large group of "lysins" or "diastases" (digestive enzymes); immunization merely induced "specific lysins," more efficient than the nonspecific ones found in the nonimmunized animal.[13] Maurice Nicolle, another French pioneer of immunology, agreed: for him, "specific or not, antimicrobial sera act in an identical way."[14]

The broad perception of immunity as a physiological phenomenon that included all the mechanisms of resistance to infection—specific and nonspecific, humoral and cellular—disappeared in the 1910s and 1920s. At that time the study of immune mechanisms came to be identified with the investigation of "specific resistance," which itself became synonymous with the study of specific antibodies that appear in serum following disease or vaccination. Studies of the "natural resistance to infectious disease" and of the cellular aspects of immunity were abandoned because of the technical and conceptual difficulties involved in this kind of research. The terms "natural immunity" and "resistance to infectious disease" covered a wide range of poorly defined pathophysiological phenomena, very difficult to standardize and to quantify with existing immunological methods. By contrast, it was relatively easy to apply quantitative, reproducible methods to the study of specific antibodies induced by the well-defined microorganisms or chemical substances. Specific antibodies in the serum were a much more rewarding subject of study than elusive, nonspecific cellular "defense mechanisms." The efforts of immunologists in the 1910s and 1920s centered on the elaboration and calibration of quantitative methods for studying specific antibodies in the test tube. These quantitative methods also had practical applications: serodiagnosis (identification of pathogenic microorganisms using specific antibodies) and serotherapy (treatment of infectious diseases with specific antibodies).[15] These practices led to the integration of immunological techniques into the hospital laboratory and to the creation of a new professional community: the serologists. Serologists, who studied antibodies, not pathologists, who studied tissues and cells, became identified with the investigation of immune reactions. This was the so-called chemical period of immunology.[16]

The discovery of the role of lymphocytes in destroying tumors was made within the broad physiological framework of immunological studies. In 1911 a young pathologist, Dr. James Baumgardner Murphy, joined the cancer laboratory of the Rockefeller Institute in order to assist its director, Dr. Peyton Rous, in the study of a "filterable agent" (supposedly a virus) able to induce malignant tumors in fowl.[17] Looking for ways to keep chicken tumors alive in the laboratory, Murphy developed a method for grafting tumors onto the embryonic membranes of fertilized eggs. He had noticed that although tumor grafts in adult animals were always species-specific (that is, it was impossible to graft, say, a mouse tumor onto a rat), it was possible to graft tumors onto embryos in differing species. Not only was he able to graft fowl eggs with tumors from other birds, but he also managed to grow mouse and rat tumors in chicken embryos.[18] The grafted tumor thrived until the last two days of embryonic life. At that time a "resistance reaction" occurred that was closely connected to the accumulation of small "round cells"—lymphocytes—around the graft. This reaction was not unique to embryos; Murphy observed a similar reaction in adult animals' rejection of previously established tumors. He concluded that the "lymphocyte reaction" was probably a physiological mechanism by which the body got rid of unwanted cells and tissues.[19]

Murphy was not the first to observe the "lymphocyte reaction" and to link it to the rejection of a transplanted tumor. Similar observations had been reported in 1910 by Dr. C. Da Fano, who worked at the Imperial Cancer Research Fund in London, one of the first institutions dedicated to cancer research.[20] However, whereas Da Fano merely described the phenomenon, Murphy undertook to prove his ideas experimentally. He monitored the changes in rat or mouse tumors grafted onto chicken embryos during the acceptance and rejection phases and demonstrated a close correlation between the extent of "lymphocyte reaction" and the fate of the grafted tissue.[21] Later he was able to show that when a lymphocyte-rich tissue (such as spleen or bone marrow) from an adult fowl was injected into a fertilized egg together with the tumor, the embryo—of any age—promptly rejected the graft. When such adult issue was treated by X rays, which selectively destroy lymphocytes, it lost the ability to induce the embryo's rejection of grafted tumors. Adult tissues that did not contain lymphocytes (such as liver or connective tissue) failed to induce rejection.[22]

If lymphocytes were indeed able to destroy malignant tumors in the body, Murphy reasoned, an increase in the amount and the activity of lymphocytes should improve the body's ability to fight malignant growth. In 1915 Murphy and Dr. John J. Morton started a series of experiments aimed at demonstrating that a nonspecific stimulation of lymphocytes in a tumor-bearing animal could stimulate its resistance to tumors. They showed that it was possible to increase the number of lymphocytes in the blood of mice by treating them with low doses of X rays.[23] The mice showed increased resistance not only to grafts of transplantable tumors (comparable to the resistance of mice pre-injected with mouse blood or tissues) but also to the re-implantation of their own, spontaneously generated tumors. The last results, Murphy believed, indicated that the nonspecific stimulation of lymphocytes might lead to a cure of cancer in humans.[24]

Murphy first announced his discovery in a paper read before the National Academy of Sciences in Washington, D.C., on August 15, 1915. The paper described experiments in mice and only briefly mentioned the possible role of lymphocytes in resistance to human cancer. However, Dr. Simon Flexner, the director of the Rockefeller Institute, made the paper's content public at a special press conference.[25] The press greeted the study as an announcement of a breakthrough in cancer studies, with headlines such as "John D. Doctors Believe Cancer Prevention Found," "Cancer Foe Discovered: Rockefeller Institute Scientists Find Immunity Guaranty," "Rockefeller Aides See Immunity from Cancer: Institute's Investigators Discover Means They Hope Will Make Man Proof against the Disease," "Can Prevent Cancer Now: Rockefeller Institute Investigators Say by Increasing the Number of Lymphocytes the Cancerous Growth Is Prevented."[26] The implicit promise that the new science of immunity would be applied to "vaccinate" against cancer clearly appealed to the public imagination.

Over the next seven years Murphy and his collaborators confirmed and extended their findings, showing clear-cut correlations between the stimulation (or inhibition) of lymphocytes and the development of experimental tumors. They were unable, however, to augment their understanding of the mechanisms of lymphocytes' antitumor activity and had to content themselves with the vague statement that these cells "play an important role in 'resistance' to cancer."[27] But Flexner did not wait for progress in experimental studies; as early as October 1915 he declared that "the work in this field is so hopeful that the Board of Scientific Directors have felt justified in applying the results to the study of cancer in man."[28]

The transition to the clinics was swift. Clinical tests of the new approach started in 1916. Breast cancer patients were treated with low doses of X-ray radiation immediately after tumor removal in the hopes of stopping the progress of their disease (in today's medical terminology, they received an adjuvant therapy). Murphy followed the blood counts of patients who were given X-ray treatment, hoping to find a correlation between the amount of lymphocytes in the blood and the clinical progress of the disease. Unfortunately, no such correlation was found. The clinical experiment lasted until 1922, with no noteworthy results: there was no improvement in patients' health, and no relevant connection was found between clinical manifestations of cancer and patients' lymphocyte counts. In his final observations on the clinical experiments Murphy noted that the number of cases was too small, follow-up was inadequate, and the data obtained in the human studies did not justify publication.[29] In his 1920 report to the Rockefeller Institute directors, Flexner no longer stated that the goal of Murphy's clinical studies was to find a cure for cancer. Much more modestly, Murphy's research was redefined as a study of the biological effect of X rays on the human body aiming at the elaboration of guiding principles for the use of radiation treatment in humans.[30]

In a 1925 monograph Murphy summed up his views on the role of lymphocytes in resistance to grafted tissue, to cancer, and to some infectious diseases such as tuberculosis.[31] This was his last contribution to the study of lymphocytes. Thereafter his research interest shifted from natural tumors transplanted in laboratory animals to artificially induced malignant growths, and from attempts to find a cure for cancer to the search for the causes of malignant transformation of cells. In a 1926 article he affirmed that investigation of "resistance to transplanted tumors" had neither advanced the understanding of the causes of cancer nor helped to find a cure. A new approach was needed, one centered on basic research in cell biology, because "when the cause of cancer is discovered it will be found to be some agent or force most intimately associated with the mechanism of growth of the cell, and will be a discovery of equal importance for those studying normal cell phenomena and to the cancer investigator."[32]

Murphy successfully implemented a shift from the muddled ground of pathology to the better-defined and more prestigious realm of basic biological research.[33] Moreover, his assertion that studies of cancer would make important contributions to cell biology was partly vindicated in the 1940s, when efforts by one of his collaborators led indirectly to a better understanding of the ultramicroscopic structure of the cell.[34] But his suggestion that nonspecific stimulation of lymphocytes might play a role in a cure for cancer was gradually forgotten. Basic researchers in immunology turned in the 1920s to quantifiable and reproducible studies of specific, antibody-mediated reactions. Nor were cancer specialists interested. Cancer pathology textbooks in the 1920s and 1930s regularly mentioned the "lymphocyte hypothesis" and cited Murphy's main publications, but studies of the possible role of lymphocytes in the destruction of malignant tumors were neglected for the next fifty years. The failure of Murphy's clinical studies contributed to this oblivion. Murphy's own move to chemical investigations of the cancer cell, an indirect disavowal of his earlier work, exemplified this trend.

Experimental Studies of Cancer and Tumor Immunology, 1900–1960

The observation, made in the early twentieth century, that selected tumors can be transplanted to other animals made possible the studies of resistance to cancer. Having noted that although some tumors could be successfully transplanted, most failed to thrive, investigators became interested in the mechanisms responsible for rejection. Two theories attempted to explain the "natural resistance" to transplanted tumors.[35] The "atrepsia" theory, developed by Paul Ehrlich, proposed that the transplanted tumor perished because grafted cells lacked the proper receptors to combine with the food elements of the recipient.[36] The vascularization theory, developed by researchers at the Imperial Cancer Research Fund, maintained that tumors were rejected because they failed to be properly vascularized, and thus nourished, by the host.[37]

Studies of acquired resistance to tumors were stimulated by the observation that laboratory animals that spontaneously rejected a tumor graft after a long period of acceptance often promptly rejected a second graft of the same tumor. This phenomenon could be artificially reproduced by injecting the recipient with living tumor cells before making the tumor graft.[38] The parallel with a specific immunization was incomplete, however, because it was not possible to detect specific anticancer antibodies in the serum of the "immunized" recipients. Moreover, investigators at the Imperial Cancer Research Fund found that the resistance phenomenon was not specific to the tumor: similar "immunization" was observed in hosts injected with normal cells of an animal of the same species.[39] The last observation had led to numerous attempts to reproduce and to quantify the resistance phenomenon and to understand its mechanism. These studies were undertaken with the hope that they would lead to possible therapeutic or prophylactic applications, but their results were highly variable, and no practical applications were found.

The main difficulty in studying the resistance phenomenon stemmed from the genetic heterogeneity of animals and tumors used in different laboratories and from the confusion between resistance to tumor and rejection of grafted tissues. The two problems were closely related. Mouse tumor grafted to a different, unrelated mouse would be rejected not because the grafted tissue was malignant, but because it was foreign. In contrast, if the donor and recipient had the same genetic makeup (for example, were genetically identical siblings), the graft should not have been *a priori* recognized as foreign: if rejection still occurred, it could be legitimately attributed to the fact that the transplanted tissue was malignant. At the time researchers had no notion that cells or tissues from a genetically different individual are invariably rejected. They did know that it was possible to vaccinate an animal with proteins from a different species but not with proteins from the same species: thus a rabbit could produce antibodies against horse or dog albumin (a serum protein) but not against rabbit albumin. This phenomenon, some researchers believed, explained why one animal could produce antibodies against the intact cells—and not only the serum proteins—of an animal of a different species: the immunized animal was reacting to species-specific proteins contained in the injected cells and liberated from those cells in the recipient's organism. The logical—but unproven—conclusion was that normal cells transplanted into an individual belonging to the same species should not induce a resistance reaction, since they do not contain foreign proteins. The rejection of a tumor transplanted to an animal of the same species, the investigators assumed, was specific resistance to malignant cells.

In the 1910s some investigators studying tumor transplantation in mice concluded that "race" (that is, affiliation with a given subgroup within the same species) influenced the acceptance of a grafted tumor. They affirmed that the chances of success in the transfer of malignant tumors were directly proportional to the degree of genetic proximity between donor and recipient. Other researchers disagreed. Some reported a failure in the uptake of transplanted tumors in different strains of mice, and only partial success with first-generation hybrid (that is, highly inbred, and thus genetically close) mice, while others affirmed that tumors could be easily transplanted to a different race of mice. This inconsistency in results was attributed to the complexity of the resistance process.[40]

Around 1910 some researchers arrived at the conclusion that the phenomenon of resistance was not restricted to malignant tissues: normal grafted tissue was rejected too. The pioneer of organ transplantation, Dr. Alexis Carrel, observed in 1910 that whereas a kidney removed from an animal and regrafted into the same animal was nearly always accepted, kidneys exchanged between two individuals belonging to the same species were invariably rejected through an unknown biological mechanism.[41] In the same year Dr. Peyton Rous injected normal cells and tumor cells into mice and noted similarities in the pattern of rejection for both kinds of cells. This observation led him to a systematic comparison of the fates of a transplanted tumor and of transplanted normal tissue.[42] Rous concluded that many of the phenomena subsumed under the heading "resistance to transplanted tumor" were in fact the expression of "a resistance directed against the graft as a strange tissue," regardless of the qualities of that tissue.[43] But Rous's experimental conclusions and Carrel's transplantation data had a limited influence. Most studies of transplanted tumors in the 1910s continued to confuse rejection of foreign tissue and resistance to malignant growth.

In 1913 William Woglom summarized the contradictory results of studies on resistance to transplanted cancer in laboratory animals, but he provided very little commentary or critical appraisal.[44] There was no attempt to elaborate clear bases for comparison among experiments made in different laboratories or in different countries. In most of the studies that involved mice, the animals were described solely in terms of their geographic origins ("Paris mice," "New York mice," "Danish mice"), and the tumors were very loosely characterized ("a slow-growing tumor," "a poorly differentiated carcinoma," "a naturally occurring tumor"). The heterogeneity of experimental systems and the absence of agreement upon methodology and criteria for acceptability of evidence reflected the lack of institutionalized structures in experimental cancer research.

The situation of experimental cancer studies in the 1910s contrasted markedly with that of bacteriology, a science rapidly institutionalized between 1880 and 1900 through the development of a network of internationally recognized experts and centers. Centers such as the Pasteur Institute in Paris and Koch's Institute for Infectious Diseases in Berlin elaborated standardized experimental techniques to study bacteria and established certified procedures for the transmission of bacteriological knowledge (apprenticeship in an appropriate institution, participation in professional courses organized by leading specialists).[45] Accepted norms for practice were refined through debates in specialized journals and confirmed at international conferences, then codified in textbooks. No similar institutional structures existed in experimental cancer studies. Research in this domain was viewed as a part of experimental pathology. It was conducted in a disorganized and uncoordinated manner by pathologists coming from different backgrounds, with no common socialization pathways and no group identity. Woglom's 1913 study mirrored the state of experimental cancer studies: a random patchwork of isolated small groups.[46]

The failure of cancer specialists to obtain reproducible results for the transplantation of malignant growths led to the gradual abandonment of transplanted tumors as a model of human cancer in studies of experimental cancer. Disappointment with this model was already perceptible immediately after the First World War, and it intensified in the 1920s.[47] The observation, made in 1918, that tar may induce tumors in laboratory animals opened the way to studies of the genesis of cancer.[48] Murphy's 1925 decision to abandon studies of the role of lymphocytes in resistance to grafted tumor and his shift to the study of artificially induced tumors and, later, to the biochemical mechanisms of the malignant transformation of the cell reflected a general trend.[49] There was a growing conviction among cancer specialists, especially those who worked in prestigious teaching and research institutions, that the future of cancer studies depended upon the progress of basic biological research. Microscopic observations and pathological investigations were therefore frequently replaced with genetic and biochemical studies.

In the 1920s resistance to malignant tumors continued to be studied in numerous pathology laboratories, but these investigations lost much of their earlier prestige. Woglom's 1929 review of 600 experimental studies conducted since 1913 reflected this change. The 1929 review, unlike the earlier one, spelled out well-defined criteria for valid evaluation of studies of immunity to transplanted tumors and used them to stigmatize many of the investigations as inadequate. Many researchers had ignored the importance of working with genetically homogeneous mice and the necessity of including a large number of animals in order to overcome the problem of diversity in individual responses. In addition, numerous studies had failed to take into consideration the great variability of transplantable tumors. Racial and individual differences among laboratory animals, as well as differences among tumors, Woglom affirmed, could account for many of the contradictions in earlier studies. In addition, many researchers had misrepresented their results by neglecting to indicate the number of animals used in their experiments: an 80 percent rate of positive results might seem imposing at first glance, but not if it represented only four of five animals. Other studies had defined the virulence of the grafted tumor by only a single parameter, the duration of survival after inoculation, and overlooked other important criteria such as rapidity of increase in the tumor's mass, degree of ulceration of the tumor, and frequency of metastases.[50]

After discarding all the experiments that he viewed as badly planned and poorly executed, Woglom asserted that studies in this domain nevertheless established some valid general conclusions. They demonstrated that the transplantability of tumors was usually dependent on the genetic makeup of the donor and the recipient and that the majority of tumors could be propagated only in the strain of animals in which they were first described. The conclusions also indicated that in animals not belonging to genetically homogeneous strains, the so-called natural immunity to tumors was nearly always a resistance to a grafted tissue, and the acquired immunity or acquired resistance to transplanted tumors was a poorly understood phenomenon related to the presence of round cell (lymphocyte) infiltration around the tumor.[51] These general findings, however, had not shed any new light on the problems of therapy and prevention in human cancer.[52] The few methodologically correct studies that had used experimental models not too distant from real-life situations did not reveal specific antitumor immunity: "ingenuity has been exhausted in devising means of treatment of animal tumors, yet no investigator has published a method which even the most charitable and tolerant reader could regard as encouraging."[53] Woglom ended his review with the assertion that he saw no hope for successful cancer immunotherapy.

In the 1920s and 1930s the frontier of experimental cancer studies had shifted to biochemical and cytological investigations that attempted to compare normal and malignant cells. Linking cancer studies with more prestigious biological disciplines was not, however, sufficient to allow the development of a well-structured scientific domain. It was also necessary to develop tools that would permit the elaboration of efficient experimental systems and research strategies. Such tools were crafted by geneticists.

Studies of the genetic aspects of tumor transplantation started with the observation in 1916 that a tumor found in a highly inbred strain of mice, the Japanese waltzing mice, could be transplanted in this line only. Geneticists attempted to test the transplantability of the tumor in hybrids of the Japanese waltzing mice and other inbred strains of mice and were able to show that resistance to the graft of this tumor was transmitted as a combination of several inherited traits.[54] Later the same investigators also showed that resistance to the graft of nonmalignant tissue obeyed identical laws.[55] Dr. Clarence Little, one of the leading researchers in these studies, was committed to the idea that studies of genetic differences governing the rejection of foreign tissues in mice might yield important clues to the causes of cancer. In 1929 he founded the Jackson Memorial Laboratories in Bar Harbor, Maine. Thanks to his efforts and later those of his collaborator, Dr. George Snell, in the 1930s and 1940s these laboratories developed numerous inbred strains of mice, which became an important tool for genetic research and for well-controlled studies of the genetic component of resistance to transplanted tumors.[56] It also promoted methodological uniformity among such studies.[57]

In 1938 a Danish investigator, Dr. Johannes Clemmensen, summed up the new findings in the domain of immunity to tumors, giving a central place to genetic considerations. Clemmensen noted that most studies of resistance to transplanted tumors had made a distinction between "primary resistance" (previously called "natural resistance") and "acquired resistance." Such a distinction, he asserted, was artificial and unnecessary: both reflected genetic differences between the grafted tissue and the host tissue. In contrast to Woglom in 1929, Clemmensen attributed the unreliable results of earlier studies to a single cause: the genetic heterogeneity of laboratory animals.

> Nearly all the studies made so far with regard to acquired resistance have been made with animal material of unknown genetic constitution and can therefore hardly be brought into relation to the ge-

netic theory. There can be little doubt, however, that in the future investigations will have to take this theory very largely into consideration. It would seem that there is a possibility here of creating order in a field which, at present, confounds the vision of the worker in the same way as did the consideration relating to the subject of natural resistance before the genetic theories were set forth.[58]

Clemmensen's assertion was vindicated by studies made with the inbred strains of mice developed at the Jackson Memorial Laboratories. These studies confirmed that phenomena previously lumped under the heading "resistance to transplanted tumors" were in fact manifestations of the body's resistance to genetically different tissue.[59]

In 1942 Dr. James Murphy, who had returned to physiologically oriented studies of cancer, employed inbred strains of mice to prove the hypothesis that "acquired resistance" was similar to "natural resistance": he observed no accelerated rejection of a grafted tumor by an animal injected with living cells from another individual belonging to the same species when both the donor and the recipient belonged to the same inbred strain. Instead, Murphy affirmed, the phenomenon reflected a reaction to cells of a genetically different individual.[60]

In the 1940s and 1950s studies of links between cancer and immune mechanisms focused on biochemical processes. The introduction of inbred strains of laboratory animals allowed researchers to look for chemical structures that were specific to the malignant tissue and were not expressed (or at least not expressed in large quantities) in normal cells. Such "cancer antigens," if discovered, would allow early diagnosis of malignant tumors and would facilitate the development of immunological methods to prevent and fight cancer.

The shift from studying a hypothetical physiological mechanism of resistance to studying chemical structures in the cell followed—though with a significant delay—the general direction of immunological and biochemical research. Immunological studies first centered on function (mechanisms of resistance to infectious disease) and later on structures (bacterial antigens and specific antibodies). The search for possible tumor antigens attracted specialists in biochemistry and immunochemistry to cancer studies. These specialists introduced new techniques for studying proteins (ultracentrifugation, electrophoresis, radiolabeling, and fluorescent labeling) which allowed more detailed studies of antigenic structures (that is, chemical structures that are recognized as foreign by the body and are able to elicit the formation of specific antibodies).

Review articles published in the 1940s and 1950s reflected the new trends in studies of tumor immunology. Dr. R. R. Spencer's 1942 review of this field focused on new developments in cancer genetics but also included a description of methods used to search for sera that would identify malignant cells.[61] These early attempts at serodiagnosis for cancer employed traditional serological methods such as precipitation and agglutination. Ten years later a review of the state of the art in cancer immunology by Dr. Theodore S. Hauschka reported numerous studies that applied the latest biochemical and immunochemical methods to the search for possible cancer antigens. The importation of new biochemical and immunochemical methods did not, however, lead to any breakthroughs. Ultramicroscopic investigations and chemical studies (studies of ribosome density, nucleic acids, levels of intracellular enzymes) revealed quantitative differences between normal and malignant cells, but all these differences could be explained by the rapid rate of proliferation of malignant cells. Only in virus-induced tumors had it been possible to identify specific viral components in the malignant tissue.[62]

Despite the lack of more concrete results, studies of the relationship between tumors and immune mechanisms continued to shift toward basic biological research. In the 1950s the rapid accumulation of data on cell-mediated immune mechanisms promoted more and more studies of relationships between immunity and experimental tumors in laboratory animals. Some specialists continued to wonder, however, if these basic and preclinical studies could be related to the therapy of human tumors. Dr. Chester Southam, who reviewed the field of experimental tumor immunology in 1960, again focused on the problem of the existence of specific tumor antigens and of immune mechanisms able to fight naturally occurring malignant tumors. The hope of finding such mechanisms, Southam asserted, had a reasonable basis: there were well-documented though rare cases of spontaneous regression of cancer in humans and in laboratory animals; white blood cells could be found around some malignant tumors; and hosts with advanced cancer often had impaired immune functions. Researchers in the 1950s had hoped that the perfection of immmunological methods of detecting even minute amounts of antigen would lead to a description of tumor-specific antigens or to a demonstration of the involvement of immune mechanisms in the control of malignant growths. But the state of the field had not changed since Hauschka's 1952 review. Southam expressed strong doubts about the future of tumor immunology.[63]

Southam judged tumor immunology from the point of view of its (problematic) past and its current (practically nonexistent) contribution to human cancer therapy. His diagnosis was right, but his prognosis was wrong. Ten years later tumor immunology and cancer immunotherapies had become rapidly growing subspecialties respectively of immunology and clinical oncology. Southam did not take into account that a domain on the boundary between immunology and oncology and between basic research and bedside medicine might possess strength by virtue of that location. It was vulnerable only so long as the two adjacent professional communities remained separate and uninterested in cooperation. Oncologists were in principle interested in collaboration with immunologists, but until the mid-1960s many cancer specialists estimated that results (either positive or negative) obtained in experimental systems were not necessarily relevant to human disease. They believed that cancer immunotherapy would be developed through clinic-based, not bench-based, investigations. Consequently, methods that had failed to cure cancer in laboratory animals were nevertheless tested in patients. The history of human cancer immunotherapy in the first half of the twentieth century reflects this separation between laboratory and clinic.

The Tinkering Period

Between 1894 and 1960 nearly every theoretically conceivable approach to applying immunological methods to cancer therapy was tried at one time or another on patients. Most were small-scale experiments, conducted by one or a handful of investigators, and usually motivated by a desire to "do something" for otherwise incurable patients. These attempts were characterized by great heterogeneity in experimental design, in criteria of inclusion, and in patient follow-up. Even the most successful of these methods, namely the application of bacterial toxins to cancer therapy, never reached the stage of standardization and was applied by individual doctors in a variety of ways.[64] Tinkering is not unusual in clinical trials, and it may lead to the development of clinical innovations. This was not, however, the case for cancer immunotherapy; nearly every approach tested was presented by some experimenters as successful, but no single approach became an accepted therapy.

Early clinical experiments with cancer immunotherapy focused on a search for specific anticancer vaccines (active immunization), the

production of anticancer antisera (passive immunization), and stimulation of the hypothetical mechanisms of resistance to malignant tumors (nonspecific immunostimulation). Attempts to produce specific
anticancer vaccines or antisera were linked with the early studies of
cytotoxic antisera. These studies proceeded from the observation,
made by Jules Bordet in 1899, that immunization using the blood of
different species elicited the formation of specific antibodies to red
blood cells.[65] When such antibodies were incubated with the immu-
nizing red blood cells, they induced the destruction (lysis) of the red
blood cells. Building upon Bordet's observation, many immunologists
injected animals with tissue extracts in an attempt to elicit antibodies
against a given tissue, then to study their properties. Such cytotoxic
sera, it was hoped, might be able to specifically inactivate a given tissue
and thus permit a better understanding of the function of the tissue.
The observation that an antiserum may selectively kill specific categories of cells also opened the theoretical possibility of specific cancer
immunotherapy through active vaccination with cancer cells or
through passive administration of specific antisera produced in different animal species. Numerous researchers attempted to produce anticancer antisera, then to use them to cure experimental cancer in animals. But the results were disappointing; no adequately controlled
study was successful.[66] The failure to produce antisera directed against
tumors in laboratory animals was consistent with earlier observations
on the absence of specific anticancer antibodies in animals carrying
either natural or transplanted tumors.[67] After an initial wave of enthusiasm for the new method, most immunologists concluded that
presumably tissue-specific antisera were in fact species-specific and
were usually directed against foreign serum proteins or red blood cells.
In the 1910s they quietly abandoned the search for specific cytotoxic
antisera.[68]

The difficulties of demonstrating the existence of tissue-specific
cytotoxic antisera and the failure of attempts to cure cancer in laboratory animals with such antisera did not discourage clinicians, who
persisted in trying to apply specific anticancer vaccines and sera to the
treatment of human cancer. Some investigators claimed that the treatment worked, and the occasional publication of an anecdotal positive
result encouraged other doctors to attempt specific immunotherapy
on their otherwise incurable patients. Indeed, clinical experimentation
with specific vaccination against cancer continues to this day.[69]

Attempts to use specific antisera in cancer therapy started in 1895, when Drs. J. Hericourt and C. Richet injected patients with serum prepared in a laboratory animal and claimed that they observed some alleviation of symptoms.[70] Other investigators applied similar methods, with variable results: some reported no measurable effects; others affirmed that they obtained a few objective positive responses or, more frequently, subjective positive responses.[71] The first attempt to vaccinate against cancer was made in 1902, when Drs. E. von Leyden and F. Blumenthal injected two patients suffering from advanced cancer with a filtrate of their own tumor tissues.[72] They claimed that although it was not possible to demonstrate any objective effects of the treatment, the patients reported an alleviation of their symptoms. Other attempts at specific immunization with cancer vaccines were made in the 1910s; again, some researchers did not observe any clinical effects, while others reported marked clinical improvement in selected patients. Both methods—active vaccination and passive cancer serotherapy—continued to be used occasionally from the 1910s on.[73]

Early attempts at nonspecific stimulation of resistance to cancer took a different course. This therapy, based on the use of bacterial products, was born in the clinics, the fruit of an unexpected clinical observation, and was tested early on a relatively large number of patients. In 1891 Dr. William Coley, a surgeon at the Memorial Hospital in New York, first observed a spontaneous regression of residual inoperable sarcoma in a patient suffering from a severe streptococcal infection, erysipelas. Intrigued by this phenomenon, he screened the literature and found 38 earlier descriptions of regression of cancer following a bacterial infection. He decided to attempt to cure cancer by artificially inducing an attack of erysipelas. The therapy proved dangerous: among the first four patients artificially infected, one was cured, and three died of complications from the infection. Coley thus shifted in 1894 to using killed cultures of streptococci, later mixed with toxins of another microorganism, *Bacillus prodigiosus* (today *Serratia marcescens*), a mixture later named "Coley's toxins."

Coley tried his new method on more than 100 patients and claimed to have obtained positive results in numerous cases of inoperable sarcoma.[74] He interpreted the antitumor effects of toxins in terms of stimulation of the body's resistance to cancer, and viewed the antitumor effects of the toxins as a possible indication of the bacterial origins of human malignancies. He was less interested, however, in the way these toxins worked than in clear proof that this method could cure cancer.[75]

Other physicians confirmed that occasionally, and unpredictably, Coley's toxins induced regression of advanced cancers. Coley's method never reached a stage of systematic testing and was not regularly employed in a major hospital (except in Coley's own department at the Memorial Hospital), and its application was never rigorously codified. The therapy remained controversial, but at the time it was one of the few treatments that could be proposed to a patient suffering from inoperable cancer. Doctors were therefore willing to use it as a last resort. Coley's toxins were at first prepared at the Memorial Hospital laboratory, but from 1899 on a commercial preparation was distributed by the Parke-Davis Company. Experiments with laboratory animals confirmed their antitumor effects but failed to reveal the possible mechanism of such effects.[76] The earlier explanation that the toxins enhanced nonspecific resistance to cancer was increasingly viewed as too imprecise, the efficacy of the therapy remained low, and its results were highly variable.[77] The advent of radiation therapy in the 1920s greatly reduced the clinical application of Coley's toxins.

Interest in Coley's therapy revived briefly in the late 1930s. The variability and the lack of predictability of the anticancer activity of Coley's toxins, some researchers then reasoned, might be explained by variability in the amounts of unknown anticancer substance(s) in different preparations of the toxins. A research program initiated in the late 1930s by Dr. Murray Shear and his colleagues at the U.S. Public Health Service Office of Cancer Investigations at Harvard University attempted to isolate the active compounds of Coley's toxins and to study their pharmacological properties. This project was a part of a screening program aimed at studying the anticancer properties of substances of bacterial or vegetal origin.[78] It successfully linked laboratory and clinics insofar as substances such as the polysaccharide of *Serratia marcescens*—the active compound of Coley's toxins—were purified by chemists, tested in laboratory animals, and then in humans. It was not, however, an immunotherapy program but a chemotherapy one, because it aimed at finding molecules able to selectively kill tumor cells in the human body. When screening of substances isolated from bacteria, fungi, and plants failed to uncover efficient anticancer drugs (for example, the polysaccharide of *Serratia marcescens* was found to be too toxic for clinical use), Shear's program shifted to large-scale tests of synthetic chemical compounds with potential anticancer activity. It became one of the first screening programs for chemotherapies

of cancer, and the forerunner of the National Cancer Institute chemotherapy programs.[79]

Sporadic attempts at human cancer immunotherapy continued in
the 1940s and 1950s. These attempts benefited from the development
of new biochemical and immunological methods following the Second
World War. Adjuvants (substances that stimulate immune responses)
and fragments of cancer cells were used to increase the efficacy of
immunizations with malignant cells. Doctors attempted to develop a
more efficient serotherapy by replacing complete antitumor sera with
the purified gamma globulin fraction of these sera, that is, by more
concentrated preparations of antitumor antibodies (antibodies are
mostly gamma globulins, and purified preparations of serum gamma
globulin are therefore enriched in specific antibodies). Finally, partly
purified preparations of bacteria were substituted for crude filtrates of
bacterial cultures employed in the early preparations of Coley's toxins.
Progress in immunological techniques made it possible to evaluate the
effects of cancer immunotherapy on the patient's immune responses.
But the advent of new techniques did not lead to important changes
in clinical experimentation with cancer immunotherapies, which remained uncoordinated. The number of enrolled patients was usually
very small, patients often suffered from a vast array of tumors, and
clinical evidence was mainly anecdotal (that is, the number of cases
was too small to allow a valid statistical analysis).

In 1961 the organizers of an international symposium on immunology and cancer asked Chester Southam to evaluate the current
status of immunotherapy of malignant growths. His judgment was as
pessimistic as his earlier views on fundamental research had been: so
far, "attempts to apply immunology to the treatment of cancer in man
. . . [have] contributed nothing to applied immunology . . . [and have]
failed to give any indication of a cancer specific antigen . . . there is
no proof that they have ever influenced the course of cancer of any
patient."[80]

Southam failed to mention an additional problem: some of the clinical trials of cancer immunotherapy in the 1940s and 1950s were ethically doubtful. This omission may have been deliberate, for the group
led by Southam at the Sloan-Kettering Institute was involved in such
experiments. To study immune reactions to cancer cells in human beings, Southam and his colleagues injected living cancer cells into
healthy volunteers such as prisoners at the state penitentiary in Co-
lumbus, Ohio, and also into invalid, sometimes mentally deficient,

patients at the Jewish Chronic Diseases Hospital in Brooklyn.[81] The volunteers knew that they were participating in a study on cancer, but they were not informed that they were being injected with live cancer cells. Biomedical ethics was not an officially recognized domain in the 1950s, but some physicians considered experimentation on prisoners and sick persons as unethical.[82] Southam argued later that he had not informed the volunteers in these experiments that they were being injected with live cancer cells in order to avoid unnecessary and, in his view, irrational fears evoked by the word "cancer."[83] His belief in the innocuousness of these experiments was based on the assumption, central to the newly created domain of transplantation immunology, that grafted cells are always rapidly rejected by a genetically different donor (no human beings, with the sole exception of identical twins, are genetically identical).[84] This basic rule of transplantation immunology was based on sound experimental and clinical studies. These studies, however, had involved normal cells. The application of this general rule to the transplantation of malignant cells from one person to another entailed an additional assumption, namely that malignant cells too are always recognized as genetically different by every potential host. This assumption was unproven, and in fact evidence to the contrary existed. Early studies on transplantation of malignant tumors, made in genetically nonidentical animals, supplied evidence on tumor transplantability across genetic barriers, especially in blood-related individuals. These studies were, however, often dismissed in the 1950s as belonging to a "prescientific" period of transplantation studies.[85]

The conviction that human tumor cells could not be successfully transplanted to a genetically different individual was disproved in 1965 by a case in which doctors—in a desperate attempt to "do something" to save a young patient dying of melanoma—tried to produce antimelanoma serum by injecting living melanoma cells from the patient into her healthy mother. The patient died before the serum was ready, and her mother developed a malignant growth in the injection site a few weeks after the graft of cancerous cells. The growth was quickly removed, but the mother nevertheless died a year later from a generalized melanoma.[86] This case, published in major medical journals, may have moderated doctors' enthusiasm for the improvised application of immunological methods to cancer therapy. In any event, small-scale bedside tinkering with immunotherapies of cancer became an outmoded approach in the 1960s, when cancer immunotherapy became part of the culture of clinical experimentation in oncology in the era of coordinated large-scale multicenter clinical trials.[87]

Cancer Immunology and Cancer Immunotherapy, 1960–1979

Articulating Laboratory and Clinics: Cellular Immunology and Bacterial Vaccines

The 1960s witnessed an exponential growth in experimental cancer studies.[88] Tumor cells, which—unlike normal cells—can be easily cultivated in the test tube, became a favorite research tool of biologists. Scientists who employed this tool to study cell biology were also able to claim—and to believe—that they were contributing to a solution to the problem of cancer. The expansion of studies in cell biology to include research on malignant cells allowed investigators in basic cell research to compete successfully for resources destined for cancer studies.[89] Immunological research also expanded rapidly in the 1960s. This parallel development favored links between immunology and experimental oncology: a growing number of cancer researchers turned to immunological studies, while numerous immunologists became interested in malignant tumors.[90]

In March 1961 the American Cancer Society sponsored the first international meeting on the role of immunology in cancer. The organizers of the conference recognized that cancer immunology was, for the moment, a heterogeneous and controversial domain, but they were convinced that it was a very promising one.[91] This conviction was not based on new clinical data, for there were none; but it may have been rooted in the assumption that the growing influence of immunology in the clinics would affect cancer studies too. Until the 1950s serology—the study of antibodies in the blood—was perceived mainly as a subdivision of medical bacteriology. The advent of antibiotics after the Second World War reduced the importance of diagnostic and therapeutic uses of sera while it increased interest in chronic afflictions with an immune component such as allergy and autoimmune diseases, and then in cellular mechanisms underlying these pathologies.[92]

In the 1960s the practical success of kidney transplantation got immunologists interested in the cellular mechanisms of graft rejection. The unraveling of the role of specific subsets of lymphocytes in the destruction of grafted foreign cells led to the hypothesis that similar cellular mechanisms might also play a role in the killing of "deviant" cancer cells. In addition, the development of new methods for the study of human immune responses made possible the observation that cancer patients were immunosuppressed—that is, their immune responses were less efficient. Some specialists viewed this immunosuppression as a consequence of the disease, but others perceived it as a possible cause of pathological manifestations. The dysfunction of immune mechanisms, these investigators proposed, favored the spread of malignant tumors, and the restoration of these mechanisms should contribute to a cure.

There was a sharp rise in the number of clinical trials of cancer immunotherapies in the late 1960s and early 1970s.[93] This trend was probably related to a general increase in clinical trials of new anticancer therapies and to the development of medical oncology as a trial-oriented professional segment. Institutions that conducted clinical trials of anticancer drugs were already organized for testing other anticancer therapies, and they established patterns of collaboration with other specialists and other institutions. Several "old-new" approaches were tested again, including active immunotherapies (vaccination with tumor cells) and passive immunotherapies (the use of antitumor sera). But the quantitative and qualitative transformation of the domain of cancer immunotherapy was the result of large-scale tests of nonspecific active immunotherapy—that is, attempts at nonspecific stimulation of immune mechanisms, usually with bacterial vaccines or their derivatives.

In most clinical trials of nonspecific immunotherapy, the stimulating agent was a living, attenuated strain of the tuberculosis bacillus, the BCG (Bacillus Calmette-Guerin). Although the BCG itself was far from being a new substance (it had been developed in the 1920s), its introduction to cancer therapy was directly linked with studies in transplantation immunology. The hypothetical antitumor properties of BCG were first described in 1959, when Drs. Lloyd Old, Donald Clarke, and Baruj Benacerraf observed that mice infected with BCG were more resistant to a graft of a transplantable murine tumor. They deduced that the BCG had stimulated the graft rejection, and they then demonstrated that BCG-infected mice indeed reject skin grafts more rapidly.[94] These findings were in agreement with the known property of certain bacteria or bacterial extracts to amplify immune response to other, unrelated antigens. This property, called "adjuvant activity," had been known to bacteriologists as early as the 1920s and was routinely applied to the practical goal of obtaining higher levels of desired antibodies. Moreover, in the same period James Murphy had already described the stimulation of an antitumor "lymphocyte reaction" with tuberculosis bacilli.[95] Murphy's findings on this subject, however, like his other experimental findings, had been made in the adverse context of diminishing interest in physiological approaches to studies of immune mechanisms, and the growing importance of immunochemistry and serology. The rediscovery of BCG's ability to enhance cellular immune reactions in the late 1950s and early 1960s occurred in the much more favorable context of heightened interest, stimulated by the practice of organ grafts, in subpopulations of white blood cells that destroyed foreign or "deviant" cells. This interest led to the development of quantitative methods for the study of the cell-killing properties of white blood cells in the test tube. These methods in turn allowed a convincing demonstration that white blood cells from a BCG-treated animal had an increased capacity to destroy tumor cells in the test tube. The next step—modeled on the steps in the search for anticancer properties of a chemical substance—was the demonstration of the antitumor effects of BCG in a tumor-bearing animal. This demonstration, made in standardized experimental models of cancer used in chemotherapy tests, opened the way for large-scale clinical experimentation with the new therapy.

In the mid-1960s a large group of French investigators, led by a hematologist, Dr. Georges Mathé, started to treat leukemia patients with a combination of BCG and specific tumor vaccines. Mathé had a long-standing interest in experimental studies of hematological cancers and was a pioneer of clinical trials of drug treatment of leukemia in France. In addition Mathé had had a part in the widely publicized— and partially successful—attempt in 1958 to transplant bone marrow in order to save the life of an accidentally irradiated Yugoslav atomic scientist.[96] His conjoined familiarity with experimental cancer research, with the organization of chemotherapy trials, and with tissue transplantation constituted a promising framework for the development of a new approach to immunotherapy of cancer. Mathé's main aim in his immunotherapy trial was the prolongation of chemotherapy-induced remission in leukemia patients.

The results of the first series of experiments, published by Mathé and his collaborators in 1969, were very impressive. Patients suffering from acute immunoblastic leukemia and treated with a combination of BCG and specific cancer vaccines had much longer remissions and lived significantly longer than controls treated with chemotherapy alone. These results, obtained in 30 patients who participated in the first, randomized trial,[97] were later confirmed by Mathé and his co-workers on a sample of 200 patients treated in several French hospitals.[98] The results of BCG therapy in leukemia, Mathé claimed, opened the way for a radically new approach to cancer treatment. The development of such a new approach was necessary, he explained, because the perception of cancer as a localized disease was no longer valid:

> two of every three patients with an apparently localized tumor have a few cancer cells outside the area where the tumor seems localized. In cases of "apparently complete regression" or even an "apparently complete remission" induced by chemotherapy . . . an imperceptible residual tumor persists, the growth of which will eventually make it perceptible again . . . There is therefore an urgent need for a new technique capable of killing the last cell or cells.[99]

Mathé's assertion challenged the prevailing view, fostered by cancer specialists and cancer research institutions, that cancer always started as a localized and treatable disease, and that only failure to detect it early led to a generalized, incurable condition.[100] The rapid development of cancer chemotherapy in the 1950s and 1960s, however, modified this view. Because chemotherapy was first introduced for the treatment of hematologic malignancies (leukemias, lymphomas), many of the pioneers of cancer chemotherapy were hematologists. As specialists in the treatment of nonlocalized malignant diseases, they were not particularly attached to a representation of cancer as a secondary extension of a localized pathology. They were also trained to solve problems through large-scale clinical experimentation. The relative importance of the localized versus systemic aspects of cancer became a subject of debate and competition between the new specialists of cancer therapy (the chemotherapists and, later, medical oncologists), who emphasized the role of systemic treatments, and the traditional specialists (surgeons and radiation therapists), who stressed the importance of local therapies.[101] This debate was enlarged by the advent of immunotherapy and attempts by clinicians and scientists specialized in the new approach to secure a place for themselves as cancer specialists. The advocates of immunotherapy accepted the assumption of chemotherapy specialists that cancer was often a systemic disease, but they claimed that in most cases chemotherapy alone was not sufficient to get rid of disseminated disease. "Active immunotherapy," Mathé explained, "is now the fourth method of curing cancer. The time is now ripe for it to be used in attempts to eradicate the imperceptible residual disease left by the surgeon, the radiation therapist, or the chemotherapist."[102]

The publication of the results of Mathé's group and the claims, made by Jordan Gutterman and D. L. Morton and their associates, that treatment with BCG prolonged the survival of patients with malignant melanoma, launched a period of enthusiasm for cancer immunotherapy.[103] Numerous clinical trials tested the effects of nonspecific immunostimulating substances or of a combination of nonspecific stimulants and specific tumor vaccines on the survival of cancer patients. The clinical trials of immunotherapies were closely modeled on chemotherapy trials. The proximity with chemotherapy allowed flexibility in the appropriation of the new therapy: while promoters of the new approach stressed novelty and attempted to carve themselves a niche as specialists of the "fourth modality of cancer treatment," clinical trials of immunotherapy were often conducted by medical oncologists who viewed this treatment as supplementing traditional drug therapies.

The combined support of specialists interested in the promotion of novelty and of medical oncologists aspiring to improve existing treatments favored the diffusion of immunotherapies. Multiauthored books dealing with immunotherapy of human cancers proliferated in the 1970s.[104] In November 1972 a group of investigators from the National Cancer Institute recommended the creation of an NCI-sponsored international registry of immunotherapy trials. The data collected by the registry document the increase, from 50 protocols submitted in 1973 to 347 in 1976. The great majority of these protocols were attempts at nonspecific stimulation of immune mechanisms by bacterial vaccines. Thus out of 347 protocols in 1976, 198 used BCG as the stimulating agent; 38, a methanol extract of BCG; 69, another microorganism, *Corynebacterium parvum*; and only 8, specific tumor vaccines.[105]

The rapid diffusion of clinical trials of BCG and other bacterial vaccines in the 1970s were not paralleled by an increase in the testing of their precursor, Coley's toxins. This "oldest immunotherapy" had a dedicated and efficient advocate, Coley's daughter, Helen Coley Nauts. In 1953 Nauts had founded the New York Cancer Research Institute (from 1973 on, the Cancer Research Institute), which became an important charity specialized in financing research in tumor immunology.[106] Besides her activity promoting research on links between immunity and cancer, Nauts published meticulously researched monographs documenting numerous cases of regression of advanced tumors in patients treated with Coley's toxins. Her efforts, however, did not convince Western oncologists to conduct large-scale clinical trials of Coley's toxins. One reason may have been the difficulties of studying the antitumor activity of Coley's toxins in the laboratory.[107] Another may have been Nauts's insistence that only a faithful replication of the original Coley's therapy led to promising clinical results.[108] A therapy based on injection of high doses of crude bacterial extracts can be improved only through trial-and-error bedside investigations, not through further laboratory studies. Moreover, clinical trials of an empirical therapy are evaluated solely in terms of their contribution to cancer cure, not in terms of their contribution to fundamental knowledge. Western oncologists thus preferred clinical experimentation with bacterial vaccines that had been carefully legitimated through preclinical research. In contrast, Chinese oncologists were attracted by the low cost and lack of technical sophistication of Coley's toxins. Coley's method was tested in several cancer hospitals in China, and its promoters claimed very promising results, especially in curing sarcoma in children.[109]

Cancer immunotherapy rapidly achieved high public visibility as a result of continuous media coverage. It was also explained, and often dramatized, in popular science books.[110] "Professor Mathé," one of these books explained,

> is one of the geniuses of present-day cancer research. He is restless, impatient with delay, anxious to see results. I said to him during our talk, "What strikes me is that you move faster from the laboratory to the human being than, say, your American counterparts." He replied, "Yes. That is our aim. We want to move fast. And we want the same doctor who treats mice to treat human beings, because if you have different people working on mice and human beings you lose a lot of time, a lot of time. Our people work on mice, on monkeys, on human beings. They must be able to work on *any* animal, studying the same problem . . . I am a professor of experimental oncology," he said, "and for me experimental oncology is not only oncology on animals but oncology on animals *and* human beings that cannot be cured by conventional methods . . . We have about twenty thousand mice, we have ten thousand rats, we have guinea

pigs, we have hamsters, we have rabbits, we have sheep, we have pigs, we have monkeys; but we also have five patients." *"Human patients?"* "Yes. In an aseptic room. They are there for investigations" . . . I asked, "Are these patients volunteers?" "Yes," Professor Mathé replied. "We asked their permission. But in France patients are very courageous and they readily give permission. It is, after all, for their benefit."[111]

The second wave of cancer immunotherapy employed the same methods—application of bacterial products to stimulate immune mechanisms, attempts at vaccination with tumor antigens—as the first. The main difference was organizational—the switch to large-scale, multicenter clinical trials and successful cooperation with the laboratory, both in the preclinical testing of immunostimulatory substances or vaccines in animal models of cancer and in the monitoring of responses of treated patients by immunologists. The rapid development of new immunological methods, in particular the expansion of *in vitro* assays of cell-mediated immunity, allowed the collection of quantitative data on the immune status of the patients before, during, and after therapy. Such evaluations had been attempted in the 1950s, but the scope of those studies had been limited. The rapid development of cellular immunology in the 1960s and 1970s, together with the increasing integration of clinical immunology laboratories into hospitals, enlarged the possibilities of investigating patients' immune responses. Many researchers believed that the introduction of new immunological monitoring methods would radically transform the practice of cancer immunotherapy, adding "a strong, rational, scientific basis to this field."[112] The historian of science June Goodfield affirmed in 1975 that "of all the scientists working on cancer, immunologists gave me the strongest impression . . . [of] being able to focus precisely on a series of intellectual and therapeutic targets. Here I finally sensed, for the first time, just where T. H. Huxley's physician, the 'blind man hitting out with a club,' will metamorphose into the sniper picking off intruders with lethal accuracy."[113]

Intellectual targets were easier to hit. Experimental studies of cancer immunology had flourished in the 1970s and led to rapid extension of the domain of tumor immunology. Therapeutic targets were more elusive. Mathé's first optimistic reports on the impressive clinical results of immunotherapy were not confirmed in larger, multicenter clinical trials organized by the British Medical Council: immunotherapy and chemotherapy were not found to be superior to chemotherapy alone.[114] Mathé's protests notwithstanding, in the late 1970s most researchers agreed that the efficacy of BCG in leukemia therapy had not been proved.[115]

Many clinicians continued to apply immunotherapy as a last resort for patients unable to benefit from conventional therapy. Different approaches were tested, usually on a small number of patients and in uncontrolled and nonrandomized trials. Not surprisingly, the results varied widely. Some investigators reported encouraging but statistically insignificant results and described rare individual cases of dramatic improvement, such as complete regression of pulmonary metastases of malignant melanoma.[116] But others had difficulties in confirming these results.[117] Even partisans were obliged to conclude that "immunotherapy as presently practiced seems to be a relatively ineffective way to treat human tumors."[118]

In the late 1970s promoters of cancer immunotherapy continued to affirm their faith in the new approach. "Negative results are not only predictable but are absolutely anticipated when you initiate clinical applications in a field of this complexity," wrote Dr. William Terry of the NCI. He and other cancer immunotherapy specialists insisted that this treatment, all its problems notwithstanding, was already the fourth major modality of cancer treatment and would soon achieve clinical efficiency as well.[119] They warned against the danger of allowing temporary setbacks in the clinics to put a premature end to research. The "childhood problems" of the new approach, experts maintained, should not mask the important achievements of this domain. The continuation of laboratory studies and the enlargement of the alliance between the clinics and biological disciplines, such as immunogenetics, immunochemistry, viral oncology, biochemistry of antigens, and clinical oncology, would necessarily lead to clinical progress.[120] Organizational innovation—efficient linking of distinct domains of activity—would lead to technical innovation and therapeutic efficacy. Thanks to new developments in basic sciences, Terry affirmed in 1978, the prospects for immunotherapies would be considerably different within five years: "there is no question that clinical immunotherapy is here to stay."[121]

Debate on the Relevance of Laboratory Models

Experimental cancer studies, once a low-prestige subspecialty of pathology, were gradually transformed into a prestigious domain of biomedical research. The development of genetically uniform strains of laboratory animals and the diffusion of standardized laboratory tumors permitted greater reproducibility of experiments, better quantification of results, and comparison of results obtained in different laboratories. It was an essential step in the institutionalization and consolidation of a prestigious international community of experimental cancer researchers. The standardization of experimental systems also facilitated the integration of cancer studies into the mainstream of advanced biological research and allowed, among other things, the forging of links between cancer studies and immunological investigations.

There was, however, another consequence of the methodological standardization of experimental oncology: a growing difference between the models used for the study of cancer in the laboratory and the human disease they were supposed to represent. The standardization of models led to a better understanding of experimental cancer in laboratory animals. Human cancer, however, continued to occur in a broad spectrum of individualized and unpredictable forms in a population highly heterogeneous from genetic and immunological points of view. The progressive reliance on experimental models of cancer thus increased the distance between studies made in the laboratory and "the odd mouse out"—the cancer patient.[122]

Early immunotherapies of cancer were not developed in the laboratory. They were either attempts to apply the principles of anti-infectious immunity (vaccination, serotherapy) or practices derived from clinical observations. In contrast, in the 1970s immunotherapies of cancer were first studied in the laboratory. The introduction of BCG and other bacterial products into the clinics was preceded by a demonstration of the efficacy of these substances in laboratory animals. Advocates of immunological approaches to cancer therapy were able to argue—as chemotherapy specialists had in the 1950s—that results obtained in animal studies justified large-scale clinical trials.[123] The conviction expressed by numerous specialists in tumor immunology in the late 1970s, that cancer immunotherapy was already an established domain that only needed to find a solution to the technical problem of efficient stimulation of antitumor immune mechanisms in humans, was grounded in studies made in experimental models of cancer.

A small number of radical critics challenged the two basic assumptions underlying this claim: that naturally occurring human cancers were sufficiently different from normal tissues to allow their destruction by immune mechanisms, and that immune responses against the tumor would necessarily benefit the cancer patient and would ultimately lead to a cure. These assumptions, they explained, derived from observations made in standardized animal models of cancer. In the absence of evidence demonstrating the validity of extrapolating from these models to naturally occurring human tumors, such assumptions should be seen at best as not yet proven. There was no self-evident link between the laboratory and the clinics.[124] As one pioneer of experimental immunotherapy, Dr. Graham Currie, explained, "most test systems for the evaluations of non-specific immunological stimulants as potential anticancer agents involve pretreatment of the experimental animal before the challenge with tumor. This situation has little relevance to therapy."[125] Another pioneer of cancer immunotherapy, Dr. David Weiss, pointed out that studies made with malignant cells cultivated in the test tube also used artificially constructed laboratory products: "the extent to which lines of tumor origin maintain a semblance to neoplasia in nature after passage [that is, transfer] for years in animals and tissue culture is highly questionable ... we can do better than delude ourselves that we really are studying leukemia when we work with EL4 cells."[126]

The advocates of cancer immunotherapy legitimated their approach by citing the measurable increase of immune responses in patients treated with bacterial vaccines. But as Currie explained, they tended to conflate the ability to elicit an immune response with the ability to produce a cure. Another assumption underlying cancer immunotherapy was the belief that the new treatment would do no harm. Immunologists recognized, however, that indiscriminate tampering with poorly understood immune mechanisms could be dangerous: "agents such as BCG may even enhance tumor growth when given alone to tumor-bearing animals ... much caution will have to be exercised before this approach can be safely tried in man in order to avoid the theoretical danger of immunological enhancement."[127]

In the 1970s, however, cancer immunotherapy was not characterized by extreme caution. The atmosphere of high excitement and feverish activity that accompanied the birth of the "fourth modality of cancer therapy" led to the rapid introduction of large-scale clinical experiments. "More often than not," Weiss warned, "immunotherapy has been carried out in ignorance, if not in actual defiance, of the recognized principles of immunology and tumor biology: the approach has been taken with a shotgun. Perhaps we should be as much surprised by the fact that any positive results have been obtained as we are by their smallness."[128] The wide diffusion and frequent replication of clinical trials did not make them more efficient. "During the last decade," stated British cancer specialist Dr. Harold B. Hewitt in 1983, "over 400 clinical trials of immunotherapy have been conducted, exposing many tens of thousands of cancer patients to treatments that are usually distressing and occasionally dangerous. The result of this highly contagious endeavour . . . has been the failure to establish immunotherapy as a useful treatment." Hewitt argued that this trend reflected the persistence, since the early nineteenth century, of an irrational faith in the ability of the human body's defense mechanisms to control malignant disease:

> The persistent recommendation of immunotherapy has this in common with the promotion of "unconventional" treatments for cancer, such as laetrile: its effectiveness has been confidently presumed before its potential value has been proved by suitable investigation. But whereas a single multicenter trial of laetrile organized by the National Cancer Institute was sufficient to quiet its vociferous lay advocates, over 400 "discouraging" trials of immunotherapy have failed to shake the conviction of its academic proponents.[129]

Hewitt's acute analysis of the role of "emotional dispositions" in attempts at cancer immunotherapy points to the importance of cultural representations of disease in the diffusion of medical innovations. But he does not extend that analysis to the undeniable linkage between the popular belief in the body's ability to fight malignant cells and what he himself describes as "the very large financial, institutional, and personal commitment to cancer immunology."[130] The rapid development of a large-scale clinical research enterprise in the 1970s occurred in response to the conjunction of several events: the growing importance of immunology as a leading biomedical discipline (symbolized by the success of organ grafts), the significant increase in funding for cancer research following passage of the Cancer Act in 1971, the impatience of the lay public and politicians with the dearth of spectacular achievements in "the war on cancer," and the contrast between the impressive success of medical oncology as an independent professional specialty (especially in the United States) and its limited practical success in curing common cancers in adults. After a decade of rapid growth, the domain of cancer immunotherapy had failed to fulfill the initial high hopes for it. But in the meantime it had become a political and social enterprise: cancer immunotherapy had created new institutional links, professional alliances, and legitimation strategies, had attracted special budgets, and had acquired the image of being at the cutting edge of cancer therapy. Once established, such structures are difficult to dismantle: it is easier to "recycle" them, that is, to find a new content for the already existing institutional and social forms.

At the end of his 1974 review of human cancer immunotherapy, Currie wrote: "Southam (1972) has pointed out that the current atmosphere of excitement generated by recent work in tumor immunology is often associated with such 'naiveté' that it resembles the narrow bias of religious fanaticism or the transient fads of women's fashion. It is to be hoped that such bias and transience will be absent from the next stages in the application of immunology to the clinical management of cancer patients."[131] Currie's last sentence is revealing. In the 1970s even an outspoken critic of existing cancer immunotherapies did not doubt that the "next stages" were close at hand. He was right. A "next stage"—the introduction of interleukins to cancer therapy—became a highly visible trend in the early 1980s. It was supported by the same professional groups that had introduced immunotherapies to the cancer clinics in the 1970s—medical oncologists and immunologists—joined by a new one, molecular biologists. In addition, cancer immunotherapy was shaped in the 1980s by a new and important development: the alignment of the interests of immunologists, medical oncologists, and molecular biologists with those of the biotechnology industry. This alignment launched the third wave of cancer immunotherapy, the subject of the next chapter.

CHAPTER THREE

Cancer Immunotherapy and Mass Production of Biological Agents, 1980–1990

Interferon

The late 1970s were a period of rapid growth for basic and preclinical studies in tumor immunology.[1] Immunological concepts and approaches became increasingly popular among physicians because they facilitated translation of the notion of biological individuality (used by doctors to account for, say, differences in individual reactions to pathogenic microorganisms) into the language of modern biology. Immunological explanations that stipulated the existence of complex regulatory networks were particularly attractive to cancer specialists, allowing them to account for otherwise inexplicable individual variations among tumor-bearing patients, while the search for the influence of a malignant tumor on immune mechanisms opened a new field of inquiry in clinical oncology. Studies of immunological parameters in cancer extended the scope of intervention for immunologists and oncologists and promoted contacts between the two groups. These contacts rapidly led to the expansion of the domain of cancer immunology and immunotherapy and to the founding, in 1976, of a scientific journal devoted exclusively to that subject.[2]

One of the important new findings in tumor immunology in the 1970s was the description of a new class of cell-killing lymphocytes, the natural killer (NK) cells. NK cells destroyed malignant cells in the test tube, and high levels of these cells in the blood of tumor-bearing laboratory animals were correlated with inhibition of tumor growth. Some investigators affirmed that such a correlation could be found in humans too.[3] NK cells were initially studied by cellular immunologists and by specialists in tumor immunology. The classification of these cells as a new immunological mechanism was, however, problematic. The destruction of tumor cells by NK cells closely recalls the destruction of foreign or malignant cells by "killer" T lymphocytes—a phenomenon that was defined as a cellular immune mechanism. But the cytotoxic activity of NK cells is different from that of T cells. The elimination of a tumor cell by a "killer" T cell is a specific reaction (that is, T cells of a given individual "learn" to recognize a particular tumor and later selectively destroy cells originated from that tumor), whereas the destruction of the malignant cells by NK cells is nonspecific and, unlike "classical" immunological reactions, does not depend on a learning process. It was therefore possible to argue that the killing of tumor cells by NK cells was not an immune process.[4] The debate over whether the destruction of tumors by NK cells should be classified as an immune phenomenon was not a purely semantic one; it had a direct effect on the definition of the limits of immunological inquiry and the distribution of domains of professional competence. The destruction of tumor cells by NK cells was, some specialists claimed, one of the principal mechanisms of elimination of malignant cells by the body. Consequently, the classification of NK activity as an immune phenomenon was an important factor favoring the inclusion of immunologists in the jurisdiction of cancer therapy.

The classification of NK cells was only one of several problems related to determination of the limits of immunological inquiry. From the 1920s on, immunologists defined their specialty as the study of specific defense mechanisms. Specificity was viewed as a hallmark of immune phenomena, and the specificity of a given "defense reaction" legitimated its study by immunologists.[5] Thus graft rejection, long viewed as a poorly understood pathological event, was recognized as a bona fide immune reaction when Sir Peter Medawar was able to show the strict specificity of the rejection reaction.[6] The role of specificity in studies of immune phenomena, however, became less central in the 1970s, when immunologists became interested in nonspecific factors that amplified immune reactions.[7] These "amplifying molecules" (interferons, interleukins, growth factors) have numerous physiological effects, not all of them connected to or explicable by their effects on classical immune mechanisms such as the production of specific antibodies or the specific rejection of grafts. The growing interest of immunologists in cells and molecules that did not fit the classical definition of immunity blurred the limits between immunology and other domains of biological inquiry (cellular biology, physiology, biochemistry, pathology) and later opened the way to debates on the attribution of specific practices to a given specialty or subspecialty. Immunologists had an important advantage in these controversies: the "ownership" of a specific set of laboratory techniques employed in studies of cells and substances that kill other cells. These techniques, first developed to study specific phenomena such as graft rejection, were later extended to the study of nonspecific phenomena such as NK cell activity. The ownership of methods for the study of cytotoxicity (cell killing) in the test tube favored immunologists' continuous control of research on biological mechanisms that eliminate malignant cells. It did not, however, automatically ensure the extension of that control to attempts to test these mechanisms in the clinics.

In the 1970s cancer immunotherapy was viewed as the undisputed domain of immunologists because these studies employed materials (bacterial vaccines, bacterial products) and methods (skin tests, measures of levels of antibodies in the blood) firmly rooted in the immunological tradition. The introduction of a "natural" regulatory molecule—the interferon—to cancer therapy complicated the debate on ownership of the new approaches to cancer therapy. Interferon is an intracellular protein that interferes (hence its name) with the multiplication of viruses. It was discovered in 1957 by Alick Isaaks and Jean Lindenmann.[8] At first the newly described molecule aroused the interest of virologists, but interferon studies were hampered by the difficulties of obtaining reproducible and coherent results, and in the 1960s they became a relatively marginal field, although many virologists continued to view interferon as a highly promising antiviral treatment.[9] In the 1960s and early 1970s there was heightened interest in the relationship between viruses and cancer. After the enactment of the Cancer Act of 1971, one of the principal axes of research developed by the NCI was the Virus Cancer Program, centered on the study of tumor-inducing viruses.[10] Scientists who believed that viruses played an important role in the etiology of human cancer looked for ways to inhibit the proliferation of viruses in the cell and became interested in interferons as a potential anticancer therapy.[11]

In 1972 the virologist Ion Gresser showed that in mice interferon inhibited not only virus-induced tumors but also other transplantable tumors (for example, tumors induced by chemical compounds such as tar). Inhibition was usually attributed to the indirect effects of the molecule.[12] In the late 1970s scientists found that there are several families of molecules with interferon activity and consequently divided interferons into three principal subgroups—alpha, beta, and gamma. At the same time specialists also showed that in addition to their antiviral activity, interferons had numerous other physiological effects, including a regulatory influence on immune mechanisms. In particular researchers found that the interferon gamma stimulated the activity of NK cells. That potential effect of interferons on immune mechanisms provided a plausible explanation for the antitumor effects of interferons, although it did not invalidate other hypotheses such as the possibility that it was directly toxic to malignant cells.[13]

In the 1970s the antitumor effects of interferons were confirmed in several experimental models and looked promising enough to stimulate attempts at large-scale production of human interferon and the beginning of clinical studies in humans. Interferons are species-specific, and only human interferon is efficient in humans.[14] Around 1970 Dr. Kari Cantell at the Finnish Red Cross developed a method for extracting large quantities of partially purified interferon from human white blood cells.[15] The method was labor-intensive and time-consuming, and the final product contained at most 1 percent pure interferon, but the quantity obtained was sufficient for a small-scale clinical trial. In the early 1970s Dr. Hans Strander in Stockholm used Cantell's interferon to treat a small number of patients suffering from osteogenic sarcoma. His preliminary results seemed to indicate that the new treatment reduced mortality from this highly virulent cancer from 80 percent to 60 percent. The evidence was, however, anecdotal. Moreover, the patients treated with interferon were compared with historical controls, not with an untreated control group, because Strander believed that it was unethical to deprive young, desperately ill patients of a potentially beneficial treatment. The use of historical controls to demonstrate the efficacy of a cancer treatment is, according to some experts, problematic. The diagnosis of a given type of cancer and the classification of borderline cases may (and often do) change over time, and these differences may account for the perceived improvement in survival. Nevertheless, some specialists received Strander's results with enthusiasm.[16]

In April 1975 Dr. Mathilde Krim of the Sloan-Kettering Institute organized a conference on the use of interferons in cancer treatment.[17] Although the only data on clinical effects of interferon to be presented there were the preliminary findings of the Stockholm experiment, the conference increased interferon's visibility. Leading physicians, politicians, and philanthropists were recruited to the interferon cause.[18]

In November 1975 the National Cancer Advisory Board of the National Cancer Institute recommended that the NCI Division of Cancer Treatment purchase interferon for basic and preclinical studies.[19] In mid-1976 the NCI allocated $1 million to the purchase of interferon for six clinical trials and for a greater number of basic investigations.

The first North American clinical trials of interferon did not produce cancer cures, but rumors persisted among oncologists that these trials revealed the capacity of the new drug to dramatically affect commonly occurring solid tumors; only the scarcity of interferon prevented the demonstration of more spectacular therapeutic effects.[20] These rumors fueled pressure to obtain more interferon—and thus to spend more money on its purchase. In October 1978 the Board of Scientific Counselors of the NCI Division of Cancer Treatment recommended that the division review the data on interferon and establish a Biological Response Modifiers Program.[21] In 1978 Dr. Frank Raucher, then the vice-president of the Research Division of the American Cancer Society, convinced the ACS to spend $2 million on the purchase of interferon for clinical trials. As a result of this decision, interferon received wide coverage as the new cancer treatment in newspapers, magazines, and television programs. The cover of the March 31, 1980, issue of *Time* magazine showed a drop of bright yellow liquid hanging at the end of a pipette with the headline: "Interferon: The IF Drug for Cancer." The highly predictable result was a surge of pressure from desperate patients and their families begging hospitals and doctors to give them the new miracle drug.[22]

Following the 1979 recommendations of an NCI subcommittee, the NCI allocated $13.5 million in its 1980 budget for the new Biological Response Modifiers (BRM) Program. The choice of name may have reflected a desire to dissociate it from earlier attempts at nonspecific stimulation of immune mechanisms with bacterial products. On the other hand, most promoters of the BRM Program were researchers in tumor immunology who had been involved in earlier cancer immunotherapy efforts.[23] The new project was closely modeled on NCI screening programs that aimed at uncovering compounds possessing antitumor activity, such as the National Chemotherapy Program, Plant Screening Program, and Fermentation Program.[24] The goal of the BRM Program was to screen large numbers of potentially active substances, to select the ones that were promising enough to be tested in preclinical studies, and finally to help organize clinical trials of the substances found to be active in preclinical studies.[25]

The search for potential biological response modifiers was defined as "the search for agents able to modify the host's response to tumor cells with resultant therapeutic benefits." This official definition was broad enough to include the study of substances (bacterial vaccines, bacterial products) employed in earlier attempts at cancer immunotherapy. But although the BRM Program did screen many natural and synthetic substances, in the early 1980s its efforts centered on interferon-related research. The interest in interferon and other regulatory molecules produced by the human organism changed the official evaluation of earlier cancer immunotherapies. These therapies had at first been presented as the results of the rigorous application to the clinics of principles discovered in laboratory studies. In the late 1970s researchers claimed that although the clinical results of immunotherapies with bacterial immunostimulants were not (yet) very impressive, these studies had been a first step in the right direction and had held distinct clinical promise.[26] Several years later the same attempts at nonspecific stimulation of the immune system with bacterial vaccines were viewed as sadly lacking in scientific rigor.

Dr. Robert Oldham, head of the BRM Program, explained in 1983 that previous attempts at cancer immunotherapy had never been efficient:

> while a small, initial, non-randomized trial would be often reported as being positive in a preliminary report, follow-up of those patients would often reveal that the study was indeed negative . . . If one looks only at the randomized studies of various human malignancies, most of the positive studies have been marginally positive, and the majority of larger studies has yielded negative results . . . In summary, the "old" immunotherapy utilized non-specific and "specific" immunotherapy in an empiric sense.

Oldham believed that recent technological advances would overcome the shortcomings of the "old" immunotherapy: "the revolution in molecular biology, the advent of computers and the improvement in hybridoma technology have combined to enable the scientists to produce the highly purified reagents necessary to begin to ask rather specific questions about immunological mechanisms involved in cancer growth, metastasis and therapy."[27] The empiricism of the "old" immunotherapy, Oldham argued, would soon be replaced by the principle of biological specificity: specificity of reagents would lead to understanding of specific pathological mechanisms, then to a specific treatment. Another specialist, Dr. John W. Hadden, similarly contrasted "primitive" therapy with the specificity and precision of new approaches: "the trend in immunotherapy has been away from the more toxic and ambivalent immunotherapy with crude bacterial and fungal preparations towards chemically defined and more selective agents."[28]

For a while interferon became a test case of the "new" immunotherapy of cancer. The expectation that interferon might cure cancer ensured the rapid flow of money from NCI, ACS, and private industry grants into studies of this molecule. Around 1980 several firms began large-scale production of interferon by traditional methods, that is, purification of interferon secreted by human cells (leukocytes or fibroblasts) in the test tube.[29] The interferon produced by that method was applied to cancer therapy in a first wave of clinical trials (1979–1982). The cloning of the human interferon gene by the Japanese scientist Dr. Tadatsugu Taniguchi in 1979 opened the way for mass production. Rapid production of recombinant human interferon (that is, interferon produced by genetic engineering techniques) became a major goal of the biotechnology industry and was strongly encouraged by the BRM Program. The increasing involvement of public organizations (NCI, NIH) in interferon studies played an important role in convincing the industry that interferon was indeed a promising investment.

The rapid rise of biotechnology firms in the late 1970s and early 1980s was directly related to the hope of developing efficient anticancer therapies that would employ molecules produced using techniques of molecular biology. Interferon production quickly became a "demonstration project" of the new industry.[30] In 1980 the Swiss-based biotechnology firm Biogen announced that one of the firm's directors, Dr. Charles Weissman, had cloned the human interferon gene in the bacterium *Echerichia coli*.[31] Other biotechnology firms also announced their intention of producing interferon, using genetic engineering methods; among them were Genentech, Cetus Corporation, Interferon Sciences, Amgen, and Flow Laboratories in the United States; Hoffman–La Roche and Cytotech in Switzerland; Hoechst in Germany; Russel-Uclaf, Institut Merieux, Sanofi, and Rhone-Poulenc Santé in France; Wellcome and Imperial Chemical Industries in the United Kingdom; Searle in the United Kingdom and United States; Ares Serono in Italy; and Toyo Jozo Corporation in Japan.[32] Many of these specialized small biotechnology firms and larger pharmaceutical firms had already been involved in the production of cell-secreted interferon. The conviction that interferon had an important therapeutic future led to an unprecedented mobilization of resources and capital and to intense competition among these concerns.[33]

Efforts to produce interferon were fueled by preliminary reports on the molecule's ability to induce shrinkage of advanced solid tumors. Shrinkage was not an unusual therapeutic effect: routine radiation therapy and chemotherapy often diminished the size of malignant growths. Advocates of the "new" immunotherapy affirmed, however, that interferon induced the shrinkage of tumors that resisted all conventional therapies. In addition, interferon and other biological response modifiers had an important advantage over earlier methods of cancer therapy: these molecules were believed to be less toxic than standard chemotherapy or radiation therapy because they acted "through physiological mechanisms."[34] A presumably nontoxic, "natural" cancer therapy was attractive to the emerging ecology- and holistic-medicine-oriented public of the early 1980s.

But interferon's lack of toxicity was only a supposition, and moreover not necessarily a well-founded one. Physicians, unlike the lay public, knew that substances produced by the organism (such as hormones) may induce severe, sometimes fatal side effects when used as drugs. Some interferon advocates also knew about its potential toxicity. In 1977 a preliminary report on the serious undesirable effects produced by administration of interferon had been presented at an international conference. Some interferon advocates, fearing that such data would hamper support for the new treatment, successfully opposed diffusion of this information.[35]

In 1983 competition in the production of interferon ended with the simultaneous success of several biotechnology firms (Biogen, Genentech, Amgen, Interferon Sciences) in bringing the new molecule(s) to the marketplace. A nearly unlimited supply of recombinant interferon became available for clinical trials. Ironically, at a time when the increased supply of interferons made large-scale testing possible, trials made with leukocyte- or fibrocyte-extracted interferon had already indicated that interferon was far from being the "penicillin of cancer." These tests had shown that only a few, relatively rare cancers—particularly hairy cell leukemia—responded well to interferon.[36] In other interferon-sensitive malignant tumors (such as non-Hodgkin's lymphoma, kidney cancer, and Kaposi's sarcoma) the proportion of positive responses to interferon therapy had been lower (between one-fifth and one-quarter of patients treated), and many of these responses had been short-term. In addition, therapeutic doses of interferon often induced significant toxicity and unpleasant side effects.[37]

At first some specialists claimed that better results would be obtained with pure and highly concentrated recombinant interferons. The arrival of these on the market allowed a sharp increase in the number of clinical trials. These trials, some critics later claimed, suffered from anarchic competition: "what has occurred with interferon to date has been an empirical thrashing about, under the stimulus of massive publicity blitz and the initial scarcity of the material."[38] The "industry" of clinical trials of interferons aimed to define clinical situations in which the molecule would become an efficient anticancer drug. But recombinant interferons never produced impressive therapeutic results. Both their efficacy and toxicity were similar to those of interferons secreted by human cells. No significant clinical responses were found in the common solid tumors of the adult, such as lung or colon cancers. Moreover, prolonged doses of recombinant interferon induced symptoms not unlike those caused by chemotherapy: decreased blood count, fever, chills, fatigue, and nausea. The toxicity of interferon was found to be the result of the activity of the molecule itself and not, as had been hoped, of impurities present in preparations of cell-secreted interferon. Toxicity and clinical efficacy were directly linked, and the first was found to be higher, and the second lower, than expected.[39]

Though not found to be a miracle drug for cancer, interferon had uncontested therapeutic effects in selected cancers. In 1983 NCI and ACS specialists claimed that its full therapeutic potential would be revealed through additional basic and preclinical research.[40] Some scientists linked with biotechnology firms that had invested a lot of money in the production of interferons and had not made rapid profits disagreed. Thus Dr. Stephen K. Carter, the vice-president for anticancer research in the Pharmaceutical Research and Development Division of the Bristol-Myers Company, stated in the mid-1980s that "interferon is clearly a failure. It is damn expensive and it is damn toxic. So how long is a doctor going to give something to a patient that makes him feel absolutely terrible, costs a fortune, and doesn't work?"[41]

In the long run, Carter was wrong. The disenchantment in the mid-1980s following the "interferon hype" recalls the period in the mid-1970s following the enthusiastic application of BCG and other bacterial vaccines to cancer therapy. But whereas BCG did not become

an accepted cancer therapy (except in the localized treatment of bladder cancer),[42] interferon was eventually included in the therapy for a
growing number of malignancies and found other clinical applications
as well (17 distinct indications of interferon therapy were enumerated
in 1994). Although the clinical efficacy of the interferons in therapy
for advanced tumors remained low except for hairy cell leukemia,
these molecules were gradually integrated into routine treatments of
Kaposi's sarcoma, multiple myeloma, melanoma, myelogenic leukemia, non-Hodgkin's lymphoma, kidney cancer, and other pathologies,
in particular chronic hepatitis. Interferon, initially a candidate "miracle drug" for cancer, was redefined as a "helpful auxiliary therapy"
for this disease, and the market for the molecule expanded from $13.6
million in 1986, to $130 million in 1989, to $1 billion in 1993. Since
the late 1980s this market has been controlled by two big pharmaceutical companies that bought licenses from small biotechnology firms:
Schering-Plough, which acquired Biogen's license; and Hoffman–La
Roche, which acquired Genentech's license. In the early 1990s interferon became an exemplary product for the biotechnology industry, a
visible proof that huge investments in cytokine research might be rewarding.[43] But its status in the early 1980s was entirely different.

Around 1983, when it became clear that interferon was not a highly
efficient therapy for cancer—and when it seemed that it would also
be a commercial failure—the promoters of the "new" immunotherapy
developed alternative strategies to legitimate their therapeutic approach. One of these was the insistence on the capacity of the new
agents to induce perceptible shrinkage of selected tumors. This ability,
argued Drs. Robert Oldham and Richard Smalley, fully justified the
definition of biological response modifiers as a "fourth modality of
cancer therapy."[44]

Advocates of the "new" immunotherapy also often stressed its close
links with the latest developments in basic biological research: mass
production of interferon was made possible by genetic engineering
methods, while new approaches to studies of cell biology and of cellular mechanisms of immunity led to progress in the understanding of
the biological effects of interferons in the test tube and in laboratory
animals; these approaches also allowed detailed studies of the effects
of interferon on immune mechanisms in humans. But the accumulation of an impressive amount of data on that subject did not lead to
a satisfactory understanding of the mechanisms underlying the physiological effects of interferon in patients. The immunological expla-

nations of interferon's antitumor activity were based mainly on the observation—made in the test tube—that interferon activated NK lymphocytes. Interferon-treated cancer patients, however, did not show significant increases in the number of circulating NK cells, and no clear-cut correlation was found between the clinical results of interferon treatment and activation of other measurable immune mechanisms.[45] Biological tests were unable to explain differences in individual reactions and could not be used to predict which patients suffering from interferon-sensitive tumors would be good candidates for the new therapy.[46] Failure to find a correlation between the activation of NK cells by interferon and clinical responses to the molecule revived the hypothesis that interferon might be directly toxic to tumor cells.[47]

After a decade of the BRM Program a major review of the "new" immunotherapy soberly stated that "the mechanisms of interferon-mediated antitumor effects are unclear,"[48] while another review acknowledged that interferon, like many other biological agents, "has more than one biological effect and may act both directly and indirectly . . . It is often extremely difficult to determine by which mechanism or mechanisms these agents are mediating their antitumor effects."[49] Recombinant interferon had been shown to be a powerful biological agent. Its chemical structure had been elucidated and its physiological effects documented in a great number of experimental systems. But in the late 1980s the understanding of interferon's therapeutic effects in humans did not seem qualitatively different from the understanding of the mechanisms responsible for the antitumor effects of the "old" immunotherapies in the 1970s.

From Interferon to IL-2

On the last page of her 1984 book, *The Interferon Crusade*, Sandra Panem reported the recent (summer 1983) cloning of a new cytokine, interleukin-2. Newspaper headlines proclaimed IL-2 as "a natural weapon against cancer" and "a new cancer drug." "For interferon watchers," wrote Panem, "the parallels are unmistakable. The soldiers have regrouped to lead the interleukin crusade."[50] IL-2 had been known to immunologists since 1976, when it was found that the molecule stimulated the growth of T lymphocytes, a subpopulation of lymphocytes that plays an important role in numerous immune mechanisms (hence the earlier name, T cell growth factor, or TCGF).[51]

TCGF was renamed interleukin-2 (IL-2) in the early 1980s, when it was found to belong to a group of substances that transmit messages between white blood cells ("inter-leukins"). Because this substance made possible the culture of specific subpopulations of T cells in the test tube, it rapidly became an important research tool for cellular immunologists. The IL-2 molecule was immediately perceived as having important therapeutic potential, and it attracted the attention of the pharmaceutical industry, interested in regulatory molecules. In 1983 the gene for IL-2 was cloned independently by several groups of molecular biologists: Tadatsugu Taniguchi's group in Tokyo (collaborating with the Japanese firm Ajinomoto); Robert Gallo's group in Bethesda, Maryland (linked with the Genetics Institute); R. Fiers's group in Gand, Belgium (collaborating with Biogen); and by R. J. Robb's group in Wilmington, Delaware (linked with DuPont de Nemours).[52]

Around 1980, when the studies that led to the cloning of IL-2 had begun, this molecule was not perceived exclusively—or even primarily—as an anticancer treatment. Researchers looked for clinical applications of IL-2 in immune deficiency states (that is, in cases of inefficient functioning of immune mechanisms), especially those in which there was a lack or a dysfunction of T cells. Such dysfunction, the specialists claimed, was often observed in advanced cancer, and it was not illogical to consider the administration of IL-2 to cancer patients. The shift toward the representation of IL-2 as the next "miracle drug" for cancer was strongly influenced by the activity of a particularly visible and dynamic group of oncologists—Dr. Steven Rosenberg's group at the Surgery Branch of the National Institutes of Health—and by the privileged relationship between that group and the California-based biotechnology firm Cetus.

Rosenberg, who had obtained a Ph.D. in biophysics before completing his surgical residency, aspired to combine the professional roles of preclinical researcher and medical practitioner. He was appointed head of the NIH Surgery Branch because the NIH directorship was interested in the introduction of modern biological research methods into that traditional, skill-oriented domain.[53] In the 1960s Rosenberg was involved in last-ditch attempts at adoptive cancer immunotherapy in terminally ill patients. He and his colleagues transfused the blood of a patient who had undergone spontaneous cancer regression to another patient. They also immunized pigs with patients' tumors and then transferred their leukocytes to the tumor donors.[54] In the 1970s

Rosenberg took part in clinical trials of BCG in melanoma and bone sarcoma. In 1982 he concluded that bacterial vaccines did not show clinical efficacy against cancer.[55] The attempts to cure melanoma and bone sarcoma with BCG, he explained, were empiric, lacked firm scientific basis, and unnecessarily increased the suffering of patients. He remained convinced, however, that immune mechanisms might play an important role in the destruction of malignant cells, and pursued studies on cancer immunotherapy in his laboratory.

In the early 1980s Rosenberg became interested in adoptive immunotherapy—the transfer, to the patient, of white blood cells that have acquired antitumor activity in the test tube. This therapy, he believed, should have multiple advantages: it should have low toxicity, because immunized cells should be capable of attacking tumor but not normal tissues; it should not limit the efficacy of natural immune mechanisms; and finally, it should be easy to combine with existing cancer treatments.[56] The last argument had strategic importance: it was easier to persuade oncologists to introduce a new therapy that could potentially extend the scope of their therapeutic interventions than to ask them to introduce a therapy that might limit them. Rosenberg's approach was, from the very beginning, strongly practice-oriented. It was also fueled by his deep commitment to contribute to a victory in the "war against cancer."[57] Although Rosenberg collaborated closely with immunologists and later with molecular biologists, this collaboration was dedicated nearly exclusively to the development, propagation, and legitimation of new therapeutic tools to fight cancer.

Adoptive immunotherapy, as we have seen, was introduced into treatment of human malignancies in the 1950s and 1960s following the observation that cytotoxic lymphocytes were able to destroy malignant cells in the test tube.[58] In early attempts at adoptive cancer immunotherapy, patients received white blood cells (leukocytes) from volunteers vaccinated with the patients' tumor cells. The failure of these attempts was usually attributed to the difficulty of generating an adequate amount of efficient cytotoxic cells. The discovery of a family of molecules (cytokines, growth factors) that would permit the large-scale culture of specific subsets of white cells in the test tube opened new horizons for adoptive cancer immunotherapy. IL-2 was found to be a particularly effective tool for expanding selected populations of lymphocytes.[59]

Rosenberg and his collaborators aimed first at the development of tumor-specific adoptive immunotherapy with IL-2-activated tumor-specific cytotoxic T cells. When they incubated blood cells with IL-2 they noticed that under these conditions normal (nonimmunized) human leukocytes spontaneously acquired the ability to destroy tumor cells.[60] The destruction of tumor cells was nonspecific and was unrelated to an immunization process. Rosenberg and his coworkers were, however, interested above all in finding an efficient way to destroy malignant tumors and were not attached to their initial hypothesis of specific adoptive immunotherapy. Their observation became the starting point of several years of efforts to introduce IL-2-activated lymphocytes into cancer therapy.

Rosenberg's group concluded that IL-2 activated a previously unknown subset of cells, which they named leukin-activated killer, or LAK, cells. The LAK cells, they claimed, were distinct from the two previously described subsets of cell-killing white blood cells: the cytotoxic T cells and the natural killer (NK) cells. Cytotoxic T lymphocytes are specific and are restricted by major histocompatibility complex (MHC) markers; that is, they are able to destroy only tumor cells that they have "learned" to "recognize" through prior contact with these cells. Moreover, such destruction is dependent on the presence of "identification" molecules—MHC proteins—on the surface of cytotoxic cells and on the surface of target cells. Like the NK cells, LAK cells were nonspecific and non-MHC-restricted. Rosenberg and his collaborators affirmed, however, that LAK cells were different from NK: they lacked the typical NK surface markers (specific proteins fixed on the cell's surface) and were able to destroy a much wider range of tumor cells. LAK cells were credited with the ability to destroy fresh tumor cells, while the NK cells were usually unable to destroy such cells, and their activity was demonstrated on cell lines maintained for a long time in culture.[61] LAK cells, Rosenberg and his coworkers proposed, were a previously unknown subset of highly efficient cytotoxic lymphocytes that would be especially good candidates for adoptive cancer immunotherapy in humans.[62]

The claim that LAK cells represented a new subpopulation of cytotoxic cells was based on two arguments: a functional one—these cells, unlike NK cells, were able to destroy fresh human tumor cells—and a morphological one—LAK cells carried surface markers that distinguished them from both NK cells and cytotoxic T cells.[63] The presence of surface markers on a given subset of cells is determined through the reaction of these cells with fluorescent monoclonal antiserum.

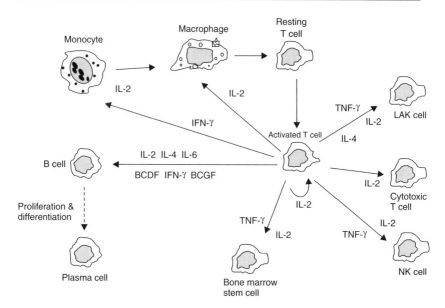

The role of IL-2 within the immune system, showing probable interactions and outcomes of IL-2 therapy. Abbreviations: BCDF = B cell differentiating factor; BCGF = B cell growth factor; IFN = interferon; IL = interleukin; LAK = lympho-kine-activated killer; NK = natural killer; TNF = tumor necrosis factor. (After Ruth Whittington and Diana Faulds, "Interleukin-2: A review of its pharma-cological properties and therapeutic use in patients with cancer," *Drugs* 46[3] [1993], 452.)

(Monoclonal antiserum is prepared by antibody-secreting cells im-mortalized by fusion with malignant cells. It has single specificity; that is, it reacts with a single type of molecular structure. Fluorescent serum is a serum marked with a fluorescent molecule to allow visualization.) The cells are put in contact with fluorescent serum, then rinsed to eliminate the excess of serum, and the amount of antibodies that react with surface antigens (antibodies that "stick" strongly to the cell's sur-face) is measured by a cell sorter, an instrument that measures the percentage of fluorescent cells in a given population and evaluates the intensity of fluorescence in these cells. The reproducibility of this method depends on standardization of scientific instruments, labora-tory techniques, reagents, and skills of laboratory workers. It may also depend on the quantity of a given marker in the tested cell population (low concentrations of a given marker increase the margin of error). The level of expression of surface markers in a given cell population, however, is difficult to standardize because studies of white cell sub-populations are made with cells taken from distinct individuals (in studies of human lymphocytes, from individual blood donors) who differ greatly in hereditary makeup and physiological status.

In functional tests, cytotoxic cells are incubated with tumor cells that have been internally marked with radioactive chromium (^{51}Cr). When tumor cells are destroyed, the radioactive chromium is released into the culture medium: the radioactivity of the medium thus measures the efficiency of cell-killing. This test may seem simpler because it does not employ complicated instruments such as the cell sorter and specially crafted reagents such as monoclonal antibodies. In fact, however, the functional tests have at least two distinct sources of irreducible variability: the previously mentioned variability of "killer" cells—the human cytotoxic lymphocytes—and the similar but unrelated variability of target cells—the tumor cells employed in the tests.[64] Both morphological and functional tests have wide margins of uncertainty, and articles discussing subpopulations of "killer" lymphocytes often present divergent results.

Rosenberg and his collaborators based their claim that LAK cells were a distinct cell population chiefly on functional arguments. Their proposal did not persuade all the lymphocyte specialists, some of whom argued as early as 1982 that LAK cells were NK cells that had been modified in the test tube by the culture in the presence of IL-2.[65] But the (minor) controversy over the nature of LAK cells did not affect Rosenberg's group's main goal—the rapid transfer of the new therapy to the clinics. The claim that IL-2-activated cells were a new, functionally important subset of cytotoxic lymphocytes probably facilitated the granting of permission to start clinical experiments. The principal argument made by Rosenberg and his colleagues was, however, heuristic: they affirmed that white blood cells activated in the test tube by IL-2 were able to destroy malignant cells in the human body. In the years 1982–1986 LAK cells were, to borrow the French philosopher Michel Serres's term, "quasi-objects."[66] The degree of certainty about their existence as an independent nosologic entity varied according to the audience to which these cells were described. The scientists who studied T-cell subpopulations (including some of Rosenberg's collaborators) described them mainly in functional terms to their colleagues, attributing to them at best only a conditional autonomous existence. In contrast, when the promoters of IL-2 therapy discussed the subject outside the esoteric circle of specialists, they insisted more on the existence of a specific cellular vehicle for the therapeutic effects of the IL-2 molecule. To the nonspecialized public (politicians, health administrators, journalists) they presented LAK cells as an unproblematic "scientific fact."[67]

To obtain permission to experiment on humans, it was necessary to demonstrate the therapeutic effects of LAK cells in tumor-bearing laboratory animals. Rosenberg and his colleagues rapidly switched to studies of the therapeutic properties of LAK cells in animal models that faithfully mirrored the clinical situation of advanced, disseminated cancer.[68] In one animal model, they investigated the effects of LAK cells on pulmonary metastases in mice induced by an intravenous injection of tumor cells. Three days later (in some experiments, 10 days later) tumor-inoculated mice received an intravenous injection of LAK cells, and these animals were compared with untreated controls.[69] In another model, hepatic metastases were induced in mice by direct injection of malignant cells to the liver; three days later tumor-carrying mice were treated by an intravenous injection of LAK cells.[70] LAK therapy led to the disappearance of established micrometastases of tumors in both animal models, but only in mice injected with very elevated concentrations of LAK cells. Rosenberg and his collaborators had found that the percentage of LAK-cell-induced cures increased if mice received intravenous injections of IL-2 together with the LAK cells.[71] However, in this case too, improvement in the therapeutic performance of LAK cells could be demonstrated only in animals receiving high doses of IL-2, a very different outcome from the one expected from the presumed physiological concentrations of this molecule.[72]

In articles reviewing the development of LAK therapy Rosenberg first described the destruction of malignant cells by LAK cells in the test tube, then the elimination of experimentally induced tumor metastases in mice by LAK transfusion and by the combination of LAK and IL-2, and finally the first experiments in humans.[73] The narrative sequence conveys the impression that the studies followed the orderly, "classical" path from the test tube, through experiments in laboratory animals, to experiments on humans. The chronology of publications of Rosenberg's laboratory, however, conveys the impression that things happened in a great hurry. Rosenberg and his collaborators simultaneously pursued studies in the test tube, experiments with animals, and preliminary clinical investigations in humans. All these studies seem to have been driven by the practical goal to rapidly develop an efficient adoptive immunotherapy of human cancer and by a strong belief in the feasibility of such therapy. The roots of that conviction may be found in an early observation, repeated frequently in Rosenberg's articles, that when peripheral blood lymphocytes of a cancer patient were activated by IL-2 they sometimes acquired the capacity to kill the cells of that patient's tumor.[74] The belief in the feasibility of adoptive cancer immunotherapy was probably also stimulated by the knowledge that enough recombinant IL-2 would be available for human experimentation, thanks to the collaboration (begun in 1982) between Rosenberg's laboratory and Cetus.[75] Indeed, it is possible to reconstruct Rosenberg's shift to LAK cell experiments in the early 1980s as the result of two events: the (unanticipated) finding that in the test tube IL-2 induced the transformation of normal lymphocytes into tumor-killing cells, and the establishment of close collaboration between Rosenberg's laboratory and Cetus. Cetus was one of the oldest (founded in 1971) and richest biotechnology companies. In 1982, however, it was in financial difficulty because the Chevron Corporation had retired from a joint project for fructose production. Cetus thereupon shifted its main commercial orientation from bulk chemicals to low-volume, high-value products in a bid for rapid profits.[76] The combination of strong faith in the antitumor efficacy of IL-2 activated cells, access to a nearly unlimited supply of IL-2, and pressure to obtain exploitable clinical results may also have guided Rosenberg's rapid switch to the use of high, nonphysiological (and thus potentially toxic) doses of IL-2 in his attempts to cure cancer first in mice, then in humans. This switch was also in conformity with the culture of clinical experimentation in oncology, strongly present at the NIH.[77]

The first experiments in humans started in 1983. The researchers observed the effects of IL-2 in cancer patients and AIDS patients suffering from Kaposi's sarcoma.[78] The purpose of these experiments was to rapidly obtain preliminary information on the physiological effects of IL-2 and to compare the biological effects of cell-secreted IL-2 with those of recombinant IL-2 (IL-2 produced by genetic engineering techniques). The similarity of the biological effects obtained with both types of IL-2 legitimated the claim that recombinant interleukin-2 had the same physiological and, by inference, therapeutic properties as the cell-secreted molecule.[79] In these experiments the injection of IL-2 into patients suffering from advanced cancer did not modify their clinical status. However, in the first series of experiments the patients received similar doses of either cell-produced or recombinant IL-2, and the scarcity of the cell-produced substance fixed the upper limit of the tested doses. A second series of experiments attempted to establish the maximum-tolerated dose of recombinant IL-2. It was found that high concentrations of IL-2 provoked fever, chills, malaise, intestinal symptoms, muscle and bone pain, and, finally, "capillary leak syndrome"— the escape of water from small blood vessels, which induces weight gain, edema, and sometimes severe respiratory and circulatory complications.[80] This last side effect was unexpected; capillary leak syndrome had not been observed in mice. But the disappointing results of the first series of clinical trials (involving 32 patients) and the observation that IL-2 had significant toxicity in humans did not delay the beginning of the second stage of the study: therapy with LAK cells and high concentrations of IL-2. That stage was guided by the assumption, derived by Rosenberg from animal experiments but also from his activist therapeutic philosophy and his experience with chemotherapy of malignant tumors, that the clinical efficacy of the new therapy would be directly proportional to the dose of IL-2/LAK used.

Clinical trials of combined IL-2/LAK therapy using the highest tolerated dose of IL-2 together with LAK cells had started in the early spring of 1985. Rosenberg later described the way he "pushed" his patients to the upper limits of their physical tolerance, and sometimes even to the brink of death from cardiac and respiratory problems.[81] This "heroic" approach was successful. In the spring of 1985 Rosenberg and his colleagues witnessed first a spectacular, partial regression of pulmonary metastases in a melanoma patient, and then a "true miracle": the complete (and stable) regression of subcutaneous nodules in another melanoma patient.[82]

In the summer of 1985 there was a widespread rumor among oncologists that Rosenberg had developed a new therapy for previously incurable advanced solid tumors. In October 1985 Rosenberg received the General Motors Cancer Research Award. The new cancer treatment was discussed in the November 1985 issue of *Fortune* magazine, and the news did not fail to have a favorable effect on the shares of biotechnology firms involved in cloning and producing IL-2 for clinical use.[83] In December 1985 an article describing the first results of the new therapy was published in the prestigious *New England Journal of Medicine,*[84] and the NCI officially announced the discovery of a new cancer biotherapy. Magazines ran cover stories about the new cancer cure, and television programs announced the first results of the LAK cell therapy experiments. The *Wall Street Journal* strongly recommended bypassing the usual FDA approval process for new drugs in order to speed up patients' access to promising therapies such as IL-2/LAK, and NCI director Dr. Vincent de Vita Jr. affirmed that the new treatment "is the most interesting and exciting biological therapy we've seen so far."[85]

The new treatment looked very promising indeed. The tumors of 11 of the 25 patients suffering from advanced, incurable cancer shrank by 50 percent or more following IL-2/LAK therapy. The new treatment induced severe toxicity and in many cases required close monitoring of patients in an intensive care unit. However, Rosenberg asserted, all toxic effects of the new therapy disappeared when IL-2 administration was discontinued.[86] Rosenberg and his collaborators ended their article with a warning about the dangers of premature conclusions and stressed that their study had involved a small number of patients who were followed for only a short time (eight months). Nevertheless, the impression conveyed by the first publication of the therapeutic effects of LAK was one of an important breakthrough in cancer treatment.

IL-2 and LAK Cells in the Clinics

Rosenberg's 1985 article led to a rapid diffusion of clinical trials of IL-2/LAK in the United States and elsewhere. An American philanthropist, Armand Hammer, donated $150,000 to the NCI for further research on the therapy, and the NCI allocated $2.5 million for six confirmatory extramural studies.[87] In addition, a clinical trial of IL-2/LAK therapy was initiated in 1985 by physicians associated with Biotherapeutic Inc., a private institute dedicated to patient-funded experimental cancer therapies.[88] Biotherapeutic Inc. was founded in 1983 by Robert Oldham, the former head of the NCI's BRM Program. In 1985 Oldham made an agreement with Cetus to employ recombinant IL-2 in cancer therapy.[89] In its publicity brochures Biotherapeutic described the advantages of individualized cancer therapy.[90] In fact Biotherapeutic clients received standardized IL-2/LAK treatment, similar in many respects to that given to Rosenberg's patients at the NCI. The most important innovation was that Biotherapeutic patients received constant intravenous infusion of IL-2 instead of bolus (single-dose) injections as in the NCI clinical trial. Biotherapeutic researchers claimed that this method of administration reduced the side effects of IL-2 therapy and enhanced its safety without limiting its effectiveness: 15 of 40 patients responded to this treatment.[91]

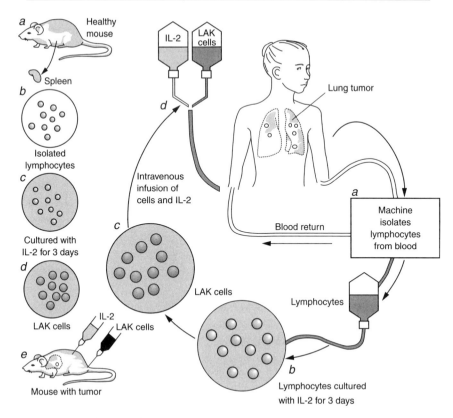

Production of LAK cells begins with removal of spleen from healthy mice (*a*, left). Lymphocytes are isolated *(b)* and cultured with IL-2 *(c)*. IL-2 causes null cells to turn into LAK cells *(d)*. LAK cells are injected into mice with tumors *(e)*. Finally, lymphocytes are isolated from the bloodstream of human subjects (*a*, right) and cultured with IL-2 *(b)* to generate human LAK cells *(c)*. Patients are infused intravenously with a dose of 50 billion LAK cells combined with IL-2 *(d)*. (Adapted from Steven A. Rosenberg, "Adoptive immunotherapy for cancer," *Scientific American*, May 1990, p. 36.)

The encouraging news about a way to limit toxic effects was moderated by the finding that early evaluations of IL-2/LAK treatment had been too optimistic. In 1986 a study by Rosenberg's group indicated that high doses of IL-2 alone might have antitumor effects.[92] But the rate of therapeutic success obtained either with or without LAK cells was significantly lower than the one reported in the 1985 article. In a commentary on the 1986 study, Dr. Charles Mortel of the Mayo Clinic noted the high costs, severe side effects, and limited clinical results of the new therapy; most of the tumor regressions attributed to it had been partial and transitory.[93] Intermediate reports on the six extramural clinical trials of IL-2/LAK therapy also indicated reduced efficacy.[94] These findings were particularly disappointing because the new clinical trials were centered exclusively on "responsive" tumors: melanoma and renal cell carcinoma. However, IL-2/LAK treatment did show undeniable effects on otherwise untreatable cancers. The new therapy also seemed to promise still more developments at the cutting edge of biomedical research. That aura of promise also supported its diffusion outside the United States.

Numerous additional clinical trials of IL-2/LAK therapy in the years 1987–1990 failed to lead to important new developments. The new trials merely confirmed the early trends: IL-2 therapy was toxic and expensive, but for 15 to 25 percent of patients suffering from melanoma and renal cell carcinoma, the total volume of their tumors was reduced by 40 percent or more. Among these cases there were a few "miracles"—that is, long-term regressions of otherwise untreatable malignancies.[95] In the years 1984–1989, 652 patients were included in the NCI clinical trials. The IL-2/LAK therapy induced regressions in 35 percent of the renal cell carcinoma cases and in 21 percent of melanoma cases, while IL-2 treatment alone induced a slightly lower percentage of regressions in renal cell carcinoma (22 percent) and a similar rate of response (24 percent) in melanoma. Among patients who achieved complete regressions (18 of 652), 14 had one lasting more than a year.[96] Comparable results were found in collaborative extramural studies of the therapeutic effects of IL-2, although in these studies the percentage of persistent complete regressions ("miracles") was usually lower than that reported by Rosenberg's group. Patients treated with IL-2 suffered from (usually reversible) severe toxic side effects. Besides fever, gastrointestinal perturbations, and the capillary leak syndrome, interleukin therapy could induce severe, sometimes fatal, cardiac or pulmonary toxicity, often linked to massive infection.[97] An important proportion (between one-third and one-half) of patients also suffered from serious neuropsychiatric perturbations during IL-2 therapy. These perturbations were attributed to physiological effects such as capillary leak syndrome, edema, impaired blood circulation, and nonspecific liberation of chemical substances by IL-2-stimulated white blood cells.[98]

The results of IL-2/LAK treatment may recall those obtained with interferon on a small number of "responsive" tumors. There was, however, an important difference: IL-2 therapy had a much stronger legitimation through immunological theories. Interferon had all along been viewed as a molecule with a wide range of physiological effects, whereas interleukin-2 was perceived above all (for some specialists, exclusively) as a substance implicated in the regulation of immune responses. The therapeutic effects of IL-2 in human cancer could therefore be interpreted (and were so interpreted by some specialists) as a vindication of the claim that cancer could be cured through immunological methods. The affirmation that interleukin therapy was an immunotherapy of cancer was translated, in selected institutions, into active participation by immunologists in clinical trials of IL-2, a participation that gave them access to the domain of experimental therapies of cancer.

Not all the experts agreed, however, that IL-2 was indeed an immunotherapy for malignancies. In 1987 an editorial by Dr. J. R. Durant in the *New England Journal of Medicine* explained that a true immunotherapy should modify the host's immune response. By that criterion, both interferon therapy (whose effect could be likened to the effect of hormones on hormonally responsive tumors) and monoclonal antibodies directed against specific tumor cells were not true immunotherapies. As for IL-2/LAK therapy, "the core of the issue is whether the reports show that cells in the human immune system can be manipulated to restore or enhance a normal function." Durant asserted that such indeed was the case and that IL-2 treatment was "the end of the beginning" of cancer immunotherapy. That evaluation was, however, dependent on proof that LAK cells were essential to the antitumor effects of IL-2. If they were, then "the results become the basis for a whole series of important biologic questions."[99]

Around 1989, reviews of the cumulative results of clinical trials of IL-2/LAK noted a lack of important differences between results obtained with and without the addition of LAK cells activated in the test tube.[100] Moreover, no significant correlation was found between the level of "LAK activity" in the blood of IL-2-treated patients and their clinical response to interleukin therapy.[101] In the meantime the meaning of the term "LAK cells" underwent important changes. Clinicians continued to employ the term to describe white blood cells incubated with IL-2 in the test tube, then injected into the patient. Cellular immunologists, however, had agreed that the LAK cells were not a distinct subpopulation of lymphocytes; rather, "LAK activity" was generated by a mixture of at least two subpopulations of cytotoxic cells:

the NK cells (usually the major component of "LAK activity") and the cytotoxic T cells.[102] The disappearance of LAK as a distinct nosologic entity did not by itself invalidate the claim that interleukin-activated lymphocytes played a key role in the regression of tumors in IL-2 treated patients. However, oncologists repeatedly failed to find significant correlations between the stimulation of well-defined subpopulations of cytotoxic cells (NK cells, cytotoxic T cells, cells endowed with "LAK activity") and the clinical results of IL-2 therapy. During the 1980s the term "LAK cells" at first described a new classificatory unit: a previously unknown subpopulation of lymphocytes. Later the same term defined a new function: IL-2-activated subpopulations of cytotoxic lymphocytes. Finally, it described a population of IL-2-activated white blood cells that were able to kill selected lines of malignant cells in the test tube and had unknown (if any) antitumor effect(s) in the body.

Many oncologists were relieved to find that LAK cells were not indispensable for IL-2 therapy. The necessity to separate, activate, then inject these cells increased the costs of an already expensive therapy and made it more labor-intensive. But the growing conviction that LAK cells were not an essential element in IL-2 antitumor activity did not lead to the conclusion advocated by Durant in his 1987 editorial, namely that IL-2 treatment, if not found to be LAK cell-dependent, could not be viewed as a "true" immune therapy of malignant tumors. Promoters of cancer immunotherapy continued to argue that the therapeutic effects of IL-2 proved that cancer immunotherapy was possible.[103] Some studies simply ignored the repeated failure to find correlations between the activation of subpopulations of cytotoxic lymphocytes and clinical results of interleukin therapy;[104] others attempted to explain the lack of correlation by postulating a migration of activated LAK cells to the tumor site (if such migration took place, the increase in efficient LAK activity would be undetectable when one measured LAK activity in circulating blood);[105] and some proposed that non-LAK-dependent immunological mechanisms (such as IL-2-dependent stimulation of secretion of other cytokines, or the stimulation by IL-2 of the expression of MHC antigens on tumor cells) might account for the antitumor effects of IL-2.[106] But although the new proposals asserted an immunological framework for explaining the antitumor activity of IL-2, the claims remained hypothetical. Elevated doses of IL-2, like elevated doses of interferon, induced numerous physiological reactions, classified by physicians as side effects of interleukin treatment. It was difficult to exclude the hypothesis that some of these physiological effects played a direct or indirect role in the reduction of the volume of malignant tumors.[107] Understanding of the hypothetical mechanism(s) of the antitumor effects of interleukin was succinctly summed up in 1989 by a pioneer of IL-2 studies and one of the leading specialists in the domain, Dr. Kendall Smith: "we still do not know which biochemical pathways the interleukins activate."[108]

IL-2 after LAK Cells: Tradition and Innovation

When clinical tests of IL-2 and LAK failed to lead to important clinical or indisputable scientific achievements, new directions in study and clinical experimentation were necessary in order to sustain the significant investments of researchers, clinicians, and the biotechnology industry in IL-2 as an anticancer drug. Such new directions were developed in the late 1980s. Steven Rosenberg's laboratory again led the way with innovative approaches to adoptive cancer immunotherapy. These approaches, like Rosenberg's earlier studies, combined faith in the future of cancer immunotherapy, rapid integration of the newest methods in biological research, and a predilection for bold and aggressive clinical experimentation. Rosenberg sought to accelerate the transfer of innovations from bench to bedside and to seek rapid clinical applications for new, spectacular developments in the research laboratory.[109]

Rosenberg's new efforts were at first guided by his long-standing aspiration to develop an adoptive cancer immunotherapy. Having speculated that LAK cells were not very efficient in the organism because they were not sufficiently tumor-specific, he had returned to his original idea of using IL-2 merely as a technical device to promote the proliferation of specific subpopulations of cytotoxic lymphocytes in the test tube. Dr. C. Da Fano had observed as early as 1912 that tumors are often infiltrated by lymphocytes.[110] Rosenberg and his collaborators assumed that the lymphocytes that spontaneously entered a malignant growth—which they named tumor-infiltrating lymphocytes (TILs)—probably contained a significant proportion of specific cytotoxic cells directed against the tumor. TILs were a heterogeneous population composed mainly of cytotoxic T lymphocytes. Rosenberg and his collaborators started to study TILs in 1980.[111] The observation that IL-2-activated peripheral blood lymphocytes (a cell population much easier to obtain than TILs) might develop nonspecific antitumor activity when cultured in the presence of IL-2 led them to shift their attention to LAK cells. But the low clinical efficacy of LAK cells brought them back to the idea of expanding selected populations of tumor-infiltrating lymphocytes in the test tube, then reinjecting these cells into patients.

In 1986 Rosenberg's group developed a method to isolate the lymphocytes that infiltrate human melanoma.[112] At the same time, they tested the antitumor activity of TILs in mice, in experimental models similar to those employed in the study of the antitumor effects of LAK cells. In the animal models, TILs were found to be up to 100 times more efficient than LAK cells.[113] Rosenberg's group also affirmed that the antitumor effects of TILs could be observed in mice even in the absence of IL-2 and were optimized by the addition of much lower doses of IL-2 than had been required for optimal activation of LAK cells. Rosenberg asserted that the low requirement for additional IL-2 during TIL therapy could substantially reduce the side effects of adoptive immunotherapy of cancer. The main drawback of the new method was the difficulty of preparing TILs. These cells were cultivated from surgically excised tumors incubated in the presence of IL-2. The tumor cells gradually died in culture, while the tumor-infiltrating lymphocytes multiplied in the presence of interleukin. The number of TILs obtained by this method was, however, small. A costly and labor-intensive long-term culture (in human tumors, six to eight weeks, and sometimes even more) was necessary to obtain enough cells for an adoptive immunotherapy.[114] Nevertheless, the method seemed promising enough to start experiments in humans.

The first series of patients treated with TILs at the NCI was composed solely of melanoma patients because TILs were particularly abundant in melanoma and it was easy to excise subcutaneous nodules of that tumor. The patients received their own TILs, an injection of the drug cyclophosphamide (which Rosenberg and his collaborators claimed potentiated the effects of TILs in mice), and the maximum-tolerated dose of IL-2. The IL-2 injection induced the same undesirable effects as standard IL-2/LAK therapy, but these effects were usually less severe because the TIL treatment was shorter. Among the first 20 patients, 9 of the 15 who had not been treated previously with IL-2 and LAK responded to the therapy, while 2 of 5 patients who had not responded to previous therapy with IL-2 responded to the new regimen. These impressive results were moderated by the observation that only one patient had a complete remission and remained disease-free after 13 months, while other remissions were partial and lasted 2 to 9 months.[115] The results of TIL therapy were thus not very different from those initially observed with IL-2/LAK therapy: an elevated percentage of responses, most of which were partial and short-lived. Other investigators confirmed that selected melanoma and renal carcinoma patients responded to TILs. No responses were observed in other solid tumors.[116]

Researchers in the Rosenberg group devised two approaches to improve the results of TIL therapy: the combination of TIL treatment with other biological response modifiers, and the genetic manipulation of TILs. The first approach was a continuation of previous studies; the second was an attempt to radically redirect adoptive immunotherapies of cancer. The first approach entered early clinical stages around 1991. TILs were injected together with other substances modulating the growth and the function of lymphocytes, such as interleukin-4, interleukin-6, interferon, and antibodies against beta transforming growth factor (beta TGF, a molecule that regulates cell proliferation). Another variant of that approach was an attempt to generate more efficient TILs in the test tube through selective culture of tumor-specific clones of cytotoxic T cells in the presence of different growth factors. The cytokines, monoclonal antibodies, and other biological reactives used in these experiments were provided by several biotechnology firms: Cetus, Genentech, Biogen, Genetic Institute, and Sterling Pharmaceutical.[117] The limited clinical success of LAK and of TIL therapies, far from restricting relations between Rosenberg's group and the biotechnology industry, had broadened and expanded them beyond the initial bilateral collaboration between Rosenberg and Cetus.

The second approach tested by Rosenberg's group—genetic modification of TILs—accentuated even more the connections between immunotherapies of cancer and biotechnologies. This approach was based on the idea that the selection of highly efficient TILs through prolonged culture of tumor-infiltrating cells was so difficult and labor-intensive that it would be easier to achieve the same goal by genetically manipulating TILs. The researchers sought to create "super-TILs" by inserting into "normal" TILs genes that would greatly increase their tumor-killing efficacy (for example, genes that code for cytotoxic molecules, such as tumor necrotic factor).[118] The first phase of the new project aimed at verifying the feasibility of this undertaking. Neutral markers (bacterial genes resistant to neomycin) were inserted into TILs. The modified TILs were then injected into patients together with IL-2, and the investigators followed their fate in the body thanks to the presence of the specific marker. Five melanoma patients received the genetically modified TILs. The modified cells were found in the blood up to two months after their administration and were also recovered from tumor deposits. No undesirable effects were observed besides those attributed to the IL-2 therapy. Three of five patients responded to the TIL treatment, one with a complete and two with partial tumor regression.[119]

The injection of modified TILs, the authors of this study contended, proved the feasibility of the genetic modification of lymphocytes and, in addition, demonstrated that at least some of the TILs migrated to the tumor site and might stay there up to two months. Rosenberg at first presented the new project as a continuation of his efforts to develop more efficient cytotoxic cells. It is difficult, however, to view that study merely as an unproblematic extension of earlier attempts at adoptive cancer immunotherapy. Indeed, Rosenberg and other commentators also stressed the potential importance of genetically modified lymphocytes in the therapy of genetic diseases.[120] The project oscillated between the relatively modest goal of searching for a better adoptive immunotherapy of cancer and the more ambitious aim of changing human heredity.[121]

While Rosenberg and his collaborators took IL-2 treatment as a starting point for innovative therapeutic approaches, other researchers attempted to improve the therapy by more traditional means. Physicians attempted to simplify the new method by reducing the dose of IL-2 administered to patients, thus allowing administration of the therapy in an outpatient setting.[122] The reported results of "low-dose" therapy were not very different from those reported with the maximum-tolerated dose.[123] These results were usually obtained in small series of patients and were viewed with skepticism by some of the main promoters of interleukin therapy, who continued to assert that the best clinical results were obtained with the highest tolerated doses of IL-2.[124]

Another approach, favored by many medical oncologists, was a combination of interleukin therapy with chemotherapy. Most of these attempts were made in cases of melanoma. Several clinical trials combined IL-2 with the standard chemotherapeutic agents for melanoma, such as dacarbazine, cisplatine, or flavone acetic acid. As of the early

1990s, such combined therapy had not been found to be significantly superior to single-agent therapies.[125] Other trials experimented with the sequential combination of several treatments: chemotherapy, interleukin-2, and other cytokines.[126] Some oncologists believed that interleukin therapy—probably combined with other therapies— would be more efficient if applied to earlier stages of cancer and not exclusively to advanced, disseminated disease.[127] The methods employed in "post-LAK" clinical trials of IL-2 therapy closely recall clinical trials of cancer chemotherapies: modulation of doses and administration methods of the active substance, attempts to find the "winning combination" of drugs, a search for the best timing for the treatment. This resemblance is not surprising. Interleukin-2 was "naturalized" by clinical oncologists, who integrated the new molecule into their routine therapeutic approaches and their "native culture" of experimentation in the clinics. A parallel effort at "naturalizing" IL-2 was undertaken by pharmaceutical firms. In the mid- and late 1980s many small biotechnology firms disappeared, and the bulk of production of recombinant biological response modifiers shifted to larger, well-established pharmaceutical firms.[128] These firms applied traditional pharmacological research strategies to substances produced through genetic engineering. The "naturalization" of IL-2 by pharmaceutical companies led to attempts at chemical manipulation of the IL-2 molecule in order to obtain less toxic and/or more effective substances and to efforts to develop more efficient ways to deliver the molecule to target cells.[129]

In the early 1990s clinicians and pharmaceutical firms continued their search for more efficient ways to employ interleukins in cancer therapy. Oncologists favored the combination of cytokines and monoclonal antibodies (the most promising combination seemed to be IL-2 with anti-CD3 monoclonal antibodies), combinations of cytokines (alpha interferon with alpha TNF and IL-2 with IL-4 were seen as potentially efficient combinations), and trials of other interleukins (beta interferon, IL-6, IL-7), while pharmaceutical firms attempted to produce combined molecules composed of parts of several cytokines, or cytokines combined with cytotoxic agents such as the exotoxin (a protein) of the bacterium *Pseudomonas*. These attempts, however, were seldom viewed as offering the promise of an imminent "therapeutic revolution" in oncology. Cytokines had not fulfilled the predictions of preclinical studies (the one notable exception was interferon therapy for hairy cell leukemia). This failure was attributed to overly optimistic interpretations of animal and tissue culture data, inappropriate methods of administration, and unexpected severe toxicities.[130] A 1992 review of cancer immunotherapy concluded that "dramatic improvements . . . cannot be expected without conceptual and technical innovations." Therapeutic uses of activated white blood cells, including TILs and genetically engineered TILs, remained problematic because of high cost, complexity, and low efficacy. Other protocols, though found to be moderately effective in patients with certain types of cancer, were unreproducible. But the main problem was the lack of predictive criteria that could ensure preselection of responsive patients, along with a growing conviction that such trials should be made in patients with a low tumor load. Imposing demanding experimental immunotherapy regimens on patients with a low tumor load, however, was considered hard to justify, because "they can be a burden on patients and clinicians alike."[131] The outlook for cancer immunotherapy in the early 1990s still seemed uncertain.

IL-2 and the Biotechnology Industry: The Cetus Story

Although several biotechnology companies were involved in the initial cloning and first clinical trials of IL-2 in the years 1982–1984, one firm, Cetus, became strongly identified with IL-2 cancer therapy. The alliance of Cetus with Rosenberg's group at NIH played a key role in the rapid development and diffusion of IL-2-based therapies. The widely publicized success of the first clinical trials of IL-2 in 1985 immediately increased the value of Cetus shares and boosted the company's financial standing.[132] From 1985 on Cetus maintained a privileged position as the main producer of IL-2 for highly visible clinical trials. Other biotechnology companies (Biogen, Amgen) had difficulties conducting clinical trials of IL-2 and gradually limited their investment in the molecule.[133]

In the years 1985–1990 Cetus' commercial strategy was centered on the promotion of IL-2. Although Cetus did develop other products such as monoclonal diagnostic kits and polymerase chain reaction (PCR), a technology that allows the amplification, then analysis of small segments of DNA, Cetus' directors saw IL-2 as the firm's main commercial asset.[134] The concern's financial viability was closely dependent on the fate of the IL-2 clinical trials. The initial collaboration with Rosenberg's group at the NIH firmly established Cetus as the leader in IL-2 production. Later, however, the interests of Rosenberg

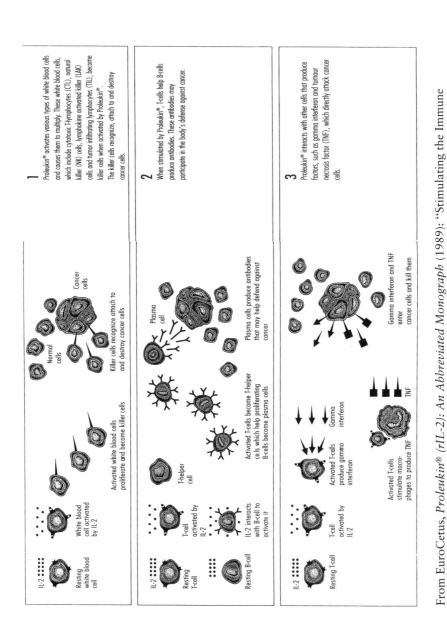

1

Proleukin® activates various types of white blood cells and causes them to multiply. These white blood cells, which include cytotoxic T-lymphocytes (CTL), natural killer (NK) cells, lymphokine activated killer (LAK) cells and tumor infiltrating lymphocytes (TIL), become killer cells when activated by Proleukin®.

The killer cells recognize, attach to and destroy cancer cells.

2

When stimulated by Proleukin®, T-cells help B-cells produce antibodies. These antibodies may participate in the body's defense against cancer.

3

Proleukin® interacts with other cells that produce factors, such as gamma interferon and tumour necrosis factor (TNF), which directly attack cancer cells.

Panel 1 labels: IL-2 · Resting white blood cell · White blood cell activated by IL-2 · Activated white blood cells proliferate and become killer cells · Normal cells · Cancer cells · Killer cells recognize attach to and destroy cancer cells

Panel 2 labels: IL-2 · Resting T-cell · T-cell activated by IL-2 · Resting B-cell · IL-2 interacts with B-cell to activate it · T-helper cell · Activated T-cells become T-helper cells which help proliferating B-cells become plasma cells · Plasma cell · Plasma cells produce antibodies that may help defend against cancer

Panel 3 labels: IL-2 · Resting T-cell · T-cell activated by IL-2 · Activated T-cells produce gamma interferon · Activated T-cells stimulate macrophages to produce TNF · Gamma interferon · TNF · Gamma interferon and TNF enter cancer cells and kill them

From EuroCetus, *Proleukin*® *(rIL-2): An Abbreviated Monograph* (1989): "Stimulating the Immune System: Proleukin (rIL-2) Fights Cancer in Three Important Ways." (Courtesy Chiron France/Cetus Corporation.)

and Cetus partially diverged. Rosenberg and his colleagues were interested in the propagation of their therapeutic method, whereas Cetus was interested in selling its product, not in the promotion of specific uses. Indeed, the high cost of cell preparation (first the selective separation of patients' white blood cells, followed by activation in the test tube for long-term culture of lymphocytes) could be viewed as an obstacle to the rapid diffusion of IL-2 treatment. Cetus thus encouraged clinical trials of IL-2 alone, or of IL-2 combined with other cytokines (in particular beta interferon, another molecule produced by the company). Beginning in 1986 the Amsterdam-based European branch of Cetus, EuroCetus, became very active in promoting clinical trials of IL-2 in Western Europe.

From 1987 on Cetus centered its efforts on rapid procurement of a marketing permit for IL-2 for the therapy of renal cell carcinoma, a malignancy for which (unlike melanoma) there is no known drug treatment.[135] Because marketing authorization procedures tend to be less stringent in Europe than in the United States, Cetus strongly encouraged the development of clinical trials of IL-2 in Europe.[136] Italy was the first country to approve the marketing of IL-2, in April 1988; nine other European countries followed suit in 1989 (the United Kingdom alone refused a permit). In France EuroCetus competed with the local biotechnology industry, which was supported by the French Research and Technology Ministry. From 1984 on the ministry subsidized a project by major French pharmaceutical firms to produce recombinant interleukin-2, a project that culminated in the first clinical trials of "French" IL-2 in 1988.[137] Cetus nevertheless obtained a marketing permit in France in 1989. Cetus also applied to the Committee for Proprietary Medicinal Products of the European Economic Community (EEC) for fast-track "high technology/biotechnology" approval to market IL-2. Approval was granted in May 1989, although it was restricted to therapy of renal cell carcinoma.[138] Cetus' hopes for the commercial success of IL-2, thus boosted by the EEC's decision, were shattered in June 1990, when an FDA advisory committee refused permission to market IL-2 in the United States. The FDA based its decision on a confusing array of clinical data. Roughly half of these were derived from studies that included LAK, which in the FDA's view failed to demonstrate the clinical efficacy of IL-2 alone in the treatment of renal cell carcinoma. Moreover, the FDA pointed out that the new therapy had not been significantly improved over time: the best results of IL-2 treatment of renal cell carcinoma had been obtained in the early clinical trials made by Rosenberg's group, and later trials had failed to surpass them. The FDA was also troubled by the unfavorable fatal toxicity/complete response ratio of IL-2 therapy: in the data supplied by Cetus, the percentage of both was about 4 percent.[139]

As a result of the FDA's decision to postpone the marketing permit and to maintain IL-2's status as an experimental drug, Cetus stock immediately plummeted, and the company's revenue projection was cut.[140] The decision also significantly weakened European support for the drug. Even before the FDA's criticism, Germany and Denmark had quietly withdrawn unconditional support for IL-2 and made it available for clinical trials only. Some observers believed that the EEC's initial approval of IL-2 had been influenced by national interests. They pointed out that EuroCetus president Filippo La Monica benefited from important political support in Italy, the country selected to prepare the report on IL-2. Cetus' products were also supported by the Netherlands, which had actively encouraged the location of Euro-Cetus headquarters in Amsterdam.[141] The FDA decision called attention to weaknesses in the European procedure for approval of IL-2. The European marketing permit was not revoked, but in several countries clinical use of IL-2 was restricted de facto to experimental or semiexperimental applications.

Difficulties in the process of introducing a new therapy are not unusual, and they do not necessarily determine the long-term commercial fate of that therapy.[142] However, unlike big pharmaceutical companies, which develop a large number of products simultaneously and are thus cushioned against such setbacks, Cetus bet on the short-term success of IL-2, and the firm was unable to survive financially the unforeseen delays in commercialization and the loss of confidence on Wall Street. In July 1991 an agreement between the biotechnology firm Chiron and Cetus put an end to the independence of the latter and highlighted the failure of its IL-2-based commercial strategy. Chiron paid Cetus' debts, while Cetus agreed to sell its most promising product, the PCR technology, to Hoffman–La Roche in order to mobilize capital for the new firm.[143] The firm's former director, Robert Fields, defended his company's earlier decision to focus its efforts on the promotion of a single product; such a policy, he asserted, had worked well for other biotechnology products, such as erythropoietin and interferon. The problem was that "no one knew in the early 1980s what any of these products would do."[144]

Interleukin-2 as a Mass-Mediated Treatment

The commercial fate of Cetus was determined by the usual economic variables: the firm's ability to mobilize capital, to avoid excessive debt, to exploit technological and commercial opportunities, and to survive market fluctuations. But it was also influenced by the public image of its product. Both the sharp drop in the value of Cetus stock (from $16 to $10 a share) the day after the FDA's decision to delay IL-2's marketing permit, and the previous sharp rise in the value of Cetus stock following the publication of the results of the first IL-2 clinical trial in December 1985 point to the importance of a company's reputation and public image for commercial strategies in the biotechnology industry.[145] At first interleukin-2 had a very positive public image. It was represented as the latest achievement of "high-tech medicine" and, at the same time, as a "natural substance" able to boost the "defenses of the body." It also benefited from the publicity given to "miracle cures" for cancer. Cetus employed all these elements in its campaign to promote IL-2. Its brochures featured photographs of huge fermenters and sophisticated scientific instruments, but also of flowers and landscapes at sunset. Johnny Noriega's story, which opens Cetus' 1988 Annual Report, sums up the "high-tech miracle" image promoted by the advocates of interleukin-2 therapy. It is worth quoting *in extenso:*

> It started with a persistent cough. Two weeks later Johnny Noriega entered the hospital for testing. On May 7, 1986, he was diagnosed with metastatic renal cell carcinoma (advanced kidney cancer). He had six areas of tumor spread in his right lung, and the prognosis for survival beyond six months was very poor. Johnny's doctors quickly referred him to an investigational program at the University of Texas Health Sciences Center in which cancer patients were receiving Cetus Proleukin (TM) interleukin-2 (IL-2). Some of these patients with the same disease as Johnny had responded well to this therapy. But disappointment followed when Johnny and his family learned that the clinical trials were full, and no additional patients were currently being admitted. Unwilling to accept such a fate, Johnny's family and friends rallied to his side. Relying on their strong faith, they organized a "Miracle Run" from San Antonio to the border town of San Juan. Their mission was to reach the Church in the Valley to pray for a miracle for Johnny. The Noriega family believes that a miracle occurred when they were notified two weeks later that there was a place for Johnny in the clinical program after

all. Under the direction of Dr. Charles Coltman and Dr. Geoffrey Weiss, Johnny was first treated with Proleukin IL-2 in August 1986. Six weeks later four of his tumors were completely gone and two others had shrunk. The following December, he underwent another course of Proleukin IL-2 therapy, and six weeks after that his doctors pronounced him free of cancer. In March 1987 Johnny returned to his job as a bus driver and remains in complete remission more than three years later. Unfortunately not every case of advanced kidney cancer ends as happily as Johnny's ... But patients like Johnny give us reason to hope. They inspire us to press even harder toward our mission of finding solutions for the devastation of cancer.[146]

The combination of high technology and miracles appeared frequently in media presentations of IL-2. Discussing interleukin therapy, journalists repeatedly employed an image of the body fighting a malignant tumor. The strength of this image derived from the assumption—implicit in popular representations of the new therapy—that demonstrating the existence of immune mechanisms able to destroy cancer cells in a test tube is identical with demonstrating its efficacy in cancer patients.[147] For example, in 1991 the Cancer Research Institute of New York produced a television ad for its fundraising campaign for research in tumor immunology and immunotherapy. As its promoters explained, this ad aimed at "exciting the public imagination." It showed "something most people will never have seen or even imagined was possible: the destruction of a human cancer cell by a human immune cell. This depiction is proof positive of the powerful cancer-fighting potential of the human immune system, and it underlines the appropriateness of our mission and the need for ever-greater support for the field of cancer immunology."[148]

Highly suggestive electronmicroscope photographs showing cancer cells "attacked" by "killer lymphocytes" became a standard feature of articles intended for the general public which described cancer immunotherapies. They promoted the image of the body destroying "deviant cells," an image that not only represented a possible cure for a concrete physical illness but also evoked the symbolic meaning of cancer as deviation.[149] The forceful image of the organism eliminating the malignancy—in both the physical and the metaphorical sense—was also promoted through the choice of certain words. In an article on the adoptive therapy of cancer published in *Scientific American,* Steven Rosenberg characterized IL-2 treatment as "the first demonstration that a therapy aimed at strengthening the activity of patients' own

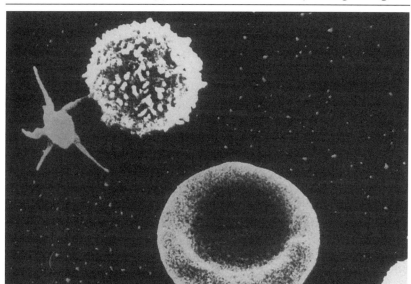

From *Le Figaro,* May 5, 1990: "Armed thanks to interleukin-2: These lymphocytes (a category of white blood cells) became more efficient against tumor cells
thanks to potentiation with interleukin-2. Lymphocytes, as well as other categories of white blood cells, red blood cells, and platelets, are found in the bloodstream." (Photo by Jean Claude Révy; courtesy of *Le Figaro Magazine.*)

lymphocytes could induce cancer regression."[150] The image of the
body fighting deviant cells was reinforced in the nonspecialized press.
A 1989 article in *Le Nouvel Observateur* affirmed that "it is definitively proven that the human organism contains all the necessary resources to rid itself of malignant cells," adding that IL-2 therapy was
"an amazing confirmation of theoretical studies."[151] In 1990 *Le Figaro
Magazine* published a lavishly illustrated article with the headline: "A
photographic feat! The wonderful adventure of interleukin. The cancer fought by the organism's self-defense forces."[152]

Most of the enthusiastic descriptions of IL-2 therapy in the media
were directly or indirectly inspired by the promoters of the new treatment. Publicity for the new therapy was an important strategic element in its diffusion, and it therefore influenced the production of new
medical knowledge. The behavior of IL-2 advocates was not exceptional. Scientists and physicians have incentives to present findings
that the media will cover and to push investigations in directions that
correspond to media priorities because publicity influences the allo-

cation of resources and the distribution of professional rewards.[153] Discussing the "interferon hype," a closely related phenomenon, Sandra Panem affirmed that "all segments of the community participated: scientists who genuinely believed that they were on the right track and that money solicited at the expense of candor would be well-used; investors and the public who wanted interferon to be a wonder drug and did not choose to ask whether the claims might be overstated; and those representatives of the media who reported anecdotes with unbridled enthusiasm." To avoid biomedical policies based on hype, she wrote, "the scientific community must do a better job of accurately portraying its work."[154] This advice would make sense if there were strong institutional incentives for scientists to avoid "hype" and to moderate their public declarations. Interferon and interleukin stories illustrate, however, precisely the opposite phenomenon: they highlight the professional rewards of hype within the scientific and medical communities.

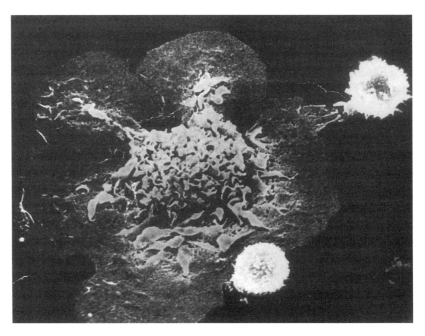

From *Le Figaro*, May 5, 1990: "The kiss of death: Here a lymphocyte is armed by interleukin-2 killing a tumor cell by adhering to it. This attack will end in the death of the tumor cell, which will disintegrate slowly and be emptied of its contents." (Photo by Jean Claude Révy; courtesy of *Le Figaro Magazine*.)

Optimistic statements by biomedical scientists stem from an inseparable mixture of genuine faith in the importance of their research and
career considerations. There is little doubt that scientists and physicians need to believe in the usefulness of their work. An optimistic
perception of the importance of one's studies may help the individual
investigator to overcome the frequent frustrations of scientific research, while faith in the efficacy of new treatments facilitates the
difficult task of caring for severely ill patients. It is important, however,
to distinguish between private beliefs and public declarations.[155] Public affirmation of the potential value of a given medical innovation by
its promoters—especially if they have already accumulated "symbolic
capital" in terms of rank and prestige—increases their visibility to their
colleagues, to the lay public, and to policymakers, directly or indirectly
boosting careers.

The professional benefits stemming from the public visibility of the
authors of a presumed "medical breakthrough" do not necessarily depend on the long-term fate of the innovation that led to public visibility. The evaluation of medical innovations is often a long and complex process. For practical reasons, it is difficult to delay granting
professional rewards for the development of a given medical innovation until clear-cut conclusions concerning its practical value have
been obtained. Moreover, the life span of medical innovations is often
short, and in some cases an innovation may be replaced by another
even before the medical community arrives at a consensus on its efficacy. In the absence of hostility of colleagues, an open scandal, or an
important controversy, professional rewards to promoters of medical
innovations (such as a tenured academic position or the directorship
of a laboratory or a hospital service) usually become irreversible upward moves. A short period of public visibility following a hype may
thus become a permanent career asset. On the other hand, the risks
of such hype are seldom high. Physicians and medical scientists—unlike businessmen—are rarely sanctioned for overly optimistic evaluations. Although Cetus lost its independence as a result of its inaccurate
appreciation of the therapeutic potential of IL-2, Rosenberg's laboratory gained strength as a result of its central role in the IL-2 clinical
trials. Moreover, despite disappointment in the wake of the "interferon
hype" in the 1980s, public support for science did not wane: people
continued to wait for "miracle drugs" for cancer, and the interferon
crusade was immediately followed by the "interleukin hype."[156] In the
1990s too, interleukin therapy continued to be presented to the lay

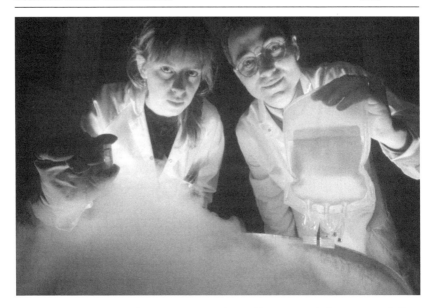

From *Le Figaro,* December 5, 1992: "A dose of hope: One billion cancer-killing cells in a bag. Four weeks ago, Nicolas Thiounn, of Cochin Hospital, and Nichole Joyeux cultivated these lymphocytes. In a few hours they will be injected into a patient to break down his tumors." (Photo by Alexandra Kobbeh; courtesy of *Le Figaro Magazine.*)

public as an important breakthrough; the promoters of the new cancer immunotherapies had little to lose from displaying enthusiasm.

Hype is not solely a superficial phenomenon, reflecting questionable public relations strategies developed by the promoters of medical innovations. It is also deeply embedded in the form and the content of scientific research, and here it may be more difficult to detect. While it is usually easy to spot excessive elements in public declarations by advocates of new diagnostic or therapeutic approaches, scientists and physicians tend to employ more restrained and neutral language when addressing their peers. The influence of hype on the content of science is nevertheless perceptible if one compares the shaping, framing, and the presentation of biomedical subjects viewed as "promising" in scientific publications with the presentation of similar subjects, perceived as "less promising." Scientific articles discussing "old" and "new" immunotherapies illustrate this point.

Consider two studies of "old" immunotherapy published in major scientific journals in the late 1980s, at the same time that the results of IL-2 clinical trials were being published.[157] The rate of success—

defined as the percentage of long-term remission or stabilization of the disease among patients suffering from disseminated cancer—was comparable for "old" immunotherapies and collaborative trials of IL-2 therapy. But the content and the style of the articles describing the "old" and "new" immunotherapies were very different. The former stressed the improvement in patients' quality of life following therapy. Patients treated with immunological methods "fared at least as well as those treated more traditionally, while complications and discomfort were less than would have been expected had only traditional chemotherapy and/or radiation been used." Therapy was described as "non-toxic and eminently feasible" and as able to bring about "a significant prolongation of survival compared with the natural history of this disease or available standard treatment."[158] The "old" immunotherapy provided "innovative, reasonable, and relatively safe treatments for cancer."[159] In contrast, articles describing interleukin therapy stressed the future promise of the new treatment. IL-2/LAK therapy, for example, was presented as "a possible new approach for the treatment of cancer, with potential applicability to a wide variety of tumors."[160] Whereas articles on "old" immunotherapy repeatedly stressed the safety and simplicity of the treatment and its role in reducing suffering and prolonging survival, those discussing the "new" immunotherapy emphasized the novelty of interleukin-2 therapy, its curative effects, and its future potential.[161]

The organization and presentation of scientific data in "old" immunotherapy and IL-2 therapy articles were also different. The former stressed the global efficacy of immunological treatment as measured by prolongation of survival and alleviation of symptoms, and provided only a limited amount of laboratory data on the physiological status of patients before, during, and after treatment. Though mentioning that in a few patients immunotherapy induced long-term regression of tumors, they did not provide detailed descriptions of these successful cases or photographs of disappearing metastases. The especially good outcomes in a small number of patients were implicitly presented as exceptions, the extreme end of a spectrum of variable clinical responses to treatment.[162]

In contrast, "new" immunotherapy articles contained numerous tables and figures summarizing the results of laboratory tests (mainly tests evaluating the activation of hypothetical antitumor immune mechanisms). They also described in detail selected cases of spectacular regression of tumors, illustrated with telling "before" and "after" photographs. The prevailing message in these articles—strengthened by the mode of presentation—was that the authors used innovative diagnostic and therapeutic methods, promoted a better understanding of the pathophysiology of cancer, and put most of their faith in the promise of "medical miracles."

In sum, the main message of "old" immunotherapy studies was care for patients, whereas that of "new" immunotherapy studies was scientific progress and the promise offered by future research. This message was reinforced by the social positioning of the respective investigations. Researchers who tested "old" immunotherapies worked alone or in small groups and employed either standard (and inexpensive) commercial products such as bacterial vaccines or substances prepared in their own laboratory (for example, "transfer factor" or activated lymphocytes). In contrast, investigators who employed "new" immunotherapies were integrated in larger professional networks, participated in cooperative multicenter programs, and collaborated with the biotechnology industry.

The close association of miracle-making medicine and high-tech biological research—present in scientific papers describing "new" cancer immunotherapies—reflected structural features of cytokine studies: legitimation through the promise of health (hence the important role of anecdotal evidence in shaping policies) and the privileged status of investigations linking basic research, clinical studies, and industrial interests. The public image of IL-2 therapy was not a distorted version of knowledge accessible to specialists, but a (relatively) faithful reflection of the process of shaping and diffusing that new therapeutic approach. There seems to be no simple solution for the problem of hype surrounding "hot" topics in biomedical research such as the search for new cancer therapies.

Cancer Immunotherapy as "Big Science" and "Big Medicine"

The story told in this and the preceding chapter may seem repetitive. Again and again the progress of basic research generated high expectations for the development of an efficient, nontoxic cancer therapy based on activation of the body's natural defense mechanisms. The successive immunotherapies of cancer were based on rational scientific assumptions, and some looked promising in animal models, in the test tube, or in both. Sometimes small-scale tests in humans seemed encouraging too. The results of bigger, better-controlled clinical trials were, however, much less impressive. Later the design of clinical trials for a given immunotherapy was strongly criticized by a limited number of outspoken specialists, while the majority of investigators first explained that the new and still imperfect treatment would soon be improved thanks to the rapid progress of basic biological research, then quietly abandoned it in favor of the next promising therapeutic approach. The impression of redundancy generated by the description of successive waves of enthusiasm for cancer immunotherapy is, however, misleading. Clinics and laboratory around 1910 were very different from clinics and laboratory around 1980, while the addition of a third actor, the industry, was not merely an extension of existing patterns but a qualitative change.

Let us look at the laboratory first. The explosion of biological and biomedical research after the Second World War had a direct and immediate effect on the growth of the community of immunologists, which in turn led to an impressive expansion of basic immunological knowledge. This expansion was not matched by parallel understanding of complex pathological phenomena, and even less so by applications of immunological knowledge to healing. Basic research in immunology was credited with important contributions to therapy, but the pace of these contributions was usually slower than the pace of cumulative basic research: detailed understanding of the structure of antibodies responsible for allergic reactions has not yet solved the practical problems of persons suffering from hay fever or asthma, the cloning of eight different interferons is for the moment of little consequence for an individual stricken by an influenza virus, and more than a decade of familiarity with the antigenic structure of the HIV virus and with the antibodies to this pathogen has not led to an efficient cure for AIDS.

Cancer immunotherapy illustrates this asymmetry between basic scientific knowledge and its medical applications. When Dr. Arthur Coca, one of the leading immunologists of his time, attempted in 1912 to cure cancer by specific vaccination, the understanding of "traditional" immune phenomena such as antibacterial immunity was not very different from the understanding of the mechanisms involved in "resistance" to cancer. Sixty years later the status of immunological knowledge was different. Rapid progress in the understanding of basic immunological mechanisms from the 1950s on led a prominent immunologist, Dr. Niels Jerne, to announce provocatively that in 1967 immunologists were "waiting for the end" of immunology—that is, they were getting close to the solution of all major immunological problems.[163] By contrast, even highly optimistic experts did not predict an imminent solution to the main problems of cancer immunotherapy. At most, experts mentioned the "coming of age" or "end of the beginning" of cancer immunotherapy.[164]

The disjunction between basic knowledge and practical applications is far from unusual. Science and technology evolved separately and often maintained only loose ties. New scientific knowledge does not necessarily yield technological applications, and conversely, practical solutions to concrete problems may be developed without appropriate scientific understanding of underlying phenomena (thus aspirin was successfully employed for 100 years to control inflammation and reduce fever before scientists developed an explanation of the physiological effects of salycilic acid).[165] Acknowledgment of the existence of a gap between the laboratory and the clinic is, however, problematic in domains, such as tumor immunology, defined through and legitimated by an alliance with medical practice, and then empowered thanks to this alliance. An important part of the activity of cancer immunologists and immunotherapists may be to close that gap—if not directly (that is, by developing efficient immunotherapies for malignant tumors), then at least through appropriate material, social, and rhetorical approaches.

The successive waves of cancer immunotherapy also reflect differences in their institutional frameworks. The first attempts at immunotherapy were isolated trials made by individual pathologists early in this century, before oncology existed as an organized and codified field. These trials, typically conducted in isolation by a small number of investigators in a single institution, were not subject to organized control by the medical community. In contrast, the interferon and interleukin trials were made in the framework of highly organized, powerful, and interdependent international communities of oncologists and of experimental cancer researchers. The centralization of research efforts is reflected in undertakings such as the NCI international registry of human immunotherapy trials.[166] Changes in the testing and diffusion of new therapeutic methods were not limited to cancer studies. The study of cancer immunotherapies in the 1970s and 1980s was shaped by powerful professional, political, and economic interests. The later clinical trials were not merely bigger and more sophisticated than the earlier ones; they were also qualitatively different. Clinical trials of immunotherapies, once a small "cottage industry," were transformed into a powerful modern industry as a result of the expansion of basic research in oncology and immunology, the rise of the culture of clinical experimentation in oncology, and the development of close connections between clinics and the biotechnology industry.

The alliance between laboratory, clinics, and industry led to the development, then the consolidation, of new institutional structures. The power of these structures in turn favored further investment in the application of recombinant molecules to the cure of human malignancies. Declarations by the advocates of biological therapies of cancer in the 1990s closely recall those of the promoters of "old" immunotherapies of cancer in the late 1970s. In the 1990s the experts explained again that the medical goals of the new therapies had yet to be achieved, "but the pioneering work is well underway and we can look forward confidently to future advances."[167] But whereas the application of bacterial vaccines to cancer therapy was brought to a halt in the late 1970s by the demonstration of their low clinical efficacy, the modesty of clinical results obtained with cytokine-based cancer therapies in the 1980s did not hamper the rapid expansion of these therapies in the early 1990s.[168]

The large-scale integration of academic scientists in the so-called biomedical-industrial complex led to important changes in immunological and oncological research. In this dense, close-knit network of cognitive, psychological, social, and political interests, members of distinct social groups coexist in a symbiotic relationship based on mutual legitimation.[169] These networks are characterized by both a certain resilience, sustained by their size, degree of professional control, and economic power, and a certain fragility due to their dependence on public funds, and thus on political factors. The existence of the biomedical-industrial complex is often directly reflected in the power structure of major medical schools, biomedical research centers, government funding agencies, and big disease-centered charities and in the career pattern of leading scientist-managers.[170] It is also mirrored in the current forms of experimentation in the clinics. It favors the funding of therapeutic innovations that efficiently articulate multiple interests: those of clinicians, basic scientists, industrialists, health administrators, and politicians.

The development of the biomedical-industrial complex is a relatively recent event. Close relationships among biologists, clinicians, and industrialists may be traced to the birth of "scientific medicine" in the second half of the nineteenth century.[171] However, before the

Second World War ties between the pharmaceutical industry and bio-medical research were seldom central to mainstream academic re-search and clinical practices.[172] Relationships among basic research scientists, clinicians, and industrialists underwent important transfor-mations in the aftermath of the Second World War, and again in the 1980s. In the late 1940s and the 1950s the conviction that the devel-opment of biological and medical research was a necessary precon-dition to the solution of major health problems led to a massive influx of public funds to academic biomedical research, but it also strength-ened selected industrial collaborative efforts (for example, in the pro-duction of antibiotics, hormones, and anticancer drugs). The organi-zational developments brought about by massive testing of anticancer drugs from the 1950s on were the consequence of these changes. In the late 1970s and the 1980s the new biotechnology industry made possible a large-scale transformation of central scientific values of bio-medical investigators into marketable assets.[173] As the anthropologist Paul Rabinow has put it: "symbolic, monetary and political capital are now in a tight feed-back loop." For this reason, he explains, "more than ever before the legitimacy of the biosciences now rests on claims to produce health. Having tilted so heavily in the direction of quasi-utilitarian ends ('quasi' in that 'health,' like wealth, is a symbolic me-dium subject to inflation and deflation), the bioscience community now runs the risk that merely producing truth will be insufficient to move the venture capitalists, patent offices and science writers, on whom the biosciences are increasingly dependent for their newfound wealth."[174]

The biomedical-industrial complex directly influences the daily practices of physicians and biomedical researchers in the Western countries. Interleukin-2 belongs to the domain of "big science" and "big medicine," but its success as an anticancer drug—and thus as a new medical practice and a commercial enterprise—was immediately linked to the (negotiated) results of clinical experiments conducted at multiple sites, and strongly influenced by a local context. The next two chapters focus on a clinical experiment that aimed to demonstrate that interleukin-2 was able or would be able to cure cancer, and in addition that an immunology laboratory was able or would be able to make a central contribution to the engineering of such a cure. The expansion of research, medical, and industrial interests at the trial's site was dependent on the success of the initial claims of the trial's promoters, or alternatively on the successful transformation of these claims into equally efficient legitimizing device(s). The "thick description" of the Cancer Foundation's IL-2 trial in the next chapters details how a small group of clinicians and scientists attempted to coordinate heterogeneous, sometimes incommensurable activities and representations in order to develop a multifunctional practice that aimed simultaneously at the construction of new biomedical knowledge and clinical practices, and at the advancement of their collective and individual goals.

CHAPTER FOUR

The IL-2 Trial at the Cancer Foundation: A Personal View

The Corridor

My participant observation at the Cancer Foundation started in a corridor. The corridor linked the research laboratories building with the main hospital building. It was long, well lighted, and freshly painted. On one side were radiation therapy rooms equipped with bulky radiation machines and computers. On the opposite side were the offices of radiation therapists, also equipped with computers. Anyone passing through the corridor caught numerous glimpses of gleaming green screens. At the hospital end, the corridor gave onto a patients' waiting room. One door in the room gave onto the hospital's hematology service. The room's decor—pastel paint, wooden furniture, magazines on low tables, colorful toys for children—was determinedly cheerful. The waiting room was often full. Some patients wore street clothes; others were in hospital pajamas and bathrobes. Nearly all the hospitalized patients had pallid gray or yellow complexions; some sat in wheelchairs and were accompanied by nurses; others carried portable intravenous infusion stands. Their drab pale blue pajamas and gray bathrobes reinforced their aura of illness. The hospitalized patients often gathered near the waiting room entrance door. Families with small children also frequently stood near that door, looking for an opportunity to speak with a passing doctor or nurse. Sometimes parents held a crying child in their arms and walked back and forth in the corridor. Outpatients often sat at the opposite end of the room from the entrance door. Many were or pretended to be absorbed in reading a book or a magazine and avoided eye contact with other patients.

The two central sites of my study were the immunology laboratory and the hematology laboratory. The immunology lab was in the research building, while the hematology lab was in the hospital building. Before the IL-2 project started, scientists from the immunology laboratory rarely passed through the corridor. The amount of traffic greatly increased, however, when the hematology laboratory became one of the centers of the IL-2 trial. One room in the hematology laboratory was dedicated to human cell studies; there researchers cultured LAK and TIL cells, studied surface markers of lymphocytes, separated cell populations, and tested the cytotoxic activity of IL-2-activated cells. Later another room in that laboratory became the center of studies of specific proteins serving as markers on the surface of human white blood cells.

The migration of human cell studies to the hematology laboratory was dictated by practical considerations. The immunology laboratory was a "mouse laboratory" and was not equipped for handling human cells, and finding space for the separate manipulation of human cells in that already overcrowded laboratory would have been nearly impossible.[1] In addition, the fact that IL-2-related studies were conducted in hospital territory displayed the links between the IL-2 project and the clinic. The distance between the human cell culture room and the immunology laboratory created complications for the researchers and technicians who worked with human cells and who frequently needed to use instruments and services located in the immunology laboratory: "hot rooms" for handling radioactive compounds, gamma and beta counters, sterilizers, computers, books and scientific journals. A steady stream of people hurried back and forth through the corridor, their hands full of tubes, pipettes, culture bottles, or computer printouts.

I was familiar with the world of this immunology laboratory, which like many others was sponsored by the Institut National de la Santé et de la Recherche Médicale (INSERM), the main public supplier of funds for biomedical research in France.[2] During my years as a full-time immunologist I had collaborated with some of the researchers there, and I had maintained friendships with several after leaving full-time immunological research. In 1985 I obtained permission to participate in the lab's weekly bibliography seminar, during which researchers commented on new scientific papers, and became familiar again with its research programs, workers, spatial arrangements, and even some of its internal problems. This familiarity, however, did not extend to the hospital. The immunology lab was situated in a building dedicated exclusively to research activities, and to get to the seminar

I usually passed through a back entrance to the Cancer Foundation used only by researchers and staff. This route shielded me from even fleeting encounters with cancer patients or their families. My first contact with cancer patients took place at the hospital end of the corridor when I started to observe the clinical trial of IL-2. During my stay at the Cancer Foundation the frequent sight of patients, doctors, and nurses in that space reminded me of the loss of my safe status as a "mouse scientist."

The immunology laboratory was crowded, chaotic, and seemingly bursting with constant activity. Staffed by young male and female researchers in about equal numbers (although most technicians were female), it contained several big multipurpose rooms, a few smaller specialized tissue culture rooms, a protected laboratory for genetic engineering experiments, a kitchen for washing and sterilizing glassware, a "hot room," a small space for researchers' desks and computers, a room for the secretaries, an office for François, the head of the department, and finally a meeting-room/library, which functioned as the center of the lab's life. Equipped with a coffee machine, comfortable armchairs, and bookcases housing stored collections of scientific journals, it was used not only for seminars, informal scientific discussions, and reading scientific journals but also for relaxation and laboratory gossip. It remained one of the few relatively uncluttered spaces in the laboratory. Other rooms and passages were densely packed with people, equipment, reagents, books, and files. Every available space became a working space. This density was visible testimony to the laboratory's good scientific reputation and its ability to attract graduate and postdoctoral students and visiting researchers. The walls were decorated with cartoons making fun of scientists, amusing or bizarre newspaper clippings, and children's drawings; there were no hints that the work space was located in a cancer hospital. Laboratory celebrations (which were frequent) took the form of drinks, potato chips, and peanuts at the end of the day.

The hematology laboratory was a different world. All its permanent staff were female, and all except Madeleine, the laboratory head, were technicians. The hematology technicians were middle-aged, some of them close to retirement. Their average education level tended to be lower than that of the research technicians in the immunology laboratory, and most had spent their entire careers at the Cancer Foundation. Several had initially been recruited as laboratory aides and had later completed evening courses to become qualified technicians. The hematology technicians wore blue-and-white striped coats faintly resembling those of salespeople in candy shops. In contrast to the immunology lab, where the dominant impression was tremendous activity and a businesslike working style, the hematology laboratory seemed peaceful, slow moving, and overstaffed. Automated blood analyses and computerized transcription of results had decreased the work load, and the technicians' narrow specialization, relatively limited professional skills, and age made retraining them for another kind of work difficult.[3] Because their job entailed great responsibility—a mistaken platelet count might lead to the death of a patient undergoing chemotherapy—the hematology technicians valued external signs of tranquility in their work routines, even on rush days. The walls in the hematology lab were decorated with color photographs of landscapes (often Alpine views) and flowers, along with souvenirs of deceased patients. Many technicians wore butterfly pins made of colorful beads, which I later learned had been made by a girl who had died in the hospital. Finally, celebrations here took the form of tea and cake at noon.

Spatial isolation between preclinical research and clinical activities is fairly common. In numerous research and teaching medical institutions, corridorlike spatial arrangements such as passages between buildings, shared entrance halls, elevators and staircases, shared cafeterias or coffee-bars, or even shared computer networks facilitate connections between the distinct spaces of research and therapy.[4] "Real" corridors, like the one at the Cancer Foundation, concretize the borders between distinct professional worlds. These boundaries were attenuated during the IL-2 trial. The human cell culture room in the hematology laboratory gradually became more like the immunology laboratory. It was crowded and was staffed by people of both sexes, many of them young, who wore standard white coats, were nearly always in a hurry, and frequently competed for space, instruments, or reagents. It did not, however, become merely a part of the immunology laboratory; its distinctness was maintained through a division of labor within the IL-2 trial: routine and semiroutine trial-related tasks were as a rule conducted in the hematology laboratory, while research tasks were confined to the immunology laboratory. Throughout my stay at the Cancer Foundation, the corridor continued to separate two different though partly intertwined social worlds.

The Setting

The IL-2 trial was a complex collective enterprise, but it started in a single, well-defined site: the immunology laboratory. Research laboratories belonged, as a rule, to the Biology Division of the Foundation. The immunology lab was the only basic research laboratory affiliated with the Medical Division. This exceptional status was the direct result of the imaginative—and obstinate—efforts of its head, François. The Cancer Foundation's IL-2 trial was affected by many variables that were independent of specific events there: the rapid development of the biotechnology industry in the 1980s, the introduction of a new class of molecules into cancer therapy, government efforts to promote funding of biomedical research in France, and international developments in oncology. It is reasonable to assume that eventually IL-2 (or a similar substance) would have been tested at the Cancer Foundation hospital. But the unique trajectory of the trial was influenced by the fact that the trial originated in the immunology laboratory and that François, the director of that laboratory, was the moving spirit behind that clinical experiment.

François was trained as an M.D. but had rapidly chosen to dedicate himself to scientific research. This decision may have been influenced by his social origins. Social skills, if possible acquired in a medical family or at least in a family of comparable social standing, have been instrumental in professional success in medicine in France. They have greatly facilitated the attainment of the status of protégé of leading doctors (the "mandarins"), an indispensable condition for a young physician's promotion to *agrégation* (professorship). François's lower-middle-class family background did not favor the acquisition of the social skills traditionally viewed as necessary for a medical career. On the other hand, after the Second World War and increasingly in the 1960s, the traditional structure of French medicine was challenged by many young and ambitious physicians from modest social backgrounds.[5] These physicians attempted to achieve prominence in their profession through internationally recognized scientific excellence (training in leading U.S. teaching hospitals, publication in recognized scientific journals) rather than through the acquisition of "appropriate" social skills. This strategy was particularly successful in science-oriented medical disciplines. But even in disciplines that placed a high value on acquiring the latest scientific knowledge—such as medical oncology—a distinguished scientific record was not by itself perceived as sufficient to secure an important professional position; social and political skills—though sometimes in a less traditional form—continued to be viewed as important assets for a successful career in medicine. Though lacking social advantages, François acquired others. As a student during the upheavals of 1968 he was active in a left-wing political movement. Although he later abandoned radical politics, during this period he developed some of the skills that later facilitated his relations with the administrators of the Cancer Foundation, with government officials, and with industrialists: the ability to speak clearly and effectively in public, to dominate tumultuous meetings, to negotiate in complex circumstances, and to propose acceptable compromises. Like many other French scientists and physicians of the 1968 generation, he also developed a pronounced gift for analyzing developments in science and medicine as power struggles and conflicts of interests.

François started his research career in the 1960s in an important immunology laboratory that studied transplantation immunity. At that time kidney transplantation was seen as one of the most advanced domains of medicine, and studies of transplantation immunity and of immunogenetic aspects of graft rejection were a prestigious domain of biological research. These studies were also perceived as exemplary cases of successful collaboration between the laboratory and the clinic.[6] Many young scientists who worked in that laboratory later occupied leading positions in French biomedical research. François left the transplantation immunology laboratory in the early 1970s to start his own research group in a middle-sized suburban research institute loosely affiliated with a big hospital. Soon afterward a collaboration with a visiting foreign scientist led him to years of study of the physiological effects of a nonspecific "factor" that regulated antibody responses in mice, together with attempts to determine its chemical structure.

François quickly acquired a reputation as a dynamic young immunologist, open to new ideas and eager to develop numerous international collaborations. This reputation, together with his skills in obtaining resources for his research, attracted gifted graduate and postgraduate students to his laboratory. The laboratory expanded rapidly, and its scientific productivity was impressive, at least on a French scale. Its growth was, however, handicapped by two elements. One was François's main research subject. The study of nonspecific regulatory factors in the immune response, central to immunological investigations in the late 1960s and early 1970s, became a less "hot" subject in the late 1970s. Immunologists described numerous such substances, but they also found that they had multiple and sometimes contradictory effects in different biological systems. It was therefore difficult to define their precise physiological role. The second problem hampering the development of François's laboratory was its unfavorable geographic location in an unattractive suburban area, far from the major centers of scientific activity in the city and from the "critical mass" of specialists in related research areas. In addition, although the laboratory was located near a major hospital, it failed to develop substantial collaborations with clinicians.

Both problems found a satisfactory solution in the early 1980s. At that time the development of molecular biology allowed the cloning and large-scale production of biologically active molecules such as the lymphokines. The difficult task of studying the biological functions of these molecules was replaced by the more feasible one of studying their structure. On the other hand, the possibility of cloning numerous lymphokines shifted the attention of scientists and industrialists to the potential medical uses of these molecules. The nonspecific regulatory molecules active in the immune system came to be perceived above all as a family of pharmaceutically active compounds able to modulate immune responses and therefore to affect pathological states. These new developments made the regulatory factor studied in François's laboratory attractive again. The large-scale production of molecules that affect the immune system also opened new possibilities for the integration of immunological research into a clinical framework. François and his collaborators rapidly grasped the new opportunities. They decided to modify their research strategy and to center their laboratory's efforts on the cloning of "their" regulatory factor. The main goal in the lab's shift in orientation was a practical one: François hoped that the cloned factor would find important therapeutic applications, and he started a collaboration with a pharmaceutical firm to explore these possibilities.

In the meantime François found a solution to his second problem. The laboratory's unfavorable location both complicated the researchers' tasks and diminished the lab's prestige. In France the distance from the city center or from important learning and research institutions is often a significant indicator of academic power and influence. The laboratory's transfer from the middle-sized suburban research center to the much bigger Cancer Foundation—the result of long and complicated negotiations—was undoubtedly an upward move. The Cancer Foundation combined the advantages of a central location and of proximity to several prestigious learning centers. In the new setting the immunology laboratory also obtained more floor space, more equipment, and specific facilities for genetic engineering. It was also directly attached to the medical division of the Foundation, and therefore had—at least theoretically—privileged access to medical resources and to collaboration with oncologists.

The Cancer Foundation, a private nonprofit institution with a long and respectable history, had an unusual structure. It was composed of three divisions: the Physics Division, which studied radioactive elements and the physical aspects of radioactivity; the Biology Division, which studied the effects of radiation on living organisms; and the Medical Division, or the Foundation's hospital, dedicated to cancer treatment. This structure aimed at optimizing the transfer of new discoveries in physics to medicine. The Foundation's hospital was established as a private nonprofit institution after the First World War in order to apply the new technology of radiation treatment to cancer therapy. It was at first a small and rather marginal institution, outside the established structures of academic medicine. For this reason it attracted physicians and scientists with unorthodox career profiles (physicians from the provinces, female physicians). These physicians developed innovative therapies of cancer such as *in situ* therapy with radioactive needles and fractionalized radiation therapies. In the 1930s the Foundation's hospital obtained impressive success rates at curing women's cancers (breast, cervix) and certain head and neck cancers. The success attracted more patients and transformed the hospital into a major French cancer treatment center. After the Second World War the Cancer Foundation hospital received massive financial support from the French Health Ministry, but because it officially retained its status as a private foundation it was able to maintain its flexible internal organization. The informal structure of the Foundation was probably one of the elements that attracted bright medical researchers with atypical trajectories, such as François.[7]

After the Second World War, research laboratories in the Foundation's Biology and Physics Divisions became increasingly dependent on government-funded research institutions such as the Centre National de la Recherche Scientifique (CNRS); the Délégation Générale de la Recherche, de la Science et de la Technologie (DGRST); and INSERM. In the 1960s most of its physics and biology laboratories were transferred to a new university campus in the suburbs. These laboratories maintained administrative links with the Foundation but in fact functioned as independent entities. The space liberated by their departure allowed an important enlargement of the Foundation's hospital. Several laboratories in the Biology Division, however, remained at the Foundation, and François's immunology laboratory could probably have joined that entity. But François had chosen a different strategy, and thanks to his efforts for the first time a research laboratory became part of the Medical Division, that is, of the Foundation's hospital. François liked to stress the innovative aspect of that move. The affiliation of the immunology laboratory with the hospital was, he explained, a first step toward new relations between basic researchers and clinicians at the Cancer Foundation.

At first François legitimated the lab's affiliation with the Medical Division through a project to study the medical applications of his laboratory's original regulatory factor. He hoped to clone the molecule in the immunology laboratory, to trigger its industrial production, and then to conduct clinical trials at the Foundation's hospital. These trials, he believed, would lead to the integration of the laboratory's preoccupations with those of the oncologists. But the cloning proved to be more difficult than expected, and in the meantime other natural substances that regulated immune responses were cloned, then produced in large quantities. These substances (interferons, interleukins, colony stimulating factors, tumor necrosis factors) were viewed as more promising therapeutic agents than the one being studied by François and his collaborators. By the mid-1980s, when François had probably realized that his original project was unlikely to lead rapidly to results that could be applied in the clinics, the laboratory was working smoothly in its new setting, and individual researchers had established fruitful collaborations with colleagues working in other research laboratories at the Cancer Foundation or in teaching and research institutions in the neighborhood. The affiliation of the immunology laboratory with the Cancer Foundation's hospital did not seem at first to influence the orientation of research in the laboratory. The only person besides François who was constantly aware of the fact that the laboratory was now directly associated with the hospital was the secretary, who negotiated financial matters with the hospital's administration.

François, however, pursued his project of integrating his laboratory into the Foundation hospital through a range of strategies. One was to involve himself increasingly in the internal politics of the hospital. Although François had not abandoned his dream of being at the source of a major biological discovery, preferably one that would also have medical applications, he also employed his political talents to come nearer to being the architect (or at least one of the architects) of a scientific turn of French oncology. The immunology laboratory joined the Cancer Foundation during a period of important transformations in the hospital. Until the 1970s, the radiation therapists had been the most powerful group at the hospital, in line with its founding by pioneers in that specialty.[8] In the 1970s a third group of physicians joined the radiation therapists and surgeons at the Foundation hospital—the medical oncologists. The introduction of drug therapy for cancer at the hospital occurred as late as the 1970s because of the radiation therapists' resistance. In the 1970s and 1980s the radiation therapists strongly opposed the oncologists' claims that radiation therapy had become a conservative medical technique and that chemotherapy represented the state-of-the-art, science-based approach to cancer therapy. The development of chemotherapy in the United States (and to a lesser degree in selected British and French centers) provided a powerful impetus for close interaction between clinical oncology and research laboratories in pharmacology, toxicology, cell biology, biochemistry, and endocrinology.[9] Without such an impetus, Cancer Foundation clinicians would not have developed sustained relationships with scientists. In the 1960s and 1970s, thanks to the activity of the Biology and Physics Divisions, the Cancer Foundation continued to be viewed as an important basic research institute. But it had lost some of its earlier reputation as a leader in preclinical and clinical investigations of human malignancies.

The "newcomers" to the Cancer Foundation's hospital (medical oncologists) and the "old-timers" (radiation therapists and surgeons) competed for control of specific jurisdictions within the hospital. This competition intensified in the late 1980s, when the construction of a new building scheduled to double bed capacity created the prospect of dramatic changes in the hospital's structure. François, an M.D. turned immunologist, did not belong to any of the competing groups at the Cancer Foundation. His neutral status helped him to acquire a privileged position in the political struggles within the hospital. In addition, François proposed a way to enhance the reputation of the hospital. The Cancer Foundation's early success, he explained, had its roots in the successful transformation of laboratory-generated knowledge (studies of the effects of radiation on living tissues) into a new and powerful therapeutic tool—radiation therapy. The fruitful collaboration between clinicians and biologists at the Foundation, however, had been short-lived: Cancer Foundation radiation therapists had become a conservative segment of the medical profession, while in the 1950s and 1960s their opposition to chemotherapy had hampered the capacity of the Foundation hospital to remain at the cutting edge of new developments in oncology. The introduction of cancer immunotherapy, François argued, might make up for the Foundation's lost opportunities stemming from its failure to take the "chemotherapy turn" in the 1950s and 1960s. It might bring biology back to the Foundation's hospital and might help the Foundation to recover its past glory as a leading institution in cancer research and cancer therapy. The IL-2 trial was part of François's efforts to promote the "biologization" of cancer therapy at the Cancer Foundation. These efforts, I learned later, accorded with the goals of the Cancer Foundation directors, who aspired to modify the power relationship within the Foundation and to promote links among research laboratories, routine analysis laboratories, the clinic, and industry.

Launching the IL-2 Trial: November 1986–March 1987

In the fall of 1986 I became aware of unusual activity in the immunology laboratory. Three new people joined the bibliography seminar: a hematologist, Madeleine; a radiotherapist, Jacques; and an intern, Daniel.[10] Madeleine was the head of the hematology laboratory at the Cancer Foundation. Her job title, I soon discovered, was more impressive than the position itself—the direction of a routine analysis laboratory. Madeleine was rather shy and rarely participated in the animated theoretical discussions in the seminar. Jacques, who presented himself as a practicing physician who was interested in clinical research, also rarely joined in the scientific discussions. Daniel, who aspired to acquire training in biomedical research, was interested in new developments in cellular immunology and eagerly demonstrated his freshly acquired bibliographical knowledge. While Daniel's participation in the seminar was easily explained by his interest in immunological research, the presence of Jacques and Madeleine was more puzzling. Yet I noticed that after the seminar Daniel and Madeleine frequently stayed to talk with François in his office.

In late 1986 I learned from overheard fragments of a conversation that the Cancer Foundation would be the first French institution to introduce a new and highly promising treatment of cancer: the interleukin-2 therapy.[11] An agreement between the immunology laboratory and a French pharmaceutical firm that produced IL-2 was about to be officially announced. Daniel would join the immunology lab and would start the preclinical studies of the new method. I was already familiar with the multiple uses of IL-2 in immunological research, but this was the first time I had heard about therapeutic uses of interleukin. Daniel provided an enthusiastic description of Dr. Steven Rosenberg's first studies and asserted that the IL-2 treatment would probably lead to a revolution in cancer therapy. Although he was reluctant to accept Rosenberg's argument that IL-2 activated a new subpopulation of lymphocytes, the "lymphokine activated killer," or LAK, cells, Rosenberg's impressive clinical results had convinced him that interleukin-stimulated cells, whatever their biological nature, were an interesting therapeutic tool for oncologists.[12] A glance at Rosenberg's first clinical publication also convinced me that the new therapy seemed very interesting. At that time I was looking for a research subject that would allow me to observe interactions between laboratory and clinic. The IL-2/LAK therapy was particularly well adapted for such a purpose because it was based on data from basic immunological research (the activation of lymphocytes by IL-2) and because by its very nature (the transfer of white blood cells activated in the test tube to cancer patients), the therapy had to be rooted in close collaboration between laboratory workers and clinicians.

I first mentioned to Daniel that I wanted to join the IL-2/LAK study as a participant-observer, that is, a part-time worker with low commitment to the experimental system. Daniel was interested because he believed that a trained cellular immunologist might help to advance the IL-2 project. The next step was to speak with François, which I did a week later. At first François was ambivalent about my participation. He was, at least in principle, in favor of historical and sociological studies of science and medicine. He was also interested in another "pair of hands" even though I was unwilling to participate actively in the research process. (Later I learned that François probably believed that I would not be able to resist the attraction of the bench and sooner or later would revert to my "true nature" as an experimental scientist.) I realized later that he might also have been interested in having a witness to the accomplishment of the first step in his project of "biologizing" oncology at the Cancer Foundation, which would be closely linked to the (prospective) success of the IL-2 trial. On the other hand, he seemed to think that my presence might be a potential source of disturbance in the laboratory and might negatively affect his relations with Madeleine and with the French pharmaceutical company. Finally, François decided that if Madeleine had no objections, he would agree to my participation. Madeleine was perplexed about my intentions and unsure about the consequences of becoming a subject of sociological investigation, but she did not oppose my plans. François and Madeleine therefore gave me permission to participate in preparatory meetings of the IL-2/LAK project, and they agreed that I would join Daniel's LAK studies as soon as possible.

I started attending the weekly meetings of the unofficial IL-2 group in February 1987.[13] At the first meeting I gave a brief introductory talk on the aims of my research: the study of the transfer of an innovation from the laboratory to the clinic and of the interaction between scientists and clinicians during that process. My talk was received with polite indifference. Thereafter I sat quietly in the meetings, taking notes. The preparatory meetings were conducted in the seminar room of the immunology laboratory, a location that underlined the fact that François was in charge of the project. The discussions centered on two subjects: Daniel's first experimental results, and the possibilities of developing an animal model of IL-2/LAK treatment.

Daniel incubated human white blood cells (supplied by the blood bank of a large general hospital) with "French" IL-2, then tested their LAK activity. These experiments were important because the French pharmaceutical company produced a chemically modified molecule of interleukin, different both from the native IL-2 molecule found in the body and from the molecule produced by an American biotechnology firm.[14] The pharmaceutical firm assumed that the modified IL-2 molecule would be as efficient as the native molecule in generating LAK cells, and Daniel's task was to prove that assumption. He was also responsible, together with Madeleine, for the practical aspects of organizing the large-scale culture of human cells at the Cancer Foundation to prepare for the repetition, in France, of Rosenberg's protocol of therapy with IL-2 and LAK cells. Daniel started to work part-time in Madeleine's laboratory and was helped by one of the hematology technicians, Dominique. I was scheduled to join him as soon as a bigger laminar flow hood (used in the sterile manipulation of biological materials) had been installed in the hematology laboratory to accommodate the presence of another worker.

The participants in the preparatory meetings discussed Daniel's early results. They also discussed a project to develop an experimental model for testing the responsiveness of individual tumors to IL-2/LAK treatment. Rosenberg was unable to predict which of his patients would respond to the IL-2 treatment. François believed that the development of an animal model that would closely mimic human tumor behavior might allow the preselection of patients who had the best chances of benefiting from the new therapy. The development of such a model, he hoped, might give the Cancer Foundation trial a competitive edge over other, similar clinical trials of IL-2/LAK.

The preparatory meetings helped me to get acquainted with the participants in the IL-2 project: the three Cancer Foundation's physicians, Daniel, Madeleine, and Jacques; a hematologist, Joseph; and two technicians from Madeleine's laboratory, Dominique and Chantal. Daniel, the key researcher of the project at that stage, aspired to work full-time on the IL-2/LAK project. In order to be able to do so, he had asked (with François's support) for a scholarship sponsored by a French cancer charity. In the meantime he was an intern in the medical oncology ward of the Cancer Foundation and became one of the (minor) links between that ward and the immunology laboratory. Daniel, though a near-beginner in scientific research, was an avid reader of scientific journals and a dedicated and enthusiastic laboratory worker.

As a radiation therapist, Jacques was a member of the oldest and probably still most powerful group among the Cancer Foundation's physicians. He was, however, atypical in that he had developed a keen interest in chemotherapy and had participated in a pharmacological study of the mechanisms by which cancer cells resist drugs. Jacques's first IL-2-related research project (strongly inspired by François's ideas) was to transplant surgically excised human tumors into a strain of mice that accepts such grafts, the "nude" mice, then to inject tumor-carrying mice with LAK cells derived from the blood of the tumor's donor.[15] Such an experimental system, it was hoped, might allow one to predict whether a given patient's tumor was responsive to that patient's LAK cells. It might also allow studies of the hypothetical mechanism(s) of the destruction of tumors by LAK cells. Jacques made a few preliminary attempts to graft tumors in nude mice, but his project soon encountered major technical difficulties and was abandoned. Later Jacques switched to a less innovative study of the toxicity of IL-2 in mice. His participation in the IL-2 project, like his previous research on tumor resistance to drugs, was only slightly related to his official professional skills. Nevertheless, François often presented him in official meetings as "our radiation therapist." Jacques was quiet and reserved. He spoke little and did not participate in the ritual exchanges of jokes and gossip during the meetings. Although his name was later included in some of the scientific publications summarizing the results of the IL-2 trial at the Cancer Foundation, his participation seemed to be motivated mainly by a personal interest in laboratory research.

Madeleine was a key person in the IL-2 project. In order to start a major clinical investigation François needed to collaborate with a physician from the Cancer Foundation hospital. Madeleine held a sufficiently high position in the hospital hierarchy to make the collaborative project credible but also was unlikely to question his leadership position. Although Madeleine was not directly involved in patients' care, her official position was "senior clinician." François patiently introduced Madeleine to immunological research and was always extremely careful to treat her as an equal. Nevertheless, she seemed hesitant during the early meetings of the IL-2 project, often blushing and stopping in the middle of a sentence. Madeleine's timidity contrasted with the self-assurance of another hematologist present at the meetings, Joseph. Joseph was invited to the IL-2 meetings because he was the director of the blood bank that supplied human white cells for the early trials of LAK. His role in the IL-2 project was relatively minor: he was mainly a provider of a product—human white blood cells— and of a service—cytapheresis. (Cytapheresis is the mechanical separation, outside the body, of white blood cells from plasma and from red blood cells. Serum and red blood cells are then reinjected into the person whose blood was separated. The process allows the collection of large quantities of white blood cells. LAK cell therapy was based on injection of large quantities of white blood cells cultivated for three to four days with IL-2—usually around 10×10^{10} cells, and occasionally up to 20×10^{10} cells. Cytapheresis was the only way to obtain such quantities of white blood cells without harming the patient.) Nevertheless, Joseph became an important participant in the preparatory discussions because of his previous research experience and his extensive knowledge of scientific literature. Chantal and Dominique, the two hematology technicians, were specialized in routine medical analyses and had difficulty following scientific discussions closely. They seemed thrilled by the opportunity to participate in a research project but, at the same time, unsure of their ability to make the transition from routine laboratory work to scientific research.

In mid-February an official preparatory meeting of the IL-2/LAK project was held in a big conference room at the hospital. It gathered all the participants in the IL-2 meetings (except the hematology technicians), several physicians from the medical oncology department, and a delegation from the French pharmaceutical firm. François presented me as one of his collaborators. The meeting started with Daniel's presentation of the results of activation of LAK cells in the test tube with the French IL-2. His preliminary results indicated that the French IL-2 was able to stimulate human white blood cells approximately as efficiently as the American IL-2. François made a short speech about the future of cancer immunotherapy, followed by a few polite questions from clinicians. The only industry representative to speak was the scientific director of the IL-2 project at the pharmaceutical firm, Diana. She was worried about the possibility of unexpected complications from IL-2 treatment (there were rumors about a treatment-induced hepatitis), and she stressed that the clinical trials of IL-2 needed to be approved by an ethics committee.[16] The Cancer Foundation did not at that time have a permanent ethics committee, and the head of the medical oncology department promptly declared that such committee would be created soon. Although the unhappy experience with interferon tests in France was never mentioned (the first clinical experiments with that molecule were stopped after a series of unexplained deaths), it was on everybody's mind.[17] The meeting ended on an upbeat note: everybody congratulated everybody else, while the industry people praised the promising preclinical results and expressed hope that clinical tests would start soon.

In the first week of March 1987 the tissue culture room in the hematology laboratory was ready for use, and I was able to join Daniel's studies. I was pleased to return to the bench and to rediscover the physical aspects of laboratory work: the pleasure of delicate manipulations of fragile biological material, the satisfaction of finding in the morning that the cells in culture looked fine, the excitement of waiting for a sheet of results near the printer of a radioactivity counter, a little talk over a morning cup of coffee. On my first work day I obtained permission to take a white coat from a closet in the immunology laboratory and then walked through the corridor for the first time to the hematology laboratory. I was amazed to discover how different it was from the world of the immunology lab. Dominique introduced me to a friendly group of hematology technicians, then started my training in methods of culture and testing of LAK cells. Dominique and Chantal were at this point relatively skilled in executing experimental protocols and gained more confidence in their ability to become research technicians, but they continued to have some difficulty in understanding the scientific principles of the experiments they were performing.[18] Daniel's duties at the medical oncology ward left him little time for discussions with the technicians. He buzzed through the laboratory in the morning, distributed tasks to Dominique and Chantal, then ran to the ward, and often came back only late in the evening to look at the results of the day's work. Daniel claimed to dislike the medical oncology ward, which he sometimes called a "dying place" or "miracle yard."[19] My impression was, however, that he was simultaneously attracted to and repulsed by this ward; although he steadily complained about lack of time for research, he spent most of his time in the clinic. The technicians found Daniel's frequent absences problematic. Dominique, who was assigned as a full-time technician to the IL-2/LAK program (Chantal divided her time between routine tasks in the hematology lab and cell culture), was particularly frustrated by her limited understanding of immunology, which reduced her to a mere executor of a long list of instructions, and was eager to learn more. During my first weeks in the lab I often explained to her the scientific background of her experiments and discussed the meaning of their results. Dominique was satisfied, Daniel was glad that somebody was taking over some of his tasks, and I felt useful.

Daniel was also pleased to have a sympathetic listener to his reflections about his research and his many new ideas; François was too busy to follow all the details of Daniel's experiments, and he was also occasionally harsh with beginners. In addition, Daniel's relationships with Madeleine were strained. He strongly resented her attempts to supervise his work, judging that, as far as immunological research was concerned, his knowledge was not inferior to hers. My relationship with Madeleine was at that point very limited. The preparatory meetings of the IL-2 project had been discontinued in the spring of 1987, and Madeleine had temporarily moved her office to another part of the hospital and was seldom present in the hematology laboratory. I tried to persuade Daniel to be more patient with Madeleine. He was professionally and financially dependent on François, and there was little doubt that in the case of an open conflict, François would support Madeleine, not him. I also had the impression that Madeleine's attempts to control Daniel were not an expression of lack of confidence in his professional skills, but rather reflected her insecurity and her ambivalent feelings about her place in the IL-2 project.

Although both Daniel and Dominique welcomed my assistance, my integration into LAK studies was not entirely smooth. The human tissue culture room quickly became overcrowded. Theoretically there were two working places under the laminar flow hood, but in practice two people could work under the hood at the same time only when they were collaborating on the same experiment. In addition, the culture room itself could accommodate no more than two to three workers at a time. A possible solution was to organize evening shifts, but Dominique and Chantal, trained as routine analysis technicians, were used to a regular nine-to-five working day and took a dim view of different arrangements. Daniel usually wanted to use the culture room in the early afternoon, and I was unenthusiastic about regularly spending my evenings at the Cancer Foundation.[20]

My first weeks at the Foundation were dominated by tensions over the allocation of time and space in the tissue culture room. These tensions spilled over into the immunology laboratory, where some of the researchers and technicians seemed reluctant to share their already crowded space and frequently-used equipment with newcomers from the IL-2/LAK group. I was also worried about the possible influence of Daniel's poor relationship with Madeleine on the LAK studies. In addition, François's mood was rather gloomy, and it influenced the atmosphere in his laboratory. My colleagues from the lab explained that François had failed to obtain an awaited professional promotion. Another candidate had been preferred, local rumor went, because newspapers had widely reported that scientist's success in developing an immunological treatment that improved the success rate of bone marrow grafts. According to the inner circle of specialists in the lab, the media's reports of a "breakthrough therapy" developed by a French scientist were not entirely accurate; the latter's uncontested practical success was an adaptation of a method first developed in the United States. Nevertheless, his work had been hailed as an original scientific contribution not only by the lay press but also by officials in the Health Ministry. It is possible that François was influenced by this episode when he started his public campaign in the spring of 1987 as the main spokesperson for interleukin therapy in France.

Preclinical Stages: April 1987–March 1988

March was a hectic month. Gradually, however, we developed an acceptable work schedule in the culture room. Usually Daniel started an experiment in the morning, I continued his work in the afternoon, and if necessary he took over the experiment when he returned from the oncology ward in the late afternoon. In my free time I helped Dominique to interpret her experimental results. Occasionally we read a scientific paper on IL-2/LAK studies together. The researchers at the immunology laboratory accepted the presence of the "LAK people," and we developed patterns of sharing space and equipment. I got used to oscillating between the immunology and hematology labs and adapted myself to the specific style of each site. In April 1987 the tissue culture room had settled into a routine of producing two to three human cell cultures per week.[21] The laboratory techniques used in the LAK studies were similar to those employed in mouse-centered cellular immunology labs. The main differences were the dependence of LAK studies on a supply of human white blood cells and the incorporation of several additional steps in preparing and isolating the cells. The results obtained in our experiments were variable. Daniel, who had hoped to obtain rapidly reproducible results, was annoyed by this variability. I was less surprised, given that the cells had been taken from a wide range of individual donors.

The progress of our scientific work seemed satisfactory, but I started to worry about the progress of my sociological research. Most of the time I saw only Daniel and Dominique. If I happened to be at the Cancer Foundation on days when Daniel discussed his results with François I saw François too, but these discussions were as a rule reduced to debates on the technical aspects of the culture and activation of white blood cells. I learned in April 1987 that the French pharmaceutical firm was having unexpected problems with large-scale production of IL-2, and that clinical trials, first scheduled for the fall of 1987, could start at the earliest in the spring of 1988. In the meantime the only "relationship with the clinic" I was able to observe was Daniel's steady stream of half-serious complaints about his work on the medical oncology ward.

In May Daniel read an article describing the increase of the LAK activity of IL-2 by gamma interferon, and proposed to look for such an increase in his experimental system. François immediately found the idea attractive. It was easy to test, and it might confer originality on the Cancer Foundation trial. François believed that this idea would also appeal to industry representatives. Several years earlier the French pharmaceutical company had invested considerably in the production of gamma interferon, but it had not become the expected miracle drug for cancer, and sales had been disappointing. The industrialists were therefore interested in potential markets for their product. They would be glad, François assumed, to give Daniel a generous supply of interferon and would perhaps also be willing to help fund research on the potential antitumor effects of the combination IL-2/gamma interferon. François was right; the industry people were enthusiastic about the project, and Daniel started on it immediately.

The interferon/IL-2 experiments were long and tedious, and their results were not very encouraging. In some experiments Daniel observed a three-to-fourfold increase in LAK activity in the presence of interferon, a far cry from the hundredfold increase described in the article that had inspired Daniel. Moreover, the phenomenon was variable and could be observed only with low doses of interferon. In the presence of higher doses, activation of LAK was systematically less efficient than in interferon-free controls. Daniel's goal at that point was to be able to publish an article as rapidly as possible. After obtaining his medical diploma he planned to join a postgraduate program in the United States (if possible at the NIH), and he needed one or two articles in order to be eligible for a fellowship. With François's . approval, Daniel therefore started to organize the results of the stimulation of LAK production by interferon into tables and graphics, hoping that by the end of the summer he would have accumulated enough data to publish an article in a minor oncology journal.

But something unexpected happened during the analysis of Daniel's experimental results. Looking at the long columns of numbers coming out of the gamma counter, Daniel experienced a perception shift. He suddenly noticed that the major phenomenon observed in these experiments was not a stimulation of LAK cells by low doses of interferon, but a steady inhibition of the activation of LAK cells by higher doses of interferon. From that time on, inhibition by high doses of interferon became his sought-after result. The shift to an inhibition study was probably less satisfactory from the point of view of the industry representatives, who hoped to develop a market for their gamma interferon. Daniel, however, was pleased by the prospect of producing an article soon. The new orientation did not bring me closer to my goal of studying interactions between scientists and clinicians, but at least the work on the bench became more interesting. At that stage of my participant observation I gave up my naive aspiration to attempt to be only a "pair of hands." I continued to refrain from discussions on the general directions of the IL-2 study, but I found it virtually impossible to pretend that I had no ideas about possible interpretation(s) of my own experiments.

In June Daniel's work became somewhat frantic; he planned to leave for the United States in the spring of 1988, and he had to finish his internship in medicine before that. He worked hard and stayed late every night, but instead of sticking to a single experimental schedule he frequently became interested in a new idea, wanted to test it right away, and modified his research projects. Dominique became wary of the constant changes in experimental protocols and asked me to try to influence Daniel to adopt a more stable direction of research. I thought that this was François's job, and anyway, I argued, Daniel would not listen to me. François's increasing involvement with the internal politics of the Cancer Foundation, however, left him little time to follow all the details of Daniel's work. Things became worse in late June and in July. The experiments became less reproducible because the tumor cell lines (malignant cells cultivated in the laboratory) used in standard tests of LAK activity became less prone to lysis, while, for unknown reasons, the peak of LAK activation, previously observed at day 5 of culture, shifted to day 7 or 8. I was relieved to depart for summer vacation.

Back at the Cancer Foundation in September, I learned that Daniel—who had worked hard all summer—had found that the inhibition of LAK production by interferon disappeared if "adherent cells" (cells that spontaneously stick to glass or plastic) were removed before the white blood cells were incubated with IL-2. The new observation was made by chance. Cells with LAK activity do not adhere to plastic. Daniel therefore hoped that eliminating all the white blood cells that adhered to plastic would increase the concentration of LAK cells and improve the results of his experiments. He was surprised to observe that in the absence of adherent cells interferon gamma did not inhibit LAK activity. Daniel and François rapidly grasped that this observation might lead to the isolation and characterization of a hypothetical interferon-activated "LAK suppressor cell" and/or its products.

Another important development was the arrival of a new participant, Pierre. Pierre became a key figure in the next stage of the IL-2/
LAK program. He had been trained in pediatrics, then switched to
immunological research. Pierre was one of the first French M.D.s
to benefit from a special government program that allowed clinicians
to spend several years in basic research laboratories. Usually, French
M.D.s who turned to fundamental research (as François had done)
lost contact with the clinic, while those who became clinicians did not
follow recent scientific developments. The new program, hailed as an
important innovation, aimed at developing in France a new, U.S.-style
brand of physicians who would simultaneously be active in the clinics
and conduct advanced scientific research. Pierre's grant had allowed
him to work in a French immunology laboratory and then spend two
years in a leading American medical school.

During his stay in the United States, Pierre had specialized in the
study of lymphocytes with hypothetical antitumor activity such as
killer T cells and NK cells. When he returned to France, he obtained
a tenure-track position as an "assistant" in the Cancer Foundation's
pediatric oncology department. Pierre negotiated an arrangement that
he hoped would allow him to continue to dedicate part of his time to
scientific research. He was scheduled to work one month full-time at
the pediatric oncology ward and then, during the next month, have a
lighter load of clinical duties that would allow him to work part-time
in the laboratory. At first Pierre wanted to continue some of the projects he had begun in the United States, but François persuaded him
to switch to the IL-2/LAK studies. Back from the United States, Pierre
became a local celebrity. He was invited to meetings sponsored by
INSERM and to medical schools to explain the advantages of dual
training in medicine and basic science. He was even interviewed by a
business journal, which depicted Pierre's career in glowing terms and
presented him, together with promising young businessmen and politicians, as one of the "representatives of France's future."

Pierre had heard about my research project from a mutual friend.
When I first met him, he expressed interest in it, and later occasionally
asked politely how it was progressing, but in fact he was more interested in talking about laboratory work and exchanging work-related
gossip. Pierre was a much more experienced laboratory worker than
Daniel. In addition, he had a large network of professional contacts.
When a chemical substance, a cell line, or an instrument was needed,
he knew immediately where it might be obtained, and thus saved him-

self and the other laboratory workers a great deal of time and effort. Pierre's search for the best conditions in which to develop LAK activity was directly related to the clinical trials of IL-2/LAK. One of his central tasks was to adapt white blood cells to a culture in serum-free media. Human cells cultivated for research purposes are usually grown in a culture medium enriched with human serum. However, the presence of human serum was a serious liability in the culture of cells destined to be injected into patients because it increased the risk of infection with pathogenic microorganisms such as hepatitis B virus or the AIDS virus. Such a risk was not merely theoretical: during the May 1987 meeting of the American Society of Clinical Oncology, doctors reported 50–85 percent infection with hepatitis B virus following IL-2/LAK treatment. The contamination was traced to two batches of human serum used for LAK culture. This incident increased the interest in the development of a method to cultivate white blood cells in a serum-free medium.

Pierre worked nearly all the time in the culture room at the hematology laboratory, but he viewed himself as affiliated with the immunology laboratory. At first he had close ties with François: they wrote several review articles together, and François chose him as co-organizer of a scientific symposium. My impression was that Pierre automatically assumed that François viewed him as an important actor in François's planned "clinical turn." Pierre's relations with Madeleine were at first indifferent, but they later became more complicated. When a cancer charity had supplied funds for the purchase of a fluorescein activated cell sorter (FACS, an instrument for the study of receptors on the cell surface) for the IL-2 project, Madeleine asked for—and obtained—the exclusive right to control access to the FACS. Pierre was unpleasantly surprised to learn that he had no right to use the newly acquired cell sorter. The restriction hampered his research projects, some of which involved analysis of lymphocyte receptors. Pierre had hoped to include me in that part of his project because cells can be frozen and their receptors analyzed later—a convenient task for a part-time worker with other professional obligations. Having failed to gain access to the Foundation's FACS, he tried to employ a cell sorter located in a different hospital, but the process was too complicated, cumbersome, and time-consuming for regular use. Pierre ended by giving up his plans to study cell receptors. After that episode he temporarily ended all communication with Madeleine.[22]

In the meantime I had learned from Pierre that the Cancer Foundation IL-2 project would not be the first clinical trial of IL-2 in

France. Physicians in another big French city were already conducting clinical trials of American IL-2 (alone or with LAK cells) in patients suffering from renal cell carcinoma. These physicians also planned to start clinical trials of IL-2 and of LAK cells in a rare childhood cancer, neuroblastoma. Pierre was particularly interested in neuroblastoma. One of the last-ditch treatments for drug-resistant, advanced (phase IV) neuroblastoma was autologous bone marrow graft. The patients were submitted to radiation therapy and to intensive drug therapy. The therapy killed the residual malignant cells but also normal bone marrow cells. The patients were then regrafted with their own bone marrow cells, which had been collected before chemotherapy. Work on that disease brought together Pierre's interests in pediatrics, oncology, immunology, and transplantation. In November 1987 he visited the physicians conducting the trials in children and returned full of enthusiasm. The leader of that group had agreed to include the Cancer Foundation in the neuroblastoma IL-2 trial in order to accelerate the enrollment of patients. François was pleased because a pediatric trial would hasten the long-delayed beginning of clinical trials of IL-2/LAK at the Cancer Foundation. The neuroblastoma trial was a part of a multicenter clinical trial of American IL-2, and Pierre was worried about a possible conflict of interest with the French producers of the molecule. François, however, believed that he could avert any problems.

Pierre was excited about the neuroblastoma experiment. He hoped for positive results, reasoning that clinical assays of IL-2/LAK in neuroblastoma, and later IL-2/LAK treatment in other childhood cancers, would bring him important professional rewards. Daniel had more doubts about clinical uses of LAK, especially in children. Preliminary reports from several clinical trials of IL-2 indicated that IL-2/LAK therapy was no better than treatment with IL-2 alone,[23] while LAK cells produced additional side effects. He recommended starting with clinical trials of IL-2 alone. Pierre strongly disagreed. He thought it was important to develop LAK therapy at the Cancer Foundation as rapidly as possible. It would take about two years to introduce it into a given hospital (that is, to establish efficient human cell cultures and to train physicians, technicians, and nurses in new therapeutic methods). Thus, if LAK therapy came to be widely recognized as safe and efficient, hospitals that had not introduced the method earlier would be at least two years behind their main competitors and might lose their reputations of being at the cutting edge of cancer treatments.[24]

In November Pierre invited me to a workshop on neuroblastoma organized by the French Association of Pediatric Oncology. During that workshop I was struck by the difference between the precise understanding of some scientific and clinical aspects of neuroblastoma treatment, and an almost complete lack of information on other aspects. For example, I learned that quantification of the number of oncogene copies in neuroblastoma cells (oncogenes are genes related to the development of cancer), using the newest methods of molecular biology, was rapidly becoming one of the standard diagnostic/prognostic tests in this disease, a basis of some clinical decisions and a necessary condition for publication in a major medical journal (more than 10 copies per cells were viewed as indicating a poor prognosis).[25] By contrast, the physicians seemed to know very little about the long-term consequences of the heavy chemotherapy to which they submitted some of their young patients. Some of the participants proposed to compare the long-term effects of several therapeutic protocols, but others pointed to the difficulty of enrolling a sufficient number of patients into a clinical trial, and to the existence of strong therapeutic preferences among the doctors.

In January 1988 the main event was the visit—organized by Pierre—of a delegation from the European branch of the American producer of IL-2 at the Cancer Foundation. The industry representatives were received by François, by the heads of the medical oncology and pediatric oncology wards, by Madeleine, Pierre, and Daniel, and by "our radiation therapist," Jacques. I was not invited. Pierre reported that the visit was cordial and ended in an agreement to collaborate in clinical trials of the American IL-2. Daniel returned to the laboratory in January 1988, following several months in the clinics, and resumed his experiments on the inhibition of LAK cells by interferon-stimulated adherent cells. At first Daniel had difficulty repeating his experiments. He attributed these difficulties to the occurrence of changes in the tumor cell lines used to test the cytotoxic activity of LAK cells (cell lines may change during long-term culture in the laboratory). Pierre knew other researchers who cultivated similar cell lines, and one of them supplied some cell lines that enabled Daniel to reproduce his earlier results. From then on, Daniel's work went smoothly. I volunteered to take over one, rather uninteresting, aspect of his investigation—the study of the kinetics of cell multiplication. This study occupied me through the spring and early summer, and I repeated parts of it into the next fall.

The kinetics studies had the advantage of being conducted mainly in the immunology laboratory. This was important, because when Daniel returned to work there was again a space problem in the human cell culture room. My work in the immunology laboratory put me in contact again with the news about recent findings in immunological research and the latest developments in Cancer Foundation politics. The latter were of interest. The director of the medical division of the Cancer Foundation resigned from his job in January 1988. In early 1988 François was nearly exclusively occupied with the hospital's affairs. At some point there were rumors that he had high hopes of becoming the new director of the medical division. At the same time, there were also rumors that an immunologist would be appointed as the head of another big French cancer treatment center. Immunology (or, more broadly, biomedical sciences) might, it seemed, move to the fore of the institutional structure of French oncology. Finally, however, the "revolution" did not happen—"traditional" clinicians were selected as directors in both institutions.

During the winter of 1987–88 the investigation of inhibition of LAK activity continued with the usual ups and downs of laboratory studies. Madeleine started collaborating with a researcher from the immunology lab, Robert. Their study was centered on a topic unrelated to IL-2: the expression of receptors on B cell lines. She obviously liked her work, got along well with Robert, and gained more confidence in her ability as a scientist. Her relations with Pierre and Daniel became more relaxed. Daniel was actively preparing for his postdoctoral studies in the United States, while Pierre became increasingly occupied at the pediatric oncology ward and spent less time in the hematology laboratory. His activity in the lab sharply increased, however, in the spring of 1988, close to the scheduled date of the first clinical trial of IL-2/LAK in neuroblastoma.

The First Clinical Trial: April–June 1988

The clinical trial of IL-2/LAK therapy in neuroblastoma started in April 1988. The aim of this trial was to give a last chance to patients who had relapsed after chemotherapy for stage IV neuroblastoma or who had not reacted to chemotherapy. For these children there was no alternative treatment. The trial was Pierre's near-exclusive responsibility. He and a doctor from the second participating hospital had written the therapeutic protocol and obtained approval from the representatives of the American firm. I learned later that the general outline and the goals of the protocol had been established by the bio-technology firm. The protocol was then submitted to the newly created ethics committee at the Cancer Foundation, which quickly approved the protocols for both the neuroblastoma trial and the future, con-stantly delayed, phase I trial of the French IL-2.[26] Pierre convincingly explained the theoretical grounds for the supposition that the IL-2/ LAK treatment might be successful in otherwise hopeless cases of ad-vanced (phase IV) neuroblastoma. The committee confirmed the prin-ciple that only patients for whom no other effective treatment was available should be included in the trials. It also scrutinized the in-formed consent forms and discussed the process of recruitment of pa-tients. By contrast, it did not discuss the technical aspects of the neu-roblastoma trial, perhaps because they were not considered to be within the committee's competence. The committee viewed the neu-roblastoma trial as an internal matter and did not discuss its place in the larger strategy of multicenter trials organized by an American bio-technology firm.[27]

The meeting of the ethics committee later gave rise to a small scan-dal. During a public debate organized soon afterward, one of the members of that committee, a philosopher, explained that whereas in some clinical trials (such as those using antidiabetic drugs) patients were given all the available information about their health status, the physicians who organized the Cancer Foundation IL-2 trial decided (unlike their North American colleagues) against explicitly informing patients that they had an incurable, terminal cancer. The philosopher's statement was not a criticism of the Foundation's doctors, but rather a comment on differences in accepted norms in different countries. Some physicians at the Cancer Foundation, however, viewed his re-marks as an unacceptable public disclosure of their private affairs. Weeks later Pierre continued to ask me: "Why couldn't your friend keep his mouth shut?"[28]

Pierre did not seem preoccupied by the ethical implications of the neuroblastoma trial, but he was worried about its technical and lo-gistical problems. Several days before the beginning of treatment of the first child (scheduled for the second week of April) there was a rush of febrile activity in the human cell culture laboratory. Daniel, Dominique, and I were mobilized under Pierre's guidance to prepare culture media, sterile plastic pockets in which the cells were to be cultivated, and the equipment necessary to test the cytotoxic activity of IL-2-activated cells. The Cancer Foundation hospital had no pediatric intensive care service, and children were scheduled to be treated by IL-2 and LAK in the intensive care ward of a nearby pediatric hospital, an additional complication in an already complicated clinical experiment. Joseph, who was to conduct the cytaphereses (separation of white blood cells), transferred one cytapheresis apparatus from the transfusion center he directed to the hospital where the children were to be treated. I learned that hematologists had limited experience of cytaphereses in children, and none whatever of IL-2/LAK treatment of pediatric patients.[29] Pierre explained to the parents of the first patient enrolled in the neuroblastoma trial that IL-2/LAK therapy was a new, experimental treatment with slim chances of success, but he did not mention that before this clinical trial IL-2 and LAK had never been injected into children. He was clearly relieved to hear that the first child treated by IL-2 and LAK at the second participating hospital was tolerating the new therapeutic approach reasonably well.

During the neuroblastoma IL-2/LAK trial the patient's white blood cells were activated with IL-2 in the test tube. Five days later the LAK cells were injected into the patient together with IL-2. Each child was scheduled to receive three cycles of injections, in accord with the original protocol developed by Rosenberg's group, followed by "consolidation treatment" with IL-2 alone. The necessity of rapidly preparing a large quantity of activated cells imposed a very stressful rhythm of work in the human cell culture room. Cells obtained through cytapheresis were brought to the hematology laboratory in the afternoon. They had to be put immediately into culture in plastic pockets together with IL-2 and tested for LAK activity (activity at day 0) and for lack of bacterial contamination. Activated cells were harvested at day 5, tested again for LAK activity and absence of bacteria, then injected into the patient. The first and last days of culture were thus times of intensive activity in the laboratory.

During the first cycle of LAK cell culture there was perceptible tension in the tissue culture room. Later, when Pierre and Daniel realized that the tissue culture equipment was working well, the cells multiplied and became activated as predicted, and no major disaster (such as massive contamination of the cultures) occurred during the preparation of LAK cells, the tension eased. The third LAK cell culture of the first patient was close to a routine task. The first two cytaphereses, then the injection of activated cells, Pierre affirmed, went fine, and although the child suffered from the side effects of IL-2 therapy, they were "no worse than expected." Both Daniel and Pierre were proud of the technical success of the culture of LAK cells.

The optimism of the first days was mitigated by the fact that the five-year-old patient developed an acute respiratory distress following the third injection of LAK cells. He was intubated (a tube was inserted into his trachea) and put under artificial ventilation. His respiratory status improved several days later, and, still intubated, he was transferred back to the Cancer Foundation hospital. Pierre was worried by this complication, but he believed that the child would improve soon, and he left for a long-overdue holiday with his family. Daniel was convinced that the first IL-2/LAK trial was a success. The respiratory accident, he explained, was predictable, and anyway it should be attributed to the child's poor general health status.

Pierre came back from vacation in a relatively optimistic frame of mind. He announced that the IL-2/LAK-treated child felt better, was no longer intubated, and had been sent home. There were also, he added, some signs of regression of the tumor. The second child in the neuroblastoma trial (a six-year-old) was scheduled to be treated in mid-May. The second IL-2/LAK trial generated less tension in the laboratory. The preparation of LAK cells was divided between Daniel, Pierre, and Dominique, with my occasional participation. It went even better than the first time. Daniel was particularly proud of the large number of well-activated, vigorous-looking LAK cells. The second child also developed a respiratory distress after the injection, but the news about the complication was received more calmly than in the first case. When Pierre told us several days later that the child was scheduled to be taken off the respirator, I assumed that he too would recover soon.

In June Daniel was very busy completing the last experiments necessary for writing an article on the inhibition of LAK activity by adherent cells. He hoped to start his work at the NIH during the summer. I helped him with some of his experiments and also worked on studies of cell multiplication. The central event in the hematology lab was the beginning of a new project: the culture of tumor infiltrating lymphocytes, conducted by Madeleine.[30] At first Madeleine was beset by technical problems, and all the cells died, but she believed that these problems would be overcome. Dominique continued to work part-time for Pierre, but Pierre himself was seldom seen at the lab. He spent nearly all his time with patients, and his center of interest shifted to the more

traditional preoccupations of a practicing physician: clinical trials conducted exclusively at the bedside. Pierre became involved in several
multicenter clinical trials of biologically active substances that stimulate the multiplication of blood cells (G-CSF, GM-CSF, erythropoietin).[31] Unlike the IL-2 trial, these trials studied biologically active substances that already had a marketing permit and were being tested in
the same way as other anticancer drugs, that is, through administration of various doses of the molecules, usually in combination with
other anticancer drugs. There were no basic researchers involved, no
complicated and unusual laboratory tests, and no expectation of dramatic results; the clinicians hoped at best to improve the results of
accepted chemotherapies.

One morning in late June I casually asked Dominique how the LAK-
treated children were doing. She was not sure, but she had heard rumors
that the second child had died from the consequences of his treatment.
I called Pierre, who confirmed the news and proposed that we have
lunch together. During lunch Pierre explained that he was so upset by
the child's death that he did not have the courage to discuss it with
other people in the laboratory. The child had died after a month of
severe respiratory distress and had been intubated the whole time. Pierre
added that the first child treated with IL-2/LAK was now dying in the
pediatric oncology ward of the Cancer Foundation. This development,
Pierre explained, added to his reluctance to discuss the neuroblastoma
trial. As to the reasons for the second child's death, Pierre blamed the
doctors at the intensive care unit, the Cancer Foundation staff, Daniel,
and himself. Pierre believed that this child was a victim of the success
of the system of LAK production at the Cancer Foundation. Pleased
with the efficiency of LAK cell production, and perhaps encouraged by
Rosenberg's affirmation that patients had to be "pushed to their limits"
if lasting therapeutic effects were to be obtained, Pierre had decided to
inject his patients with all the LAK cells generated in culture. The dose
might have been too high for a small child. One hypothesis was that
the excess of activated white cells clogged the patient's lungs and induced severe respiratory distress. Thanks to the growing technical expertise of the workers in the human cell culture laboratory, the LAK
cultures of the second child had been even better than the first; that is,
even more cells had been obtained in culture and injected, with the
result that the child suffered more severe pulmonary complications.
Children treated at a second hospital according to the same protocol
had also received a full dose of cultured LAK cells, but they

had not had respiratory complications. The staff at the other hospital had attributed the lack of such complications to better-quality intensive care service in their institution. But Pierre thought—or rather, feared—that the reason the children had not suffered from respiratory complications was probably that the activation of LAK cells at the other hospital was less efficient. Pierre was proud of his success in introducing technical innovations that increased the yield of active LAK cells; he was therefore particularly disturbed by the thought that the technical success might have been the direct cause of a clinical disaster.[32]

I was so distressed by Pierre's story that I radically departed from my role of "neutral observer" and accused him (as I see it now, entirely unjustly) of being a poor coordinator of the IL-2/LAK program. My outburst was probably an expression of anger at finding myself in what I perceived as a nearly impossible situation. The risk of failure is always present in clinical oncologists' work, and Pierre had numerous reasons to justify his decisions: the IL-2/LAK trial was a last-ditch effort to save terminally ill children who could not be treated by the more accepted but very risky autologous bone-marrow transplantation; pediatric oncologists were ready to take risks in an attempt to save a child, and the new therapy did not seem more dangerous (and in fact was not found to be riskier) than other therapies employed in such cases. I had no reasons of equivalent weight with which to justify my response. My duties in the laboratory were defined at that point as helping Daniel with his studies on inhibiting the generation of LAK activity in the test tube. I had no obligation whatever to take an active part in the clinical trial of IL-2/LAK in neuroblastoma, and such direct participation could not be justified by its importance for sociological observations. Nevertheless, I had been pleased to be invited to take a very modest part in the first clinical trial of IL-2/LAK at the Cancer Foundation, and I had shared the initial fears of "technical breakdown," then the feeling of triumph when "beautiful LAK cells" were obtained. The disastrous effects of the clinical application of these "beautiful cells" left me confused: I was not sure any more what I was doing at the Cancer Foundation or why I was there. I went back to the laboratory, finished my experiments, then decided to halt my "participant observation" at least until the end of the summer vacation.

Interlude: IL-2 Trials Abroad

From 1987 through 1990 I made several short trips to observe clinical trials of IL-2 in Israel and the United States. In 1987–88 I observed two trials in Israel. The first was a multicenter trial sponsored by an American biotechnology firm and conducted in a big teaching hospital. It tested the combined effects of IL-2 and chemotherapy. The physicians there explained that they were not interested in LAK cells, because this approach was too expensive to be seriously considered for routine cancer therapy in Israel. Immunologists and clinicians collaborated closely in the IL-2/chemotherapy clinical trial. Their collaboration was, however, less central to their professional strategies than the collaboration between the physicians and scientists participating in the Cancer Foundation's trial. Cooperation between clinical oncologists and scientists was a rule, not an exception, in the Israeli teaching hospital and was viewed by doctors and scientists alike as a routine way of improving their professional status. The IL-2 trial was only one of several collaborative programs under way in the oncology department, and it was not considered the most important.

The IL-2 trial was far from being unanimously hailed by clinicians and scientists. One of the senior scientists at the medical school did not conceal his skepticism about IL-2 therapy. He viewed its clinical results as, at best, marginally significant, and no better than those of earlier attempts at cancer immunotherapy. He also did not believe that the results of IL-2 therapy would be improved in the future. This scientist, however, did not oppose the IL-2 trial, because, as he put it, "young people need to learn from their own experience." In contrast, the scientist responsible for immunological studies in the IL-2 project believed that the efficacy of IL-2 therapy could be increased by finding the right combination of IL-2, drugs, and possibly other lymphokines. He showed me impressive experimental results obtained in tumor-carrying mice treated with a combination of anticancer drugs and IL-2, but he warned against extrapolating from these results to human cancer, because "nearly anything can cure a cancer in a mouse." A surgeon who worked in Rosenberg's group at NIH and who was involved in the clinical studies of IL-2 was the most enthusiastic supporter of the new therapy in the teaching hospital. He told me that if only the people who had doubts about the efficacy of IL-2/LAK treatment were able to *see* the tumors disappear (as he had), they would immediately change their minds.

In Israel I observed an entirely different clinical experimentation with IL-2. Researchers working in the cancer ward of a general hospital had employed IL-2 in small-scale clinical trials since the early 1980s. They injected semipurified IL-2 secreted by stimulated lymphocytes (the experiment was made before recombinant IL-2 became available) directly into tumors and affirmed that they obtained a reduction of the tumor mass. Clinical trials of IL-2, LAK, and TILs continued at that hospital in the late 1980s mainly thanks to the obstinacy of a single researcher in the hematology laboratory. The hematology lab had limited funds for research and no arrangements for large-scale human cell culture, but that researcher, a gifted "tinkerer" in cell culture, had used discarded culture medium bottles and other recycled materials to produce first LAK cells, then TILs. These cells were later employed in clinical trials conducted in collaboration with a small number of interested oncologists. Those trials had no "official" status, and their organizers had difficulty obtaining recombinant IL-2. Consequently, patients received roughly the same doses of LAK cells or TILs as Rosenberg's patients did, but much lower doses of IL-2.[33] There was no fixed therapeutic protocol, and the quantity of cells and of IL-2 injected into each patient depended on the availability of activated cells and of IL-2 and on the clinical judgment of the physician responsible for the treatment of a given patient. This "low-tech" style of LAK and TIL therapy seemed to work: the response rates obtained were similar to those obtained in large multicenter trials (20–25 percent tumor regression in selected malignancies), while the undesirable effects of the treatment were, the doctors claimed, much milder, thanks to lower concentrations of IL-2. On the other hand, results obtained through local tinkering were probably more difficult to publish and to export to different settings.

I observed three clinical trials of IL-2 in the United States. In 1987 I followed a trial, introduced by one of the leading specialists at a big cancer treatment center, that studied the effects of IL-2 alone, of IL-2 with beta interferon, and of IL-2 with cytotoxic drugs. The doses of IL-2 were much lower than those employed by Rosenberg's group, and most of the patients were treated on an outpatient basis. The trial included studies of selected "biological activities" of the patients' lymphocytes, but it was not viewed as an occasion for formal collaboration with scientists. In fact direct contact between scientists and clinicians was replaced by dialogue with a computer. Each doctor who enrolled a patient in the trial was able to obtain all the results of the patient's biological tests (laboratory tests measuring the activation of white blood cells by IL-2, such as increase in the number of lymphocytes in circulating blood, increase in LAK activity, changes in distribution of subgroups of T cells) through a shared computer network (access to the network was restricted by security codes to protect the patient's privacy). The clinical results of that trial were akin to those obtained by Rosenberg's method: regression of the tumor was observed in 15 to 25 percent of eligible patients.[34]

The IL-2 trial was conducted by a senior oncologist, but most of the practical coordination tasks were carried out by a research nurse (a former oncology nurse who had "burned out"). The coordinating nurse played a central role: she informed patients about the scientific background of the therapy and its possible side effects, was responsible for the administration of IL-2 and other substances, collected blood samples for biological tests and delivered them to the laboratory, and finally centralized the results of all the tests (both biological and clinical), making sure they were accessible on the computer network. During her work as the coordinator of the IL-2 trial, she became very knowledgeable about its technical aspects (in particular the secondary effects of the therapy and how to deal with them), but in talking to me she stressed the role of interleukin therapy in giving hope to desperate patients. Both she and the physician responsible for the trial explained that there were sufficient clinical experiments in their institution (at that time, about 25) to allow nearly every patient to be eligible to enroll in a clinical experiment. A significant proportion of the center's patients had sought help here after being told by their physicians that nothing more could be done for them. They felt abandoned by the medical profession, and their participation in a clinical trial was perceived as a way to overcome their frustration and anger.

The role of clinical trials as a coping mechanism was even more evident in the oncology department of a big medical school I visited in 1990. This middle-sized department was participating in 97 multicenter clinical trials of new therapies for cancer. Two of these included IL-2 (one in combination with alpha interferon, the other in combination with a traditional cytotoxic drug). Four more included interferon. A complete list of these clinical trials was printed on yellow index cards distributed to all the center's physicians. Each time physicians faced a patient suffering from a tumor for which no effective therapy existed, they were invited to consult the list to see if that patient was eligible for one of the trials. As a rule, the center's oncologists explained, each patient was found to be eligible for at least one clinical trial. Doctors who enrolled patients in clinical trials were also responsible for obtaining trial-related data; that is, they made the relevant clinical observations and made sure that patients' blood was collected at prescribed intervals and was delivered to the laboratory.

Later the doctors transcribed the clinical data and the laboratory data on follow-up sheets and sent them to the trial coordinators. Debates on the results of clinical trials were conducted in meetings of collaborative groups of specialists, usually divided according to medical subspecialty. The IL-2 trials lost all singularity in that hospital; they became only numbers in a long list of ongoing clinical experiments.

In 1988 I found that another oncology department in a major American medical school had a different attitude toward clinical trials of IL-2. These trials were recommended by some physicians, while other specialists were skeptical about their utility. The department was not at that time participating in a multicenter trial of IL-2, but physicians interested in the therapeutic effects of interleukin were able to join IL-2 distributing networks individually and to obtain the molecule for their patients. Both the advocates and the opponents of IL-2 therapy (there were no attempts to use LAK cells or TILs) saw the method as a pragmatic approach to the treatment of selected cancers, and judged it according to their perception of its (current) clinical efficacy. There were no systematic investigations of the biological activity of lymphocytes in patients treated with IL-2. The advocates of IL-2 therapy also believed that biological tests were expensive, time-consuming, and unproductive of new information, and that the need to perform frequent blood tests exacerbated the already hard plight of cancer patients. The exclusively pragmatic perception of IL-2 therapy and absence of research on the physiological effects of interleukin were not typical for that research-oriented oncology department. They probably reflected contingent local conditions. The department's leaders were not interested in immunotherapy, but they were involved in experimentation with antitumor drugs. Consequently, they did not collaborate with immunologists, but with other groups of scientists (biochemists, pharmacologists, cell biologists). Collaboration with the laboratory was viewed as part of the regular duties of an oncologist working in a teaching hospital.

Phase I Clinical Trials of French IL-2

Back in Paris in September 1988, I found that Daniel had been replaced by a Chinese doctor, Hoang, who had come to France to be trained as an immunologist. Hoang's task was to expand Daniel's studies on the inhibition of LAK formation by adherent white blood cells.

Though not well acquainted with cellular immunology and handi-capped by her limited knowledge of both French and English, she had a pleasant personality, learned quickly, and was an able laboratory worker. She also had a keen sense of humor, knew what she wanted, and was not easily bullied. François and Madeleine seemed slightly disappointed to discover that Hoang did not correspond to the ster-eotype of a workaholic oriental scientist. She intended to enjoy her stay in France, and she had little inclination to spend all her evenings and weekends in the laboratory.

Pierre came occasionally to the lab and maintained some small re-search projects, but he quietly abandoned his plans to be simulta-neously a pediatric oncologist and a half-time basic researcher. The neuroblastoma IL-2/LAK trial continued, and two more children were enrolled in the fall; Hoang helped Pierre prepare their LAK cells. Pierre supervised the IL-2/LAK therapy closely and controlled the number of activated cells injected into LAK-treated children. There were no major treatment-related complications, but no promising clinical re-sults either. The same was true for the children treated at the other participating hospital. A new technician, Bernard, joined the IL-2 pro-ject to help Madeleine with TIL cultures. His arrival made the space problem in the human cells tissue culture room even more acute.

Phase I of the French IL-2 trial started in the fall of 1988, a year and a half later than initially planned, and was conducted simulta-neously at the Cancer Foundation and another cancer treatment cen-ter.[35] Clinical trials of a new drug start with phase I tests, which de-termine the dose that can be safely administered to patients. During this phase it is necessary to test several concentrations of a given sub-stance, and to obtain statistically valid results each concentration must be tested on several patients. IL-2 was scheduled to be tested in pa-tients suffering from relatively infrequent tumors—melanoma and re-nal cell carcinoma. The industry representatives, who were already well behind their own schedule and who aspired to move forward fast, were interested in enlarging the trial to include another cancer treat-ment center in order to accelerate the enrollment of eligible patients. They persuaded that center and the Cancer Foundation to collaborate during phase I trials of IL-2.

Clinical trials of IL-2 were conducted at the Foundation's medical oncology ward. At first there was strictly nothing to report: the pa-tients received increasing doses of IL-2, but when they reached the doses at which, according to the experience of the American producer of IL-2, interleukin-treated individuals should start to suffer from toxic effects of the molecule, nothing happened. The patients, hospitalized in intensive care and closely monitored for physiological changes, felt well, looked bored, and did not understand the reason for all the fuss. The physicians from the medical oncology ward, who, Pierre affirmed, at first were not very interested in the IL-2 trial, joked that they were probably injecting saline solution into their patients.[36] In late November 1988, something did happen: the patients who had received higher doses of IL-2 started to demonstrate the expected physiological symptoms (fever, shivering, edema, digestive problems). Moreover, the tumors of some of those patients showed signs of shrinking. In December the physicians at the medical oncology ward underwent, in Pierre's words, a "true conversion." Former skeptics, they were transformed into "true believers" and enthusiastic supporters of the IL-2 trial.

In mid-November 1988 an international conference on IL-2 and LAK in cancer treatment summed up the results of European multicenter trials. The person responsible for the clinical trial of neuroblastoma presented the early results. He explained that no antitumor effects were observed, but he also claimed that the trial demonstrated that, if handled properly, IL-2/LAK treatment was safe in children. True, in one of the centers there had been two cases (out of four) of severe respiratory distress, one of them fatal; but in the seven cases at the other center (his own), there had been no such troubles. He blamed the problem on the inadequacy of the intensive care unit in one of the participating centers. Pierre was not very happy with this presentation but did not wish to attract undue attention to possible shortcomings of the Cancer Foundation trial, and anyway the blame was put mainly on the staff of the intensive care unit at a different hospital.[37]

The results of European multicenter trials of IL-2 roughly confirmed Rosenberg's results (20–25 percent responses in melanoma and in renal cell carcinoma), with two important exceptions: first, unlike the responses obtained by Rosenberg, which included a low but significant number of complete remissions, nearly all the antitumor responses in Europe were partial remissions; and second, the addition of LAK to IL-2 did not improve the clinical results of IL-2 therapy. Rosenberg, who was present at the conference, suggested that European investigators had obtained very few complete, long-term remissions because their therapeutic protocols were not aggressive enough. European patients had received continuous infusions of IL-2, whereas Rosenberg's patients had received single-dose injections. Continuous infusion, some researchers believed, reduced the side effects of IL-2, but bolus injection allowed the administration of higher doses of interleukin. A few days later, in a talk at the Cancer Foundation, Rosenberg restated his belief that only an aggressive approach to IL-2 therapy might lead to cures. He was convinced that the therapeutic activity and the toxicity of IL-2 were directly associated, and it was therefore pointless to look for conditions in which the IL-2 treatment would be less toxic. The leitmotif of Rosenberg's talk was that one should adopt a "heroic" approach and abandon the fear of undesirable effects of IL-2 therapy, because "the most toxic thing for a cancer patient is his/her cancer."

In December 1988 the American producers of IL-2 and the French Cancer Society organized a symposium on IL-2 and cancer therapy. Most of the papers presented discussed the scientific aspects of lymphocyte activation by IL-2. There were also several clinical reports, including an optimistic account of the first French clinical trial of IL-2 therapy in renal cell carcinoma. The head of the European office of the American biotechnology firm summed up the results of the recent international conference, emphasizing positive trends. An invited guest, Dr. Robert Oldham (formerly the head of the NCI's Biological Response Modifiers Program, and in 1988 one of the directors of Biotherapeutic), painted an enthusiastic picture of the future of biological therapies of cancer. He proposed that BRMs were not "immunotherapy" but a radically new approach to cancer treatment. French immunologists in the audience disagreed. Several of their papers stressed that the therapeutic use of interleukin was a striking example of direct (and successful) application of fundamental immunological knowledge to the clinic, and that the visible antitumor effects of IL-2 demonstrated the importance of immunological mechanisms in curing cancer. The only truly discordant note in the meeting was a report made by a Belgian physician who reported complications of IL-2 therapy in his ward, including two cases of severe and irreversible neurological symptoms (one patient remained for a long time in a coma; another was moved to a psychiatric hospital). The Belgian doctor's conclusion was that the price for the short-term improvement sometimes obtained by IL-2 therapy was perhaps too high. His talk was received with silence, with the sole exception of an approving comment from a French oncologist who added that IL-2 might repeat the interferon story: a putative "miracle drug" that finally found only limited use in cancer treatment. Nobody reacted, and Pierre, who was seated near me, whispered that the French doctor would certainly get into trouble at his hospital.

In December Pierre invited me to participate in a meeting with Joseph and with hematologists who worked in the Cancer Foundation's blood bank. The meeting was called by François in order to discuss the introduction of LAK therapy into the treatment of renal cell carcinoma at the Cancer Foundation. Several reports proposed that the addition of LAK to the IL-2 treatment in renal cell carcinoma increased the chances of achieving a complete remission. François was interested in testing that proposal, the more so because the introduction of LAK therapy could justify earlier (and important) investments in cell-culture equipment. In addition, clinical trials of LAK therapy might offer an opportunity to test the hypothesis (based on Daniel's and Hoang's work) that the elimination of adherent white blood cells would increase the efficacy of LAK cells. François hoped to convince the Foundation's blood bank specialists to perform the cytaphereses of patients scheduled to be treated with IL-2 and LAK cells at the Foundation. Joseph offered to help them with equipment and advice. The Cancer Foundation blood bank experts flatly refused to be involved in the LAK project. They viewed it as an uninteresting and unrewarding increase of their work load. Both they and François became angry, and the meeting degenerated into an unpleasant confrontation.

After Christmas vacation Pierre asked to meet me for lunch outside the Foundation. I discovered that I had unintentionally caused him trouble: after the meeting with the blood bank people, François had reproached him harshly for inviting me to be present at that meeting without first asking François's permission. The incident did not seem to me to be very serious: François was known to have occasional fits of temper, but his coworkers claimed that they seldom led to further complications. Pierre, however, was troubled; he thought that the outburst of anger was a symptom of François's negative attitude toward him. Indeed, at that point Pierre was not indispensable to François's plans: he had not developed an independent research program, the neuroblastoma clinical trial was not a success, and the human tissue culture room could function with a staff of technicians only (mainly, Pierre stressed, thanks to his own efforts the previous year). François's center of interest had shifted to IL-2 trials in adults conducted in the medical oncology ward, and to collaboration with physicians on that ward. Space was a problem too: two new research technicians were to soon join the IL-2 project. One technician was paid by the French pharmaceutical firm to study the toxicity of French IL-2; the other was supported by a cancer charity as part of its contribution to IL-2 studies.[38] There was no space in the human tissue culture room for part-time workers—either for me or for Pierre. Pierre's recommendation was to take into account the new configuration and to put an end to my participation in the IL-2 project. I was not inclined to take Pierre's advice, and preferred to stick to my original project of following the IL-2 therapy to its routine or near-routine integration into the clinic, or alternatively to its dismissal. But Pierre rightly pointed to the effects of recent changes in the IL-2 project on my status within the trial. A renegotiation of the conditions of my observation was indeed necessary.

In late January 1989, looking idly at a newspaper stand I noticed the cover of a leading French magazine: a bright yellow sun in a blue sky and above it a big headline: "Cancer—a new hope." Inside I discovered a 10-page story about the new, miraculous cancer cure currently being tested at the Cancer Foundation. The story was illustrated with color photographs: François (wearing a white laboratory coat, a rare sight) standing in front of an array of complicated scientific instruments, François together with the head of the medical oncology department near a patient's bed, Madeleine pointing to an open incubator full of tissue culture flasks. The first part of the article consisted of a synopsis of Rosenberg's method which stressed the pioneering role of the Cancer Foundation in bringing it to France, followed by a long interview with François about the future role of immunotherapy in cancer treatment. François was depicted as a daring scientist thanks to whom new, exciting developments in cancer therapy were now available to French cancer patients. The impression that the Cancer Foundation trial was a pioneering endeavor was conveyed through omission—François did not mention other clinical trials of IL-2 in France. The second part of the article was a "human interest" story about patients treated with IL-2 at the Cancer Foundation. Interleukin-treated patients were presented as "cures." One of them gave an enthusiastic account of his treatment, thanked the doctors who had "saved his life," and praised the wonderful progress of medical science. His declaration was illustrated with photos of a smiling patient surrounded in his bed by smiling doctors. Other patients were not interviewed, but several were described as persons who "made it."

I phoned my colleagues in the immunology laboratory to ask what they thought about the article. They described it as "excessive" and even "disgusting," but (unlike me) they were not particularly impressed. The most frequent comment was: "You know, that's the way François is." They regarded the entire episode as minor. They felt little interest in the clinical trials of IL-2, viewing them as François's private business. French basic scientists tend to view power struggles among doctors as "dirty," in contrast to the much "cleaner" (because better codified) competition among scientists. Those who worked at the immunology lab thought that if François was trying to obtain a powerful position in the medical milieu, he had no choice but to play according to a different set of rules. Self-promotion, they explained, may seem unsavory, but it may well pay off.[39]

The magazine article provoked a small tempest among the physicians and scientists involved in IL-2 trials in France. The relationship between François and the coordinator of the first French clinical trial of IL-2 cooled considerably. Other colleagues made ironic remarks about François's "publicity efforts." The other director (in a different center) of the phase I trial of French IL-2 reportedly said that his wife had been very impressed by the article and asked him why they did not try to do the same thing at his hospital. François commented later that the magazine article indeed became a turning point in his career. From that time on, he explained, he was obliged to function much more aggressively. But, he added, he became used to it.

The controversies around the magazine article slightly delayed the renegotiation of the conditions of my observations of the Cancer Foundation IL-2 trial. In mid-February 1989 I had a formal lunch appointment with François and Pierre. My principal goal was to obtain access to meetings of the newly established official IL-2 group. During these meetings scientists and technicians from the immunology and hematology labs gathered with physicians from the medical oncology and pediatric oncology departments (the latter was represented by Pierre) and discussed, among other things, the clinical status of patients treated with IL-2. Agreement to my participation in these meetings was not something I could take for granted. Physicians who discuss their patients often do not welcome outside observers. In addition, I had the impression that François was annoyed with my presence at the Foundation. Indeed, during the lunch François first complained that I had not fulfilled my part of our agreement. He had believed that I would become more involved in immunological research. I pointed out that I had clearly stated my goals when I first entered the laboratory (or at least I believed I had). I had come to the Cancer Foundation to do sociological research, not to return to basic immunological studies. I apologized, however, for unintentionally making a misunderstanding possible. Finally François reluctantly agreed that as long as none of the other participants objected I could participate regularly in the meetings of the IL-2 group.

Phase II Clinical Trials: February 1989–June 1990

My observation of the later stage of IL-2 trials was different from my active participation in earlier stages. I now had a well-defined external status, manifested by the fact that I no longer wore a white coat. The meetings of the IL-2 group were held every Wednesday afternoon on neutral ground, in a study room adjacent to the Foundation's library. I was formally introduced by François (most of the participants knew me already) and made a short presentation of the aims and methods of my research. The participants listened politely and did not ask any questions. François proceeded to a vote—there was no opposition—and I was officially allowed to participate in the group's meetings. Although François insisted on a formal vote, I was convinced that before the meeting he had asked the opinion of the only person who could have raised serious objections to my presence, the physician responsible for the IL-2-treated patients, Georges. Georges often arrived late at the IL-2 meetings. He spoke little and usually left the presentation of clinical cases to an intern. Sometimes, in particular during debates on scientific topics, he seemed to doze. I was surprised to discover that Georges had already participated in numerous clinical trials of new drug therapies of cancer and had an impressive record of publications on the subject. We had limited contacts only. I had also little indirect information about Georges: he was an introverted person, was seldom seen on social occasions, and was not the subject of gossip among the people I knew at the Cancer Foundation. Other regular participants in the meetings of the IL-2 group were the radiologist, Jacques, who with the new research technician, Marie, studied the toxicity of IL-2 in mice; another research technician, Bernard, who together with Madeleine was responsible for the TIL cultures; Hoang, who continued to study the mechanisms of the inhibition of LAK formation by adherent cells; Cyrile, an additional research technician who measured receptors to IL-2 on lymphokine-activated cells and in patients' serum,[40] a study made in collaboration with a researcher from the immunology laboratory, Robert; the intern who took care of patients treated with IL-2 (first Annette, then Sandra); and Pierre, when he was able to free himself from his duties on the pediatric oncology ward. The hematology technicians Dominique and Chantal at first participated in the IL-2 group's meetings, but they rapidly gave up. There were also occasional visitors such as representatives of the pharmaceutical industry or collaborators in one of the projects related to the IL-2 trial.

The meetings of the IL-2 group had a fixed structure. François, always the self-appointed chairperson, sat at the head of the table, with Madeleine and Georges near him. The "leading trio" directed the meetings and steered all the important debates. It also guided the informal part of the meetings: the exchange of jokes and isolated bits of information and gossip. These informal exchanges, usually made at the beginning and end of each meeting, were an additional means of establishing hierarchy. They were led by François and were punctuated with occasional interventions by Madeleine and, more rarely, by Georges (who specialized in black humor). Other participants in the IL-2 group (perhaps with the exception of Pierre, who had an uncertain status) participated in these meetings mainly to report the results of their work to François, Georges, and Madeleine. Animated debates and sometimes even open conflicts occurred during these meetings, but I had the impression that important topics were discussed separately by the leading trio: after the "public" meetings of the IL-2 group Madeleine and Georges often went to François's office, and they also met separately before each important event, such as discussions with pharmaceutical industry representatives or debates with collaborators outside the Cancer Foundation. I had no access to these deliberations: Pierre, my privileged informant on events "at the top" in the previous phase of my research, was often excluded from important discussions.

The meetings of the IL-2 group lasted about two hours. They usually started with a presentation by Madeleine of the results of the patient's biological tests. Next Georges or an intern from the medical oncology ward provided information about the clinical status of IL-2-treated patients. The participants (mainly François and Madeleine) commented on possible correlations between biological and clinical findings. In the second part of the meeting other participants presented the results of their research during the past week. During the year and a half I observed it, the structure of the meeting changed in only one way: at first the scientific and clinical discussions occupied nearly equal time, but gradually the time spent on patients dwindled to only a small fraction of the meeting time, often taking up no more than 10–15 minutes of the two hours.

Laboratory studies discussed in the IL-2 group meeting were viewed as directly linked to the IL-2 clinical trial. In fact their relationship with the clinic was more complex than this. These investigations could be divided into two categories: studies that directly addressed trial-related questions, and those that were perceived as potentially interesting for clinicians. The first category included Jacques and Marie's research on the toxicity of IL-2 in mice and Madeleine and Bernard's efforts to cultivate TILs. The toxicity studies investigated IL-2-induced capillary leak, a problem of great importance for the management of IL-2-treated patients. The study was, however, made in mice, and it was not certain if the mouse was an adequate experimental model for studying IL-2 toxicity in humans. The culture of TIL was an essential part of a clinical project, but was probably closer to a service provided by the laboratory than to an autonomous research project. The second category included studies such as Annette's study on autologous mixed lymphocyte reaction (a reaction in which lymphocytes proliferate following a co-culture with other populations of lymphocytes) and Robert and Cyrile's work on the expression of IL-2 receptor and other proteins on the surface of lymphocytes. These investigations used biological materials (sera, cells) derived from patients enrolled in the IL-2 trial. It was reasonable to assume that correlations might be found between the clinical status of patients and biological data uncovered in these studies. During the time I observed the IL-2 clinical experiment, however, no such correlations were found, and laboratory studies centered on investigation of the physiological effects of high doses of IL-2 in patients. Finally, there was an intermediary category: studies that at first aimed more directly at clinical applications but, as the latter became problematic, shifted toward a more fundamental orientation. Hoang's research on the role of adherent cells in LAK inhibition typifies such investigations.

Hoang successfully replicated Daniel's results and started to look for a possible mechanism of the inhibition of development of LAK

cells. François immediately evoked the possibility of the practical utilization of the observation that LAK activity could not be suppressed
in the absence of adherent cells. He thought that LAK cells prepared
by separating the adherent cells (or monocytes) before the stimulation
of white blood cells by IL-2 might be more efficient in fighting tumors
in the body.[41] The IL-2 group discussed two ways to get rid of the
monocytes: a mechanical method—separation through centrifuga-
tion—and a chemical one—the elimination of monocytes by a chemical substance, the polymyristic ester (PME). At first François viewed
the mechanical method as a safer way to treat cells that would be
injected in patients. He even discussed with manufacturers of cytapheresis equipment the possibility of integrating a mechanical separation of monocytes into a routine process of cytapheresis. But the
mechanical method was complicated and not very efficient. Utilization
of PME was seen as simpler and cheaper, and François and Madeleine
selected that method to eliminate adherent cells.

Hoang began preliminary attempts to eliminate adherent cells with
PME during the first stage of LAK cell preparation. In the meantime,
the future of the Cancer Foundation LAK project became uncertain.
The latest results of clinical trials in other centers did not indicate that
there was a clear-cut advantage to IL-2/LAK treatment as compared
with IL-2 alone, not even in renal cell carcinoma. François and
Georges decided nevertheless to stick to their original plan and to treat
some renal cell carcinoma patients enrolled in the IL-2 trial with a
combination of IL-2 and LAK. Two patients were treated with LAK
cells in January 1990. The results were disappointing. The first patient
supported the LAK injection relatively well, but his clinical condition
did not improve, and his cancer continued to grow rapidly. The second
patient developed severe, life-threatening gastric bleeding in the aftermath of the injection of LAK cells. He was given steroids by frightened
interns who suspected an immune reaction—"graft versus host"
(GVH) reaction. François was very angry when he heard about the
interns' action. GVH reaction—a frequent complication of bone marrow grafts in which a patient receives bone marrow from a genetically
different donor—is the attack of grafted foreign white blood cells
against the host's organism. Steroids are the standard therapy administered to suppress that adverse immune reaction. But the patient
treated with LAK cells had received his own blood cells, and François
therefore saw no reason to suspect a GVH reaction, while steroids,

powerful suppressors of immune responses, were not the drugs one should administer to a patient undergoing an immunotherapy.

Two failures were certainly not enough to determine the validity of a therapeutic method. But the problematic results of the first adult LAK trials diminished the clinicians' already limited enthusiasm for that method. In addition, François's relationships with the Cancer Foundation blood bank experts continued to be uneasy,[42] while Georges had to face the resistance of intensive care unit nurses overwhelmed by the difficult task of monitoring LAK-treated patients. Although, as far as I know, no formal decision was taken, the LAK trials were postponed indefinitely. Hoang went back to her previous studies and focused on a search for the hypothetical LAK-inhibitory substance secreted by adherent cells. Her studies could now be classified in the second category: biological investigations that had potential to yield clinically relevant data.

In contrast, the attempts to cultivate TILs had a direct therapeutic goal. Rosenberg had affirmed that TILs were more efficient than LAK cells in eliminating disseminated tumors. In addition, he explained, patients who became refractory to treatment with IL-2 alone or IL-2 and LAK might still respond to TIL therapy: TIL could therefore become a "second chance treatment" for patients who no longer reacted to IL-2 therapy. Tumor infiltrating lymphocytes are isolated from tumors or tumor fragments. Chunks of tumors, I discovered, were sought by many researchers at the Cancer Foundation, while the distribution of that scarce item was controlled by surgeons. Madeleine was not among the surgeons' favorites and at first had difficulties obtaining tumor fragments for the TIL cultures.[43] TILs were also difficult to grow, and it took Bernard and Madeleine nearly eight months to develop a reliable culture system that made possible the regular production of large quantities.

The first injection of TILs was scheduled for February 1990. The weeks beforehand were fraught with suspense. It was indispensable to expand the TILs to at least 10^{10} injectable cells, and until the last moment it was uncertain that the goal could be met. Madeleine had invested a great amount of time and energy in the TILs project and was looking forward to an impressive clinical result, the more so because the TILs she and Bernard had obtained were very active in the test tube. The injection of the cells themselves went without a hitch, but the patient showed no signs of clinical improvement. In the second

TIL assay, the cells were even "better" (more cells were obtained, and they had stronger cytotoxic activity). The injection of TILs again went smoothly, but the patient's clinical status worsened after the treatment. Madeleine was very disappointed. She had been convinced that the second patient would show at least temporary improvement: his cells were so active! She did not give up the TIL project, but she lost much of her initial enthusiasm. In the meantime Bernard became interested in adapting the cell culture methods he had elaborated for the preparation of TILs to the culture of other cells such as tumor cell lines. TILs continued to be applied to selected patients but had lost their status of "miracle therapy."

The TIL and LAK experiences illustrate the influence of early clinical results on the fate of a new treatment. A physician may find it difficult to continue to recruit patients for a nonrandomized clinical trial that has begun with a series of failures (such as the Cancer Foundation's neuroblastoma trial). Conversely, the occurrence of a "miracle" (that is, impressive regression of an otherwise incurable disease) in early stages of a clinical trial may sustain enthusiasm for the new method regardless of later statistical evaluation. In both Rosenberg's IL-2/LAK trial and the Cancer Foundation's IL-2 trial a "miracle"—a complete and stable regression of a disseminated melanoma—was observed among the first patients treated by the new method, strengthening the doctors' determination to pursue this therapy.

The principal goal of the collaboration among the physicians and scientists in the IL-2 group at the Cancer Foundation was to find correlations between the biological data (the activation of specific subgroups of lymphocytes by IL-2) and the clinical status of IL-2-treated patients. Most of the patients did not respond to IL-2. An efficient preselection of "responsive" patients could save time and money and reduce patients' suffering. The participants in the IL-2 clinical experiment at the Cancer Foundation assumed that "responsive" patients could be identified through their "biological response profile," that is, a specific pattern of white blood cell response to IL-2. In order to uncover such a profile, it was indispensable, they believed, to test the patient's blood for the presence of activated cells at the beginning and end of each treatment cycle. Madeleine frequently complained that nurses at the intensive care unit did not understand the importance of biological research and repeatedly forgot to provide the necessary blood samples. In addition, the staff often failed to take a blood sample at the end of a cycle of treatment. Madeleine fought hard for the adoption of a rule that IL-2-treated patients would be allowed to leave the hospital only after the last blood sample had been collected. Since treatment cycles usually ended late in the evening, and it was sometimes difficult to find a nurse willing to draw blood then, this rule sometimes made it necessary to keep patients in the hospital for an additional day or even through the weekend.

In 1986, when Cancer Foundation scientists and doctors first discussed the introduction of IL-2 to cancer therapy, the goal to correlate the stimulation of specific subgroups of white blood cells by IL-2 with clinical findings (the shrinking of tumors) seemed perfectly straightforward. Two and half years later, when they started phase II trials of IL-2 in adults, it seemed less so. At that point the Foundation's researchers were familiar with the failure to find correlations between results of biological tests and clinical data: no one was able to demonstrate a clear-cut relationship between the size of a specific subpopulation of lymphocytes and the antitumor effects of IL-2. Some clinicians abandoned the search for correlations. Nevertheless, the Foundation researchers maintained their conviction that a direct causal link must exist between the IL-2 molecule's antitumor effect and selective activation of subpopulations of lymphocytes able to destroy cancer cells, and that the identification of such a link was only a technical problem. High doses of IL-2 induce numerous physiological effects such as high fever, increased permeability of blood vessels (which induced edema), changes in the level of thyroid hormones, changes in blood pressure and the number of thrombocytes in the blood (the latter effect increased the probability of internal hemorrhages). These physiological effects were, however, invariably perceived by the organizers of the IL-2 trial as the "secondary effects" of interleukin—secondary, that is, to the molecule's primary (and therapeutic) effect, the activation of cytotoxic lymphocytes.

The researchers at the Cancer Foundation attempted to identify a "winning profile," that is, a pattern of biological response associated with good clinical response to IL-2 treatment. The dramatic disappearance of tumors observed during the phase I trial of the French IL-2 was often only a short-lived phenomenon. However, one patient, Ms. R., had undergone a nearly complete remission of her malignant melanoma and remained symptom-free for a long time (she was well in June 1990). Ms. R. became a token patient for the IL-2 trial and the iconic image of its success. Ms. R. had an unusual distribution of subpopulations of lymphocytes. Biological profiles of all other patients in the trial were therefore carefully screened for their similarities to the "R. pattern." However, the association between "R. pattern" and good clinical response was not confirmed. About a quarter of the patients had a clinical response to the interleukin treatment (usually a short-term one), but it was not possible to define a clear-cut "responder" biological profile. Nevertheless François, Madeleine, and Georges continued to describe their patients as "good" or "poor" biological responders, and were pleased when they found that a given patient had a "good biological response."[44]

In March 1990 François and Madeleine announced that they believed they held the key to the puzzle of biological response. Other researchers, they explained, were looking for a correlation between the peak of the response to IL-2 (that is, the number of LAK cells in the blood at the end of a single cycle of IL-2 treatment) and the clinical response to IL-2. They became convinced, however, that the decisive element was not the absolute size of the biological response but its persistence. Rather than pay attention to the peak of biological response to IL-2, it was necessary to look for the continuation of response at the beginning (day 0) of the next cycle of treatment (usually nine days after the interruption of administration of IL-2). Patients who maintained a reasonably high level of LAK response after nine days of "rest" were those who had better chances to show a clinical response to IL-2. François calculated that this new rule had worked in five recent "responsive" patients. Later cases, however, failed to conform to the "persistence" pattern, and the new way of looking at the biological data was not transformed into a reliable predictive measure. In addition, data that had at first seemed to sustain the correlation between continuation of biological response to IL-2 and the clinical effects of IL-2 therapy were reevaluated later. Some of the patients first viewed as "responders" were later classified as "nonresponders" because their tumors expanded rapidly after a short period of regression, while some of the patients who were first viewed as "failures" were later classified as "stable disease" or as "partial response," that is, as partial successes of IL-2 treatment.[45]

From January 1989 through June 1990 approximately 40 patients were included in clinical trials of IL-2 at the Cancer Foundation. Most were enrolled in the phase II trial of French IL-2, which tested the effects of this molecule in melanoma and in renal cell carcinoma. Several patients were enrolled in multicenter trials of American IL-2 in melanoma and of American IL-2 and alpha interferon in renal cell carcinoma. In addition, a few patients who did not meet the official inclusion criteria were given IL-2 on a compassionate basis or as a favor to a colleague. In its meetings the IL-2 group closely followed the fate of patients treated with IL-2 and was well informed about every case of tumor regression following treatment. But it was difficult to learn what happened to patients once IL-2 therapy was over. Georges practically never volunteered information on that subject. Thus, in a case of short-term therapeutic success the IL-2 group heard detailed reports for several weeks on the patient's progress, but if the disease subsequently worsened, one usually heard about it only months later, and even then often by chance. The response rate to IL-2 at the Foundation was similar to that reported in other clinical trials: 20–25 percent positive responses, mostly short-term ones.[46] The practical meaning of these numbers was that there were a few "miracles," but that most of the patients classified as "responders" relapsed several weeks or several months later.[47]

At first I was puzzled that the clinicians did not seem dissatisfied by the clinical results. The side effects of IL-2 included most of the usual effects of drug therapy for cancer: fever, diarrhea, fatigue, and nausea. But IL-2 therapy also induced more severe complications, such as cardiovascular perturbations and temporary dementia. The latter complication was particularly frightening for patients and their families. These side effects seemed to me a heavy price to pay for the clinical results of IL-2 therapy—with a few exceptions, at best a short-lived remission. Later I realized that my way of thinking differed from that of the medical oncologists. Oncologists frequently administered potent combinations of cytotoxic drugs that induced severe iatrogenic effects and usually brought limited clinical gains for patients suffering from disseminated cancer. IL-2 was not worse, and perhaps was even slightly better, than the aggressive chemotherapies that might have been proposed to many of the patients enrolled in the IL-2 trial. Moreover, the definition of acceptable side effects of a cancer treatment was dependent on a given doctor's personal outlook. The first intern who followed IL-2-treated patients, Annette, was a beginner in oncology. She provided dramatic accounts of the patient's sufferings and seemed uncomfortable with the instructions to continue the administration of IL-2 to patients who tolerated this treatment poorly. In contrast, the intern who replaced her later, Sandra, did not tell dramatic stories about the consequences of IL-2 treatment. I thought at first that the difference reflected the Foundation staff's improved ability to deal with the iatrogenic effects of IL-2. But this did not seem to be the case. Some of the side effects of IL-2 treatment, such as fever and nausea, were indeed better controlled in later trials, but the number of patients who dropped out in the middle of a treatment cycle because they could not stand the IL-2 therapy remained roughly the same. Later I learned from Sandra that before coming to the Cancer Foundation she had worked at a ward specialized in the treatment of leukemia with bone marrow grafts. The side effects of these grafts were at least as severe as, and sometimes more severe than, the effects of IL-2 therapy. Sandra's familiarity with iatrogenic effects of oncologists' intervention helped her to face with equanimity the consequences of IL-2 therapy.

The interest in links between the persistence of biological response at day 0 of the second cycle of IL-2 treatment and the patient's clinical reaction to that treatment was the last surge of enthusiasm I witnessed during the Cancer Foundation's IL-2 clinical trial. Biological tests measuring the cytotoxic activity of white blood cells in patients treated with IL-2 became just one of the numerous routine or semiroutine tests performed on patients' blood. The LAK cells were abandoned for the time being. Madeleine continued to perfect the culture of TILs, but this approach became only a rarely used variant of IL-2 therapy, itself partly routinized. The word "routinized" should not be misunderstood, however. IL-2 therapy remained an experimental treatment, submitted to all the restrictions of such therapeutic approaches. One might speak about the "routinization" of that therapy only in the sense of the loss of its special status as an unusual and exceptionally promising treatment, and its transformation into an experimental therapy of cancer among many others. Interleukin treatment continued to be proposed to eligible patients, but the organizers of the IL-2 trial did not hold their breath anymore.

In the spring of 1990 the IL-2 group's meetings were dedicated mainly to the analysis of scientific results obtained by various investigators. The liveliness of debates about these results contrasted with the nearly complete absence of discussions about patients. The IL-2 group gradually became mainly a group of immunologists and physicians who shared an interest in basic and preclinical immunological research. The participation in meetings of a group of scientists, even scientists studying biological materials derived from cancer patients, did not, I felt, advance research dedicated to the study of interactions between clinicians and biologists. The choice of the precise moment to end my observations at the Cancer Foundation—early July 1990—

was influenced by external considerations (the end of the school year, the slowdown of research activity during the summer, travel plans), but my decision to leave reflected my conviction that my observations at the Cancer Foundation had failed to bring to the fore new and interesting data.

Postscript, January 1993: The Disappearance of the Corridor

Halfway through the writing of this book I decided to discuss the IL-2 project once more with some of its organizers. After two and a half years of absence I returned to the Cancer Foundation. I arranged a meeting with Madeleine, assuming that her office would be in the same place. When I crossed the immunology unit and headed to the corridor that had led to the hematology laboratory, I found myself unexpectedly among busy and noisy construction workers. The new hospital, until recently under construction, was now open. Its inauguration had led to important changes at the Cancer Foundation. All the rooms in the old hospital building, including the radiation therapy rooms along the corridor and the patients' waiting room at its end, had been transformed into laboratories. The hematology lab, I finally learned, had been temporarily moved to another building. That building—which had housed some of the less prestigious hospital wards—was also destined to be renovated and transformed into a laboratory complex. The original plan of the Foundation's directors was to encourage well-known biological research groups to join the Cancer Foundation. That plan, however, had been postponed because the French government, faithful to its decentralization policy, which encouraged the dispersion of research and teaching institutions, had vetoed the project to develop an important cluster of leading biological laboratories in the center of a big city.

The temporary rooms of the hematology laboratory were much bigger than the old ones. They were half-empty, dark, and without decoration. There were only a few technicians around, all wearing standard white laboratory coats. The laboratory, Madeleine explained, continued to participate in the IL-2 project. Previous clinical trials of IL-2, such as the trial of American IL-2 in kidney cancer and the phase II trial of French IL-2 in melanoma, had ended, with results similar to those obtained in the first year and a half. A new clinical trial was testing the effects in melanoma of therapy that combined either a drug (cisplatine) and IL-2 or IL-2 and alpha interferon. It was the first randomized trial of IL-2 therapy in melanoma in France. (A randomized trial of IL-2 in renal cell carcinoma—that is, a trial using internal, not historical, controls—had started in France a year earlier.) It was organized by the French Federation of Cancer Treating Centers, and theoretically all centers belonging to the federation could participate. In practice, however, the number of centers that tested biotherapies of cancer in France had been restricted through direct intervention by the French Ministry of Health. A newly created "biotherapy committee," which distributed government funds for clinical trials of new biotherapies of cancer, had decided that only four leading cancer treatment centers would receive such funds. All the centers selected to test biological products had already conducted clinical trials of biotherapies of cancer. The government decision thus made official a preexisting situation.[48] In order to conform to the more stringent norms of control over Health Ministry funds and to maintain contact with the "biotherapy committee," the Cancer Foundation had created its own "biotherapy commission," headed by François. François had also become the head of a "biotherapy unit," an internal collaborative structure that coordinated all the biotherapy trials conducted by the Foundation's physicians and scientists.

In 1990 and 1991 the Cancer Foundation specialists tested a non-randomized therapeutic protocol according to which melanoma patients received high doses of IL-2 alone for two weeks. The clinical results obtained with that protocol were similar to those obtained in earlier phases of the IL-2 project. The newest attempt to improve IL-2 therapy for melanoma, the IL-2/cisplatine protocol, had been introduced in the summer of 1992. It was too early, Madeleine explained, to evaluate the clinical results. The new protocol included certain biological tests: the survey of surface markers of patients' lymphocytes and the systematic measurement of the levels of soluble IL-2 receptors in their serum. Studies of the cytotoxic activity of the patients' lymphocytes (LAK activity, NK activity), central to the earlier efforts to correlate biological activity with clinical activity, had been abandoned. The IL-2 employed in the melanoma trial was bought from its American producer, but the pharmaceutical firm was not actively involved in the trial and was viewed solely as a supplier of an active—and expensive—drug. Madeleine was also participating in a clinical trial of IL-2/TIL therapy in renal cell carcinoma. This trial employed the French IL-2 and was conducted in a different hospital. Madeleine and her collaborators prepared TILs from tumors of all the patients who underwent surgery for renal cell carcinoma, then froze them and waited for future developments. Patients who developed metastatic disease were treated with IL-2, and if they reacted to interleukin, they were later injected with their own TILs. Up to this moment, Madeleine had prepared TILs from about 20 patients, and 4 of these patients had been inoculated with their cells. Here too it was too early, she explained, to estimate if TIL therapy was effective. In the meantime, in late 1992 the French TIL trial had benefited from press coverage reminiscent of the coverage of the IL-2 trial three years earlier. TILs were described as efficient weapons against malignancy which might (and probably would) lead to a "vaccine against cancer."

The low, noisy, overcrowded, and brightly lit rooms of the immunology laboratory contrasted with the high, silent, and partly empty rooms of the hematology lab. The immunology laboratory looked exactly as I remembered it, but in fact the impression of continuity was entirely misleading. My colleagues explained that radical changes were imminent. In a few months the laboratory would move to new, more spacious rooms in the old hospital building. The immunology laboratory would be lodged near the clinical laboratories, also headed by François. The important news was that François had recently been appointed director of a newly created Clinical Biology Division.[49] The new division was the culmination of a long-standing project of some of the Foundation's directors, a project that coincided with François's aspirations. The Clinical Biology Division would include all the Foundation's clinic-oriented "service" laboratories (hematology, pathology, cytology, clinical immunology).[50] Under the new arrangements, Madeleine's laboratory would officially be supervised by François. In addition, the main focus of research in the hematology laboratory, a new subunit dedicated to the study of immunological reactions in cancer patients, was soon to become an autonomous laboratory. The Foundation's directors hoped that later the Clinical Biology Division would also include research laboratories that would use the latest techniques in biological investigation to study biological materials (blood, secretions, solid tissues) collected from the Cancer Foundation's patients.

My colleagues at the immunology laboratory stressed that it would continue its research-centered orientation and would be only marginally involved in clinical studies. On the other hand, it was already involved in an important collaborative project with industry: the development of a semiautonomous unit dedicated to biological research with potential industrial applications. The new unit (directed by Robert) would be considered part of the immunology laboratory but would be financed entirely by pharmaceutical firms. The relationship between the new unit and the immunology lab was to be modeled on the relationship between the immunology laboratory and the IL-2 project. Geographic proximity was expected to generate occasional collaborations, but each entity would preserve its autonomy and its distinct domain of activity.

I was impressed by François's success in obtaining the direction of the Clinical Biology Division, an additional step toward his goal to "biologize" cancer clinics and to promote investigations that would translate clinical questions into biological ones, thus opening new avenues for research at the Cancer Foundation.[51] During the last three years François's ability to negotiate directly with politically powerful people and with important industrial partners had greatly increased. Although his projects to develop preclinical and industrial research at the Cancer Foundation were just starting, he had already firmly established himself as an important player in France's "big biomedical science." François's new position reflected the growing importance of laboratory studies at the Cancer Foundation's hospital.[52] The new spatial arrangement at the Cancer Foundation also mirrored that change. The new status of laboratories in that institution was directly reflected in the fate of the corridor that had previously linked the research building with the cancer hospital. The corridor, which exemplified for me invisible boundaries between the distinct social worlds of scientific research and cancer therapy, had been transformed into a small segment of a big new laboratory complex that would gather together under one roof routine analysis laboratories, research laboratories, and laboratories dedicated to preclinical and industrial research.

CHAPTER FIVE

Making the IL-2 Trial Work: Professional Cultures, Jurisdictions, and Practices

Frameworks: IL-2 as "Immunotherapy" or "Anticancer Drug"

The Cancer Foundation's IL-2 trial was defined—as Dr. Steven Rosenberg's original study had been—as an attempt at "immunotherapy of cancer."[1] The definition of IL-2 treatment as immunotherapy played a central role in the Foundation's trial, initiated by immunologists. That definition, however, was not shared by all researchers who organized clinical trials of IL-2. Consent forms given to patients enrolled in some clinical trials of IL-2 presented interleukin-2 as a new anticancer drug. For example, a consent form for a 1989 phase I study of sequential administration of recombinant IL-2 and recombinant TNF (tumor necrotic factor) at the Fox Chase Cancer Center in Philadelphia explained that "drugs used to treat cancer often have side effects. The drugs used in this program may cause all, some, or none of the side effects listed." The consent form did not supply any explanation of the unusual character of this "drug."[2]

The perception of IL-2 as a drug was consistent with the practical uses of the new therapy. Patients treated with IL-2 received highly toxic doses of interleukin and were "pushed" to the limits of their tolerance of the treatment, exactly like patients treated with intensive chemotherapy. The perception of IL-2 as a drug was also consistent with industrial strategies. Industrialists were not particularly interested in the demonstration that IL-2 activity is mediated by the activation of immune mechanisms. Their main interest was to show that IL-2, alone or with other products, had antitumor properties. An introduction to a multicenter protocol drafted by the American producer of IL-2 in 1987 started with the statement: "Interleukin-2 has a far reaching effect on the cells of the immune system *and* on the ability of the tumor-bearing host to resist neoplastic disease" (my emphasis). The careful wording of that statement eluded the question of whether there was a causal relation between the activation of cells of the immune system by IL-2 and the influence of the molecule on malignant tumors.

The claim that a direct causal link existed between the effect of IL-2 on the cells of the immune system and its antitumor activity was, however, central to the Cancer Foundation's IL-2 trial and to several other French trials of the molecule. Scientists who initiated and conducted the first clinical trials of IL-2 in France were either immunologists or physicians who had developed a strong interest in immunology.[3] The important contribution of immunologists to interleukin trials probably reflected the important role of immunology in the reorganization and modernization of French biomedical research.[4] In the 1970s French scientists were recognized internationally for their success in two practically oriented domains of biomedical inquiry: the introduction of tissue groups to kidney transplantation (by Jean Dausset and his collaborators) and immunotherapy of malignant tumors with bacterial vaccines such as BCG (by Georges Mathé and his collaborators).[5] Immunology became central to biomedical research in major French hospitals, and from the 1970s on, immunologists occupied many important positions in the French research establishment.[6] Hospital-based immunology laboratories, however, were dedicated mainly to basic and preclinical research. Immunologists sometimes collaborated with physicians (for example, in the 1960s transplanters and immunologists elaborated together the criteria of tissue compatibility and developed a kidney exchange organism, France-Transplant).[7] On the other hand, although immunologists were often physically present in the hospital—and frequently influential in its internal politics—they usually had limited contacts with the clinic.

Immunologists' efforts to initiate and develop clinical trials of interleukins in major cancer treatment centers may be viewed as a part of their attempts to consolidate the important role of immunology in the French medical establishment. The introduction of interleukins into cancer therapy, some immunologists believed, would modify the "professional landscape" of French oncology. But the replacement of Rosenberg's original protocol of adoptive immunotherapy using LAK cells with protocols using IL-2 alone restricted the definition of IL-2 therapy as immunotherapy in France. Some organizers of IL-2 clinical trials in France remained faithful to an immunological explanatory framework. Others developed a more pragmatic attitude, centered on the practical effects of IL-2 therapy, not on its theoretical background. The differences in these two approaches were reflected in the role of the immunological explanatory framework in shaping therapeutic protocols (for example, strict adherence to immunological explanations favored the proliferation of immunological tests in the laboratory) and influenced the interpretation of results of clinical experiments.

Two meetings dedicated to uses of IL-2 in oncology mirrored the changes in the perception of this treatment in France. The first meeting (December 1988) was organized by the French Association for Clinical Oncology, and the second (January 1990) by the American producer of IL-2. In 1988 few clinical trials of IL-2 were being conducted in France. The 1988 meeting was divided into two parts: the first was dedicated to basic and preclinical studies of the effects of interleukin-2 on the immune system, and the second to clinical trials of that molecule.[8] All the French speakers in the clinical segment of the meeting firmly located IL-2 therapy within the immunological paradigm and stressed the contribution of the new treatment to the establishment of immunotherapy as an alternative approach to the treatment of human malignancies.[9] In contrast, the 1990 meeting was dedicated exclusively to the clinical aspects of IL-2 therapy (in the meantime, IL-2 had been tested in several other French hospitals) and was not dominated by the immunological paradigm. Some of the talks in the 1990 meeting discussed the relationship between therapeutic effects of IL-2 (or their absence) and the effects of that molecule on the immune system, but numerous other papers—in particular those discussing the clinical management of IL-2-treated patients—presented IL-2 as an additional antitumor drug. These distinct framings of IL-2 therapy partly reflected divisions between institutions and between medical specialties. An immunological framework was usually emphasized in reports from institutions in which clinical trials of IL-2 were organized and conducted by immunologists, while it was played down in reports from institutions in which interleukins were tested by medical oncologists. But this rule was far from being rigid: local contingencies and investigators' personal preferences also influenced how IL-2 activity was viewed.

The dual framing of interleukin therapy as immunotherapy or anticancer drug was observable during the Cancer Foundation IL-2 trial. Because the immunology laboratory played a central role in the introduction of IL-2 to the clinics at the Cancer Foundation, the trial was strongly rooted in the immunological paradigm. The actual conduct of the trial, however, was not entirely restricted by that paradigm. Grant proposals and research reports written by the Foundation's researchers in 1986 and 1987 stressed the role of LAK cells in IL-2's antitumor activity. Cancer immunotherapy, François had explained in an early proposal, was a brilliant approach from the intellectual point of view, but up until then it had often been disappointing from the practical point of view. Recombinant lymphokines were "a revolutionary innovation" because these molecules "allow the stimulation of particularly important cells in the immune system, the LAK cells." By 1988, however, LAK cells had lost their central place in the IL-2 trial. Later grant proposals written by Cancer Foundation researchers no longer emphasized the innovative aspects of adoptive immunotherapy but instead stressed the therapeutic effects of IL-2.

Some of the collaborators (who were often, at the same time, direct competitors) in the Cancer Foundation IL-2 trial held different views of the importance of the immunological explanatory framework. The researcher who organized the first French clinical study of IL-2 and his coworkers attempted to explain all the clinical observations made during the IL-2 trial by modifications (stimulation or repression) in specific subpopulations of lymphocytes, in particular of the natural killer (NK) cells. The strong immunological orientation of one of the main competing groups stimulated efforts by the Foundation scientists to find immunological explanations for the phenomena observed in the clinics. On the other hand, the (comparatively) less rigid adherence of the Cancer Foundation's researchers to the immunological paradigm allowed them to present themselves as more "serious" researchers who were committed to open-minded interpretations of experimental data, not to dogmatic views and preconceived ideas. For example, in an IL-2 group meeting in November 1989 Pierre mentioned that another French group participating in clinical trials of IL-2 had concluded that a correlation existed between the ratio of cytotoxic T cells to NK cells and the reaction to IL-2 therapy, and added that the other group "was speculating on the basis of two cases. That's easy. We are also able to propose numerous speculative interpretations of our data."

By contrast, during a meeting in the spring of 1989 with Israeli investigators who had a more pragmatic approach to interleukin therapy, François and Madeleine insisted on the importance of their theoretical framework. An Israeli scientist explained that while he accepted the principle that the therapeutic effects of IL-2 were mediated by the immune system, "it will take at least ten years to unravel what is really going on in an interleukin-treated patient." Anyway, he added, "when we study immunological mechanisms, the more experiments we do, the less we understand."[10] He proposed making the system work first, rather than trying to find out why it worked. Rosenberg's method, another Israeli researcher affirmed, was in fact a clinical failure. However, he added, Rosenberg merited respect because he had persisted with his clinical experiment until he was able to demonstrate that IL-2/LAK therapy could affect chemoresistant tumors. François strongly disagreed. In his view, Rosenberg's greatest merit was to have provided definitive proof that stimulation of the immune system could have antitumor effects. François also occasionally stressed the difference between his attitude—stemming from sincere, long-standing faith in cancer immunotherapy—and the opportunistic behavior of some of his colleagues. Thus, François described one of the organizers of an IL-2 clinical trial in another French hospital as a "guy who in private always explains that IL-2 treatment has nothing special [to offer] and is not qualitatively different from routine chemotherapies of cancer, but is always eager to appear on TV and to talk about the latest breakthrough in the treatment of malignant disease: immunotherapies of cancer."

Resources: Negotiating with Industrial Sponsors

The project to test French IL-2 at the Cancer Foundation had strong governmental support. The Ministry of Industry encouraged the local production of recombinant, biologically active molecules, while the Health Ministry actively promoted collaboration between government-sponsored research laboratories and industry. The official agreement between the immunology laboratory (supported by INSERM), the Cancer Foundation hospital (a private, nonprofit foundation), and the French manufacturer of IL-2 was therefore hailed as an exemplary endeavor that paved the way for future developments in French biomedical research. Nevertheless, in the years 1987–1990 government agencies did not contribute directly to the funding of the Cancer Foundation IL-2 trial. Most funding for the trial came from industrial partners and cancer charities; additional expenses linked to clinical studies (beds in intensive care, additional nursing care, drugs that controlled the side effects of IL-2) were financed by the Cancer Foundation hospital's regular funds.[11]

The cancer charities did not play an important role in the shaping of the Cancer Foundation's IL-2 trial. The small size of the French oncological milieu and its close ties to cancer charities transformed the distribution of cancer charity funds into almost a family business. Leading researchers in prestigious cancer treatment centers who are at the same time main scientific advisers for the cancer charities often reach an unofficial (approximate) agreement on the distribution of funds among institutions and laboratories, then confirm this agreement in formal committee meetings. The contacts of the organizers of the IL-2 trial with the cancer charities were limited to occasional discussions with charity administrators and to the annual writing of grant proposals and research reports. By contrast, contacts with the French and American producers of IL-2 were frequent, sustained, sometimes difficult, and influential in the dynamics of the IL-2 trial.

The IL-2 trial started with a single, French industrial partner and with one source of interleukin. It also started with the tacit assumption by Cancer Foundation researchers that they were the sole clinical partners of the French industrialists. Both sides in the initial agreement probably wanted more independence and more flexibility. In the spring of 1987 François discussed the possibility of presenting the results of Daniel's studies in a meeting on lymphokines, and added that "we are not allowed to show our results without obtaining the agreement of our industrial collaborators. And anyway, they will be at the meeting." At the same time François stated, in a different context, that "if they [the French pharmaceutical firm] are not able to fulfill all our need . . . Well, we will look elsewhere. We are free, aren't we?"

The Cancer Foundation researchers indeed started to look elsewhere and negotiated with the American producer of IL-2. Pierre was worried that collaboration with a competing company might harm relations between the Foundation and the French producer. François, however, doubted that such a risk existed, because the French firm was legally obliged to collaborate with a cancer hospital to test its product, and the Cancer Foundation was the only French cancer treatment center sufficiently advanced with IL-2 studies to provide such a service.[12] In the spring of 1989 François and George accidentally discovered that the French pharmaceutical firm had developed contacts with other hospitals in several cities; several groups of physicians were simultaneously studying the effects of French IL-2 on cancer patients. After an initial reaction of surprise and uneasiness, the Cancer Foundation researchers adapted to the loss of their presumedly unique status.[13] They were comforted by the conviction that "their" trial was the only serious one: their competitors were merely adding IL-2 to a long list of substances administered to patients suffering from advanced cancer; in contrast, they were involved in an innovative attempt to understand the scientific basis of the new therapy, then to improve it.

In the fall of 1987 the Foundation's researchers started to use American IL-2 in addition to French IL-2. The decision was stimulated by the French pharmaceutical firm's difficulties in producing IL-2 and by the fear that another major French cancer treatment center—one allied with the American firm—would become the sole "owner" of the new treatment. It was also motivated by material considerations (the prospect of entering an existing multicenter trial, the likelihood of recruiting a sufficient number of patients, the existence of adequate material resources to implement the protocol at the Foundation) and explicitly by political considerations, including the progress of a given trial in a competing institution and the necessity of producing clinical results rapidly.

In 1987 and 1988 the Foundation's researchers participated simultaneously in several clinical trials that tested either the French or the American IL-2. In the fall of 1989 seven of these were under way: two trials (one with French and one with American IL-2) of IL-2 in melanoma, two (one each with French and American IL-2) in renal cell carcinoma, a phase I trial of French IL-2, and two pediatric trials with American IL-2. All these trials were small (most involved fewer than 10 patients); in 1988 and 1989, a total of approximately 50 patients were enrolled.

In 1987 and 1988 the competition between biotechnology firms did not play an important role in shaping therapeutic protocols. Moreover, the existence of parallel clinical experiments allowed for considerable flexibility in the management of individual patients. Physicians who participate in a clinical trial are asked to conform to rigid preestablished criteria of enrollment. Although the decisions to enroll patients in the IL-2 trial were made by the physician locally responsible for the trial, those decisions were reviewed by the trial organizers, who were authorized to reprimand—and nullify—improper enrollment.

This tight control over enrollment contrasted with the attitude toward decisions about the interruption of a given patient's treatment or ways of dealing with severe, life-threatening complications of therapy. The therapeutic protocols of both the French and American IL-2 clinical trials specified that these decisions were the exclusive responsibility of the oncologist directing the trial and were not subject to external scrutiny; they thus highlighted the importance of individual doctors' clinical judgment and therapeutic skills.

The coexistence of several similar clinical experiments in the same hospital enlarged the physicians' ability to make individual decisions based on their clinical skills. For example, it made possible the inclusion of a patient who did not fit the enrollment criteria of one trial's therapeutic protocol in a different trial. In a particularly telling case, a patient suffered from a severe iatrogenic complication (Quincke's edema) while treated with French IL-2.[14] Her therapy was immediately stopped, and, in accordance with the rules of the French IL-2 trial she was definitively excluded from that clinical experiment. Her doctors, however, believed that before the accident the patient's response to IL-2 had looked promising and that she should not be denied a last-chance attempt at a cure. They therefore decided to include her in the American IL-2 trial, omitting to inform its organizers that she had been excluded from the French trial following a severe iatrogenic effect of IL-2 treatment.[15]

In 1989 clinicians became more aware of the direct relationship between the choice of an industrial partner and the structure of a clinical trial. The debates preceding the adoption of the "consolidation" protocol of bone marrow grafts in children with IL-2 illustrate how competition between industrialists and conflicts among the doctors shaped experimentation in the clinic. The consolidation protocol followed the failed attempts to cure advanced neuroblastoma with IL-2 and LAK cells. The organizers of the neuroblastoma trial looked for different therapeutic uses of IL-2, aiming at improvement of the long-term effects of autologous bone marrow transplants (ABMT). Children over one year of age who suffer from advanced (stage IV) neuroblastoma generally have a poor prognosis. Recent studies proposed to treat such children first with usual chemotherapy (which induces an initial remission), then with high-dose chemotherapy (vincristine and melphalan) and total body irradiation—both aimed at destroying all the malignant cells in the body. Immediately after the intensive chemotherapy and radiation therapy the patient receives an autologous bone marrow transplant of marrow cells collected before irradiation/chemotherapy, to replace those destroyed by drugs and radiation. According to 1987 data, this therapeutic approach allowed 40 percent survival at two years, and 20–25 percent survival at five years (compared with 8 percent survival in historical controls.)[16]

Pierre and some of his colleagues thought that interleukin-2—known to activate cells of the immune system—might stimulate the bone marrow's ability to eliminate residual malignant cells, and increase the chances of bone marrow graft recipients to achieve complete remission. The rationale behind this proposal was that IL-2, a substance known to stimulate the proliferation of lymphocytes, might activate cytotoxic cells able to eliminate malignant cells. In addition, it was hoped that IL-2 would stimulate the proliferation of the grafted bone marrow cells and thus accelerate postgraft recovery.[17] They tentatively tested this approach in four bone-marrow-grafted children. The consolidation protocol was addressed to relatively stable patients. The expected result was improvement in the survival rate of grafted children (measured in long-term survival statistics), not dramatic and immediately visible changes in their clinical status: the number of patients was therefore much too small to provide statistically valid conclusions about the efficacy of IL-2 therapy. The authors of that study found, however, that IL-2 treatment was well tolerated by the children, and that it induced high levels of circulating natural killer (NK) cells.[18] These preliminary results, they believed, were promising enough to warrant a clinical trial centered on the "consolidation" of ABMT by IL-2. They also proposed to enlarge the study to include children who suffered from drug-resistant acute lymphoblastic leukemia (ALL) and who had been treated with autologous bone marrow grafts. Children with ALL who relapse during treatment have a poor prognosis and as a rule cannot be cured by chemotherapy alone. Bone marrow graft is the therapy of choice for such children. Such a graft brought a cure rate of about 50 percent if the donor was a tissue-compatible sibling, 20–25 percent if the donor was an unrelated compatible individual, and about 10 percent if no donor could be found and the child was treated by ABMT.[19] The physicians hoped that IL-2 therapy would improve the low rates of cure of ALL by ABMT.

In the summer of 1989 Pierre and one of his colleagues drafted a consolidation protocol proposing that children grafted with their own bone marrow be treated afterward with IL-2. They sent the draft to all the members of the French Pediatric Oncology Group, consisting of specialists from 15 hospitals in the French Oncology Association, then to the American producer of IL-2. Researchers at the American firm responded by producing a different, much more complicated therapeutic protocol. According to the industrialists' proposal, each grafted patient would receive IL-2 twice: first together with the heavy chemotherapy and total body irradiation preceding ABMT (a "preparation treatment"), then several weeks after the graft together with a different combination of anticancer drugs (a "consolidation therapy"). The proposal made by the French pediatric oncologists aimed exclusively at studying whether IL-2 could improve the outcome of ABMT, whereas the protocol proposed by the American manufacturer of IL-2 had two distinct goals: to study the feasibility and toxicity of joint administration of IL-2 and high levels of anticancer drugs, and to study the influence of IL-2 on the survival of ABMT recipients. The clinical trial, the American firm's experts added, should be made at the same time in children and in adults who received ABMT. The protocol proposed by the American industrialists reflected their preoccupation with the physiological effects of a combination of IL-2 and other anticancer therapies. In 1989 it was generally accepted that IL-2 alone had a limited efficacy in treating cancer. The American producers of IL-2 hoped that if they were able to show that IL-2 improved—even if marginally—the efficacy of routine and semiroutine drug therapies for cancer, the molecule could still become a commercial success. Their hypothesis was that the increase in the permeability of blood vessels by IL-2—the capillary leakage previously viewed exclusively as a harmful side effect—might be redefined as a "therapeutic effect" that might improve the performance of chemotherapy. In this context they abandoned the definition of IL-2 treatment as immunotherapy and replaced it with a conception of IL-2 as auxiliary anticancer drug. The American industrialists were interested in the rapid testing of the joint effects of administering IL-2 and a wide range of anticancer drugs in different categories of patients. They therefore proposed a trial that would rapidly evaluate the effects of a combination of IL-2 and several anticancer therapies in children and adults.

Pierre and his colleagues viewed the proposal of a single trial for adult and pediatric patients as the most problematic aspect of the American firm's project. Pierre immediately informed his correspondent in the American company that he and his colleagues strongly objected to unification of adult and pediatric trials. He argued that ALL in children is not the same disease as ALL in adults, and therefore that the criteria for enrolling children in a clinical trial should be different from those for enrolling adults. Indeed, many oncologists view the (frequently curable) ALL in children and the (seldom curable) ALL in adults as two distinct diseases. There was probably an additional reason for Pierre's strong opposition to a single clinical trial for children and adults: the initiators of the consolidation protocol (including Pierre) saw it as a way of strengthening the Pediatric Oncology Group. They may also have seen it as an indirect way of reinforcing their own prestige (since all were young doctors) within the group. The inclusion of adult patients in the IL-2/ABMT trial could hamper these goals, especially because in France the treatment of ALL in adults was "owned" by a powerful professional segment—the hematologists. On the other hand, Pierre did not strongly object to other important changes in the experimental design of the American IL-2/ABMT protocol, and proposed only some minor technical changes.

The representatives of the American biotechnology firm agreed to separate adult and pediatric clinical trials. In the meantime, however, other members of the French Pediatric Oncology Group submitted a draft of the original consolidation protocol to the French producer of IL-2. The French pharmaceutical firm adopted the broad outlines of that proposal but asked that in addition the consolidation protocol test the effects of various doses of IL-2 on therapy of ABMT in children. A member of the Pediatric Oncology group sent a letter to all the other members of the group, strongly advocating collaboration with the French producer of IL-2. The American industrialists, he explained, were rigid and "difficult," whereas the French producer of IL-2 was more flexible and more open to the clinicians' suggestions. Physicians who favored collaboration with the American firm (including Pierre) replied that both the French and American producers of IL-2 were following a commercial line of reasoning. The American industrialists were interested mainly in assessing the effects of combining IL-2 therapy with chemotherapy or with total body irradiation. They had produced their IL-2 several years before the French and had already completed all the tedious and time-consuming phase I tests. In contrast, the French producers of IL-2 still needed to test the toxicity of their product and were interested in trials that tested the effects of different concentrations of the molecule.

Pierre and his colleagues proposed to give priority to the American

IL-2 trial, and to include in the French IL-2 trial (which had less restrictive enrollment criteria) only those patients who could not be enrolled in the American protocol. The supporters of the French firm strongly disagreed. The American trial, they asserted, was confusing because it tried to study simultaneously two different effects: those on pregraft "conditioning" and those on postgraft "consolidation"; consequently, it was bound to generate uninterpretable results. In contrast, the French protocol asked a single question and made it possible to obtain an interpretable answer.

The French and American protocols involved two opposing types of clinical experiments: a multicenter trial that offered greater international exchange and enhanced visibility for participating doctors but imposed a rigid experimental structure, and a locally controlled trial that was smaller and less visible but more flexible and more attuned to the physicians' demands. But the heated debate within the French Pediatric Oncology Group about the relative merits of the trials soon subsided. The small number of pediatric patients eligible for ABMT/IL-2 trials (12 in 1990) reduced the importance of the clinical experiment. Moreover, the preliminary ABMT/IL-2 trials had shown that patients who received IL-2 treatment were no better (and no worse) than patients treated with a well-adjusted intensive chemotherapy. These results indicated that the choice of IL-2 treatment in ABMT might depend on local arrangements, on physicians' individual preferences, and, above all, on financial considerations.

Negotiations between clinical researchers and industrialists over the design of therapeutic protocols sometimes continued during the clinical trial. The small scale of the trials of French IL-2 and the close personal relationship between Cancer Foundation researchers and investigators working for the manufacturer encouraged such continuous negotiations. At first the Foundation researchers and IL-2 producers agreed upon a therapeutic protocol for phase I and II trials of French IL-2: patients were to receive an "induction treatment" consisting of three cycles of five-day infusions of the near-maximal tolerated dose, separated by a week of rest (a $5 \times 5 \times 5$ formula); if no positive results (significant reduction of tumor mass) were obtained at the end of the third cycle, treatment was to be discontinued. The clinicians quickly found that the severe iatrogenic effects of IL-2 therapy (circulation and blood-clotting disorders, high fever, digestive troubles, neurological disorders) prevented many patients from completing a full cycle of treatment. The high number of dropouts from the original protocol endangered the principal aim of the French manufacturers of IL-2: the collection of a complete and uniform set of clinical data necessary to obtain a marketing permit for their interleukin. They therefore proposed a different schedule: five days of IL-2 therapy, then four days, and finally three days (a 5 × 4 × 3 formula). Industry representatives hoped that the new protocol would allow more patients to complete their treatment cycle and thus preserve the validity of the trial's clinical results.

The clinicians participating in the IL-2 trial agreed to the changes proposed by the industrialists. François and Madeleine, however, were not consulted. When François learned about the new protocol, he strongly opposed it, arguing that it would probably diminish the clinical efficacy of therapy. Biological tests, he claimed, had revealed that a strong stimulation of the patient's cytotoxic lymphocytes was often obtained only at the end of the 5 × 5 × 5 treatment cycle; a shorter cycle would not lead to strong stimulation of the patient's antitumor responses. François's argument was grounded in the assumption that a direct correlation existed between the level of activation of cytotoxic lymphocytes found in the blood of IL-2-treated patients and the clinical status of those patients. This supposition was not supported then or later by experimental data. His argument, based as it was on immunological reasoning—however weak—probably aimed at stressing the importance of asking the immunologists' opinion before making changes in a protocol. The conflict, which revealed uncertainty about the precise role of immunologists in the IL-2 trial, ended in a compromise. The new protocol was maintained, but the pharmaceutical company representatives promised that in the future all participating senior researchers would be consulted before changes were made in a therapeutic protocol.

Jurisdictions: Institutional Contexts

The definition of IL-2 as new drug therapy or as immunotherapy was but one aspect of debates on the division of tasks and distribution of rewards during the Cancer Foundation's IL-2 trial. The IL-2 trial was conducted in three distinct sites: the immunology laboratory, the hematology laboratory, and the oncology clinic (the medical oncology ward and the pediatric oncology ward). The distribution of jurisdictions—who did what and where, who was responsible for a given segment of work, and who got the credit for results—was negotiated either in semiofficial settings—first the meetings of the trial's preparatory group, then the meetings of the IL-2 group—or in private conversations among senior investigators. Jurisdictional divisions were established, then consolidated or modified, in debates over the control of space, equipment, biological materials, subordinate workers (technicians and students), enrollment of patients, and the allocation of representational tasks.

Control over Space

The decision to conduct an important part of the IL-2 trial in the hematology laboratory was probably influenced by material constraints (it would have been difficult to find space for a human tissue culture room in the immunology lab) but also by strategic considerations (the trial was thus sited in "real" hospital space). The researchers who worked in the human tissue culture room (first Daniel, then Pierre), however, perceived the room's location in the hematology lab as purely accidental and viewed themselves as attached exclusively to the immunology lab. Both Pierre and Daniel acknowledged François's right to supervise their work. In contrast, they saw themselves as practicing immunologists, and thus as professionally equal, if not superior, to Madeleine. Daniel had a fellowship attached to the IL-2/LAK trial, and one might have argued (and indeed Madeleine tried to argue) that he should be accountable to both Madeleine and François because they were (at least formally) equally responsible for the trial; but Daniel strongly resisted that idea. The perception of the human tissue culture room as an "annex" of the immunology lab was not shared by Chantal and Dominique, who moved back and forth between routine work in the hematology laboratory and LAK studies. Chantal and Dominique spent a significant amount of their time with their colleagues in the hematology lab, and whenever possible (for example, during a long incubation period) they helped the hematology technicians with their routine work.

   The hybrid status of the human cell culture room and its close links with the immunology lab were maintained during the first phase of the IL-2 trial (study of LAK activity, inhibition of LAK by adherent cells) and the second phase (IL-2/LAK therapy in neuroblastoma). It changed, however, in the fall of 1989. At that time Daniel left for a postdoctoral position in the United States, and Pierre was busy at the pediatric oncology ward and maintained loose links only with the IL-

2 trial in adults and with the studies of LAK activation. The only researcher who worked full-time in the tissue culture room, the Chinese postdoctoral student, Hoang, had weak claims to expertise in immunology and more readily accepted Madeleine's authority. The technicians hired to accomplish IL-2 trial-related tasks, Jacques and Cyrile, worked directly with Madeleine. In addition, the shift from preclinical studies of LAK to clinical trials of IL-2 in adults (in the fall of 1988) reduced the volume of exchanges between the immunology and hematology labs. The integration of the tissue culture room into the hematology laboratory accentuated the "routine analysis" aspect of studies made there.

Control over Equipment

The IL-2 trial was guided by the hypothesis that the antitumor activity of IL-2 was mediated through the activation of cell-killing lymphocytes that eliminated malignant cells. If that hypothesis was correct, correlations should be found between the clinical status of IL-2-treated patients and the presence in their blood of specific subpopulations of activated cytotoxic lymphocytes. The organizers of the IL-2 trial assumed that once a way was found to link the measurable pattern of activation of lymphocytes in the patient's blood with clinical data, it would become possible to identify the best candidates for the new therapy and then to monitor their antitumor response.

Subpopulations of cytotoxic lymphocytes can be studied through a functional approach and through a morphological one. The first approach investigates the capacity of the patient's white blood cells to kill malignant cells in the test tube, while the second studies the expression of specific receptors on the cell's surface. The functional approach—the evaluation of the "tumor killing capacity" of lymphocytes—is based on techniques that were first elaborated by immunologists, and it is usually viewed as belonging to the immunologists' jurisdiction. Cytotoxicity is studied with the standard equipment of a biology laboratory (radioactive compounds to mark target cells, radioactivity counters to measure the radioactivity released by killed tumor cells). In contrast, morphological studies of receptors on the cell surface are as a rule conducted with complicated and expensive equipment—the fluorescein activated cell sorter (FACS), an apparatus that automatically quantifies the number of fluorescent cells in a given population.[20] The FACS was developed by immunologists, but it is not viewed as their exclusive "property" and is employed by other specialists as well (cell biologists, cytologists, biochemists, pharmacologists, hematologists).

In the late fall of 1987 a cancer charity provided funds for the acquisition of an advanced model of FACS, destined for the IL-2 trial. Madeleine, a hematologist, had a particular interest in studies of subpopulations of white blood cells. She conducted the negotiations with the firm that manufactured the FACS, and played an important role in the purchase of the apparatus. The FACS was placed in the hematology laboratory, and Madeleine declared that the right to use it would be limited to her and to her technician, Chantal. The FACS, she explained, was a very delicate apparatus and could not be used indiscriminately by unqualified workers. Other researchers affiliated with the trial argued that they needed to use the FACS in their investigations, some of which were directly related to the IL-2 trial. Pierre, who was particularly interested in studies of subpopulations of lymphocytes, asserted that he possessed the required technical expertise. Other investigators agreed to use the FACS only under the supervision of a trained technician. Madeleine refused to yield, and insisted on her exclusive control over the use of FACS. Both sides employed technical arguments: practical working arrangements, allocation of machine time, acquisition and evaluation of skills. All the interested parties clearly understood, however, that the true issue of the debate was Madeleine's aspiration to wield exclusive control over a specific segment of the IL-2 trial.

François supported Madeleine, confirming her right to supervise the use of the FACS. François's decision was probably motivated by his aspiration to maintain a harmonious collaboration with Madeleine, at that time the main representative of the hospital in a study which, its organizers repeatedly affirmed, should become a model for collaboration between the laboratory and the clinic. On the other hand, Madeleine's victory was ultimately a pyrrhic one. Madeleine's exclusive control over the FACS, combined with the paucity of autonomous research projects that employed the FACS in the hematology laboratory, may have helped to reinforce the division of labor that confined routine trial-related tasks to the hematology lab and research projects to the immunology lab. When Madeleine, together with a senior investigator from the immunology laboratory, Robert, conducted a research project unrelated to the IL-2 study, all the experiments in that project were conducted in the immunology lab. Thus in order to take part in a basic research project Madeleine had to leave her "strong-hold" in the hematology lab and become de facto one of the (junior) investigators in François's laboratory.

Control over Patient-Derived Biological Materials

The decision, made by the organizers of the IL-2 trial, to start cultures of tumor infiltrating lymphocytes brought to the fore the question of control of access to fragments of human tumors. Madeleine took on herself the task of securing tumor fragments for TIL studies. She was particularly interested in obtaining melanoma fragments, a rich source of TILs. Fragments of malignant tumors, and in particular "interest-ing" tumors—that is, malignant cells credited with the ability to yield interesting results in scientific experiments—were, however, a highly sought resource at the Cancer Foundation. Melanoma is one such "interesting" tumor, and Madeleine, who had to face fierce competi-tion over tumor fragments, often failed to obtain samples from the Foundation's surgeons. Tumors that had been promised to her, she bitterly complained, "ended up in the trash bin." François proposed to "interest the Foundation's surgeons in our research" by inviting them to inspect TIL cultures, but that project was never carried out. Madeleine was exasperated. It was unbelievable, she repeated, that researchers working in one of the biggest French cancer treatment centers were unable to obtain tumor fragments. Finally, Georges, François, and Madeleine wrote a memorandum to the Foundation's directors on the importance of developing TIL cultures. Once they obtained official support, they had no difficulty in gaining access to scraps of "interesting" tumors.

Tumors are a by-product of cancer surgery, and surgeons merely had to be persuaded to pass them along to researchers. In other cases, however, it was necessary to persuade professionals who were external to the IL-2 trial to contribute actively to it. These professionals, who could not expect any trial-related professional rewards, frequently re-sisted attempts to employ them in what they perceived as inferior, "service" tasks. One such task was the collection of blood samples for biological tests by intensive care nurses. Another was obtaining pe-ripheral blood leukocytes (PBLs), necessary for the preparation of LAK cells. To obtain human PBLs, the Foundation investigators needed access to specific equipment (cytapheresis machines) and spe-cific skills (separation of blood in these machines). During the early stages of the IL-2 trial (calibration of LAK cultures, testing for IL-2 and LAK in neuroblastoma), cytapheresis studies were the exclusive responsibility of a specialist from another hospital, Joseph, and thus outside the control of Foundation researchers. François and Madeleine were not entirely at ease with the dependence of all LAK experiments on Joseph's services. In the summer of 1987 François mentioned, during a conversation with Daniel, that it might be a good idea to obtain independent information about the quality of PBL supplied by Joseph. Madeleine added that Joseph was not the only cytapheresis specialist in the city, and hinted that it might be desirable to have an alternative source of PBLs. Daniel, however, strongly resisted the proposal to diversify the supply of PBLs or to doublecheck the quality of Joseph's services. He stressed that Joseph was a reliable and trustworthy research worker.[21]

When full-scale clinical trials of IL-2 therapy started at the Foundation's hospital it became difficult, for practical reasons, to rely on external cytapheresis services, but the physicians responsible for the Cancer Foundation blood bank at first refused to perform the cytaphereses on candidates for LAK therapy. This problem was eventually settled, probably in large part because there were so few attempts to treat adult patients with IL-2 and LAK. The cytapheresis machine that had been bought especially for the IL-2 trial was for a long time stored in a corner of a spare room, covered with a big white sheet. Ultimately it was used in a different project.

Control over Subordinates

The right to control subordinate workers (technicians, students) helped to define jurisdictions and zones of influence. Technicians were as a rule allocated to a given researcher and remained his or her "property." Chantal and Dominique were "Madeleine's technicians" and were controlled by her (and "lent" with her permission to other researchers). Other technicians were hired through special IL-2 trial-related funds to accomplish specific tasks: thus Marie was hired to study with Jacques ("our radiation therapist") the toxicity of IL-2 in mice; Bernard, to develop TIL cultures with Madeleine; and Cyrile (also with Madeleine), to extend studies of changes in immune mechanisms in IL-2-treated patients. Control was reaffirmed through the distribution of tasks. For example, François's request to Madeleine, "Would it be possible for Chantal to help with the blood separation on Wednesday?" made it clear that Chantal "belonged" to the hematology laboratory staff, while François's polite suggestion, "Daniel, wouldn't it be a good idea to test the thymidine incorporation by LAK cells at day 7?" (an offer that Daniel usually could not refuse), made explicit François's responsibility for the scientific content of Daniel's work.

Technicians accept their dependence on a given senior investigator as a part of their job description. In contrast, graduate students and junior researchers often aspire to maintain control over their investigations. Daniel strongly resisted Madeleine's attempts to control his work, and occasionally resented François's supervision as well. He attempted to demonstrate his independence by performing "unofficial" experiments (that is, experiments which he preferred not to submit to François's gaze). He strongly resisted some of François's equally strongly formulated suggestions concerning the planning and execution of experiments and the presentation of results, and he refused to be treated as a mere student. Consequently, he resented being criticized in public by François, even when privately he admitted that François was right. Daniel's relationship with François was, however, based on mutual respect—François viewed Daniel as a promising young researcher—and was not seriously disturbed by a few minor incidents.

The relationship between François and another student, Annette, was different. Annette was an intern who first worked with Georges and shared responsibility for the care of IL-2-treated patients. She found that experience distressing. Her regular participation in the IL-2 group meetings led to an interest in biological research, and she decided to join François's laboratory in order to prepare for a university degree in immunology.[22] François proposed that she study the immunological reactions of lymphocytes in IL-2-treated patients. Annette, unlike Daniel, had no previous experience in scientific research. She first learned basic laboratory methods from Dominique, then went to a different hospital to learn more advanced techniques such as the application of molecular biology methods to immunological studies. At that point her integration into the immunology laboratory went astray. Annette missed several IL-2 group meetings, then reappeared and proposed to collaborate with the researchers who had trained her in the uses of advanced immunological techniques, and to study with them the immune functions of lymphocytes from IL-2-treated patients.

François found Annette's behavior highly improper. At that stage of her training she was not supposed to propose new experimental approaches, even less to switch loyalties and decide to collaborate with another group of scientists. François criticized Annette for scientific ignorance (her new research project, he affirmed, was worthless) and for inappropriate professional conduct. He then gave her a choice between sticking to her original research project and "behaving herself" (a term that also had disciplinary overtones: it included an obligation of punctual attendance at all meetings of the IL-2 group) or leaving his laboratory immediately. During her participation as a clinician in the IL-2 trial, Annette was responsible for important decisions concerning the management of IL-2-treated patients. François might have wanted to make clear that there is a well-defined boundary between the jurisdiction controlled by clinicians and the one controlled by scientists. When Annette joined the immunology laboratory she was expected to surrender her independence as a physician and to accept a relatively humble position as a beginning researcher.

François also used the conflict with Annette to stress the rules of control over trial-originated biological material. Access to certain biological materials employed in the IL-2 trial (fragments of tumors, PBLs) was controlled by other groups of professionals (surgeons, blood bank staff), and researchers who wanted to obtain access to these materials were obliged to negotiate with the "owners" of these materials. Similarly, biological materials collected during the IL-2 trial itself (sera and white blood cells of IL-2 treated patients, LAK and TIL cells) were perceived as the "property" of the researchers who had organized that trial. By reacting sharply to Annette's "deviant behavior" François probably wanted to make clear that junior members of the IL-2 group who have access to biological materials derived from IL-2-treated patients were not allowed to share those materials with persons external to the Cancer Foundation's trial or even to discuss the possibility of such sharing without the explicit permission of the group leaders.

Control over Enrollment

The criteria for including patients in a clinical trial are as a rule established before the trial. During the Cancer Foundation IL-2 trial, however, the doctors were able to include a small number of "unofficial" patients who did not conform to the strict criteria for enrollment in a given clinical trial; these were the "out of protocol" patients. The French IL-2 producer provided a liberal supply of that substance to Cancer

Foundation researchers—a (negotiated) indication of confidence in the clinical and scientific judgment of the trial's organizers. The lack of tight control over the amount of IL-2 supplied to the trial's organizers made possible the treatment of the few "out of protocol" patients.[23] One category of "unofficial" patients consisted of "specially recommended" patients. For example, the head of the oncology department at the Cancer Foundation asked the trial's organizers (via Georges) to include in the trial one of his colleagues. The colleague, Dr. M., suffered from a disseminated melanoma, a cancer viewed as responsive to IL-2. He did not, however, meet other criteria for inclusion in the IL-2 trial. The admission of Dr. M. as an "out of protocol" patient irritated François, Madeleine, and Georges. Although his inclusion was formally presented as ultimately dependent on the trial organizers' decision, they knew that practically speaking they could not refuse him. To make things worse, Dr. M. was interested in receiving experimental treatment but not in trial-related research. He flatly refused to return to the hospital in order to give blood for biological tests (he was weakened by his disease and lived far from the hospital). Such behavior would not have been tolerated from "ordinary" patients, who before their enrollment in the IL-2 trial had signed a consent form that obliged them to submit to frequent blood tests. Dr. M., however, as an "out of protocol" patient, could not be controlled. The case of Dr. M. became a permanent source of black humor in the IL-2 group meeting. Madeleine, in particular, half-seriously expressed the fear that this "illegal" and undocumented patient (that is, a patient who could not be included in the group's publications) would respond better to IL-2 therapy than the "official" patients enrolled in the trial.

In another case, Foundation pediatricians who had treated a teenage girl suffering from terminal cancer asked for permission to include her in the IL-2 trial. The patient, who was at the end of a long and complicated disease trajectory, suffered from a malignancy (Ewing's sarcoma) that was not viewed as responsive to IL-2 therapy. There was no theoretical justification (besides the "who knows?" argument—that is, hope for a miracle) for the assumption that the patient would respond to interleukin therapy. Her doctors' request to include her in the IL-2 trial was implicitly understood as asking for "one more chance" for both the patient and themselves. At that point the physicians had a difficult time accepting their therapeutic failure, and a clinical trial could give them time to adjust to the inevitability of their patient's death. The clinicians of the IL-2 group (in particular Pierre and Georges) were sympathetic to the pediatricians' request "to do something." The IL-2 group leaders agreed to include the girl as an "out of protocol" patient notwithstanding their conviction that the chances of her responding to interleukin therapy were practically nil.

Control over Representational Tasks

Representation of the Cancer Foundation's IL-2 trial to outsiders was limited to senior investigators. François, as the group's self-appointed spokesperson, exercised a near monopoly. He frequently talked in seminars and in conferences for general practitioners, for medical students, for specialists in other disciplines, and for industrialists. He also appeared on radio and TV programs and gave numerous interviews to newspapers and magazines. In the fall of 1989 he "complained" (with evident pride) that practically every day he was invited to give a talk about IL-2. François's activity as a popularizer of IL-2 therapy may have been part of a deliberate strategy to make interleukin therapy as visible as possible. This strategy facilitated the mobilization of public and private funds and the enrollment of patients. It also reflected François's genuine enthusiasm for immunological methods of treating cancer, his equally genuine interest in the popularization of science and medicine, and his indisputable talents for the latter activity. François's status in France as one of the main spokespersons for cancer immunotherapy in 1988 and 1989 reflected not only his interest in the media but also the media's interest in him.

François's efforts to make the IL-2 trial visible were at first supported by the directors of the Cancer Foundation. In the summer of 1989, however, some of them complained about the excessive "mediaization" of IL-2 therapy. At the same time, oncologists studying IL-2 in other hospitals objected to what they perceived as exaggerated identification of IL-2 therapy with the Cancer Foundation trial, and unfair publicity for that institution (and for François). The Foundation's directors may have feared that the consequences of a conflict with powerful personalities in the French oncological milieu might outweigh the benefits of the increased public visibility of the Foundation's IL-2 trial. François's comment was that "the media are there anyway, and we are obliged to live with them, or rather we need to learn how to use them." On a different occasion he remarked that television is the "cultural revolution" of our times, and that scientists and doctors need to adapt themselves to a changing world.[24] Popularization of interleukin therapy was only one aspect of François's activities as the spokesperson of the Cancer Foundation's IL-2 trial, and though undoubtedly the most visible, it was not necessarily the most important one. Other, perhaps more important representational tasks involved relationships with external agencies: government officials (at the Health Ministry, INSERM) and industry leaders. The growing importance of the second kind of task indicated the rise of François's professional status. In the years 1987–1989 François spent a significant amount of his time in popularization. From 1990 on he spent less time on this and much more time in meeting with government officials and industrialists, which may be seen as a "private" representational task.[25]

Representations by other organizers of the trial were limited to their respective professional circuits. Thus Georges frequently presented the clinical aspects of that trial to other clinicians, for instance at meetings of the French Oncological Society. His talks were usually limited to practical details of IL-2 therapy such as doses of drugs, clinical management of patients, or ways of dealing with trial-related complications, and he avoided discussions about relationships between IL-2 therapy and the activation of immune mechanisms. Thanks to his prolonged stay in the United States, Pierre had numerous professional contacts there and often represented the Cancer Foundation IL-2 trial at North American meetings such as the annual meeting of the American Society for Clinical Oncology. He was also an active advocate of interleukin therapy within the French Pediatric Oncology Group. He gave a course on interleukins and tumor-killing cytotoxic cells to medical students. Finally, his double identity as a clinician and a part-time researcher in immunology occasionally allowed him to represent the Cancer Foundation trial at immunological gatherings. Madeleine also represented the IL-2 trial at several immunological and hematological meetings. In 1987 and 1988 she was also one of the speakers in a series of conferences organized by the Cancer Foundation for general practitioners. Although Madeleine did not have clinical responsibilities, she discussed the clinical management of terminal cancer patients. These conferences may have helped to reinforce Madeleine's image as a "real clinician" and thereby strengthen her role as the senior representative of the Foundation's hospital during the early stages of the IL-2 trial.

François explained that he—and he alone—had taken "great risks" during the IL-2 trial. At first I understood that statement as an allusion to the possibility of scientific failure or, worse, a medical disaster, such as the trial-related deaths that occurred during a French clinical trial of interferon. However, the scientific and medical risks of a clinical experiment that faithfully reproduced studies made in several other cancer treatment centers did not seem to me excessively high. François, I thought then, unnecessarily dramatized the dangers of an unexceptional clinical investigation. Now I believe, however, that François referred also (mainly?) to the political risks of his strategy in conducting and publicizing the IL-2 trial. These risks were, by contrast, very real, and François's enthusiastic and aggressive promotion of IL-2 therapy and his unorthodox ways of making the IL-2 trial visible outside the restricted circle of concerned professionals indeed generated a significant amount of hostility among his peers.[26] François was able, however, to neutralize that hostility and to limit damage to his professional status. His success in doing so may have contributed to the recognition of François's organizational talents and leadership qualities and favored his appointment as the head of the clinical biology division at the Cancer Foundation.

Articulations: The Laboratory, the Clinic, and the "Intermediary Zone"

The Cancer Foundation IL-2 clinical trial was organized around two axes: laboratory investigations and bedside practices. The coexistence of these two axes was central to the trial's structure. One of the trial's main declared goals was the demonstration of smooth and fruitful collaboration between scientists and physicians. The task was not easy. Clinicians and scientists who participated in the IL-2 trial evolved in different spheres of activity. Each professional group maintained its own distinctive structure, set of practices, and criteria for judging professional achievements. Moreover, there was no recent tradition of close collaboration between physicians and scientists at the Cancer Foundation, and research activities played only a limited role in shaping the careers of clinicians at the Foundation's hospital. However, the organizers of the Cancer Foundation IL-2 trial found an imaginative solution to the problem of articulation between the laboratory and the clinic: the development of an "intermediary zone" of trial-related semi-routine tasks that were not directly subordinated to either the clinic or the laboratory. Trial-related routine tasks such as the measurement of activation in patients' lymphocytes were, it is true, performed in many centers that conducted IL-2 trials. However, such tasks could be accomplished (and in the United States often were accomplished) by one or more technicians directly accountable to clinicians. In such cases biological tests were directly subordinated to the clinic. The development of a separate zone of activity centered upon biological tests and the culture of cytotoxic cells mirrored the important role of immunologists in the Cancer Foundation IL-2 trial. This intermediary zone served as a bridge between clinical and scientific activities and focused a significant portion of the participants' attention on the IL-2 trial. It also absorbed an important share of trial-related resources.

The intermediary zone of the IL-2 trial included the study of trial-related parameters (cytotoxic activity of LAK and TIL cells, activation of specific subpopulations of lymphocytes, concentration of soluble IL-2 receptors in the serum). These parameters were studied mainly in the hematology laboratory. Because the intermediary zone included laboratory activities directly related to the clinic, it gave scientists and clinicians access to each other's domain. It also opened space for negotiations over the boundaries of professional jurisdictions. Nobody contested the immunologists' "ownership" of basic immunological research or medical oncologists' and pediatric oncologists' "ownership" of diagnostic and therapeutic activities in their respective hospital wards. The oncologists' "ownership" of the clinical uses of IL-2 was reinforced as a result of the switch from therapy with activated LAK cells to a treatment based on the administration of IL-2 alone, akin to a standard chemotherapy. But in the early stages of the IL-2 trial, the intermediary zone opened a space for negotiations over the participants' degree of autonomy, the "ownership" of scientific and medical knowledge produced by the IL-2 trial, the right to shape and control this knowledge, and the distribution of trial-related professional rewards.

The intermediary zone did not, however, remain open. At first the researchers studying the activation of white blood cells by interleukin viewed these studies as a mixture of research activity and routine tasks. Technicians who perform routine tasks have only limited control over those tasks. In contrast, the control of researchers (including even beginning researchers) over their investigations is a negotiable item and may vary according to the personality of a given researcher and his or her supervisor(s), the institutional framework of the study, and the nature of the research itself. Daniel and Pierre attempted at different stages of the IL-2 trial to establish an autonomous research space within the intermediary zone. They tried to use the human tissue culture room, trial-related equipment such as the FACS, and trial-linked biological materials (white blood cells, LAK or patients' sera) to advance independent and semi-independent research projects. Later Annette made a brief and unsuccessful move in the same direction.

Daniel's attempts to gain autonomy within the intermediary zone were undoubtedly the most successful, perhaps because they were made early in the trial, before jurisdictions had jelled. His studies of the activation of LAK cells, at first purely practice-oriented (attempts to produce more efficient LAK cells), later became research-oriented (the mechanisms of activation and inhibition of LAK cells by adherent cells). His investigation was legitimated by a practical goal: the production of "super-LAK" to improve the efficacy of LAK treatment. Daniel's studies employed methods and approaches used in basic immunological research. This duality was a source of friction between Daniel and François. François viewed the study of the inhibition of LAK production mainly as a small-scale research centered on potential practical uses of LAK cells, whereas Daniel perceived it as a starting point for more fundamental immunological investigations. Consequently, François insisted on rapidly obtaining results that might indicate ways to obtain more active LAK cells, while Daniel—sometimes without François's knowledge—attempted to conduct experiments destined to answer basic questions concerning the mechanism behind the inhibition of LAK activity by adherent cells. Occasionally he engaged in what he himself described as a "wild-goose chase"—the verification of some far-fetched hypothesis. But his opportunities to conduct "unofficial" studies were later restricted by lack of time, by the necessity to obtain rapidly enough material to publish an article, and by François's closer supervision of the activities in the "intermediary zone."

Pierre's attempts to develop autonomous investigations in the framework of IL-2 studies were less successful. Pierre came to the IL-2 program hoping for an opportunity to work part-time in the laboratory. This opportunity did not materialize, however. He realized that he had to face a heavy work load in the clinic, and although François initially promised to help him find practical arrangements that would leave him enough time to conduct immunological research, he was either unable or unwilling to fulfill that promise. In addition François pressured Pierre to progress with studies of the optimal conditions in which to culture LAK cells (the culture of PBLs in plastic bags, the use of serum-free media). These studies were important to Pierre too, because in the meantime he had become one of the organizers of the neuroblastoma IL-2/LAK trial and was eager to find optimal conditions for LAK cell activation. The combined pressure of his duties at the pediatric oncology ward and the need to develop efficient ways to produce LAK cells prevented Pierre from developing independent research projects. For a while he tried to pursue small-scale investigations, but he finally gave up his research projects altogether. Pierre's failure to create an intermediary professional role (and not only an intermediary space) was later highlighted by the fact that when he finally obtained a leave from the clinic in order to work full-time in the immunology laboratory in the academic year 1992–93, he became an "ordinary" laboratory researcher who worked, under François's supervision, on an "ordinary" immunological investigation, only loosely related to the clinics.

In the fall of 1988 Daniel left for the United States, and his studies were taken over by Hoang. Unlike Daniel, Hoang did not seek to develop an independent research program. She gladly accepted François's instructions (or rather François's guidelines, translated into proposals for detailed research protocols by Madeleine). The search for inhibitory substance(s) secreted by adherent cells continued to employ immunological and biochemical methods, but there were no more "unofficial" experiments or other deviations from the goal-oriented pattern established by François. Hoang usually faithfully followed the directions traced by François and Madeleine. Her "passivity" may be attributed to her lack of familiarity with a Western research milieu or to her rapid understanding that she had little to gain by working hard on a project that she had not initiated and over which she had little control.[27]

Two additional technicians, Bernard and Cyrile, joined the intermediary zone in the fall of 1988. Both were qualified research technicians and, unlike Dominique and Chantal, were trained to conduct semi-independent projects. These projects (the culture and the testing of TILs, the measurement of soluble IL-2 receptors in serum) were, however, subordinated to the needs of the clinics. Except for Hoang's work, from 1989 on the intermediary zone became mainly an enlarged and upgraded "service zone" providing services for the clinics (biological tests) and the research laboratory (biological materials).

Madeleine probably hoped at first to be able to conduct independent research of her own. Her acceptance of the status of a glorified service supplier for the IL-2 trial was probably a necessary condition for her to maintain her position as an official codirector of the trial. Presumably Madeleine's options were limited because her relatively low status in the Foundation's hospital did not give her a strong negotiating position.[28] Participation in the IL-2 trial—even a de facto subordinate position—gave access to more interesting tasks (the culture of TILs, studies of receptors on lymphocytes' surfaces), to advanced scientific instruments (FACS), to interesting biological materials (patients' blood, tumor fragments), to additional—and better-qualified—subordinate staff (Hoang, Cyrile, Bernard). From 1989 on Madeleine was responsible for all the routine activities in the intermediary zone. She supervised Chantal's and Cyrile's studies of biological activity of patients' lymphocytes and sera, Bernard's TIL cultures, Dominique's tests of LAK cells, and Hoang's experiments on the inhibition of LAK activity by substance(s) secreted by adherent cells. She actively participated in some or all of these activities and followed closely the presentation of experimental results. Nevertheless, François's frequent polite inquiry "What do you think, Madeleine?" and the fact that he appreciated her technical expertise and took into consideration some of her remarks did not mask the fact that the broad lines of the investigations conducted in the intermediary zone were defined by him and by Georges (or other clinicians) and that the same persons (for immunological studies, François alone) also defined the interpretative framework of these investigations. The creation in 1992 of a clinical biology division headed by François made his control over all the IL-2 trial-related laboratory activities—and over Madeleine's laboratory—official.

The structure of the Cancer Foundation IL-2 trial might have led to the development of a zone of mixed activity combining research activity, preclinical investigations, and routine studies and representing a more substantive integration of the laboratory and the clinic. One may assume that clinicians who had scientific training and were interested in laboratory studies—the likes of Daniel and Pierre—might have played an important part in the constitution of such an active intermediary zone. Why was no independent trial-related research developed at the Cancer Foundation during the first four years of the IL-2 trial? There are, I propose, two possible answers. One is that the replacement of cell-centered adoptive immunotherapy by treatment with IL-2 alone or with IL-2 in combination with other molecules (interferon, antitumor drugs) limited the possible scope of trial-related research activities. The second is that during the early stages of the IL-

2 experiment its organizers (immunologists, oncologists, the Foundation's administrators) were not eager to develop autonomous, trial-related studies. Such studies might have jeopardized their goal of transforming the clinical experiment into a demonstration of exemplary cooperation between laboratory and clinic. Senior immunologists and medical oncologists at the Cancer Foundation wanted to display *their* ability to work together, rather than the ability of newcomers to the field to construct a distinct and dynamic new entity. Such a demonstration of successful collaboration might have been facilitated by the maintenance of the service nature of the intermediary zone. That zone, potentially a starting point for original and innovative investigations, became in the later stages of the IL-2 trial an efficient but essentially passive link between the laboratory and the clinic.

"Trading Zone" and "Boundary Objects": Linking the Practices of Scientists and Clinicians

The intermediary zone of the IL-2 trial was the main locus of interaction between scientists and clinicians. The existence of a common space is not sufficient, however, to secure common action. Oncologists and immunologists developed in addition shared practices that facilitated efficient interaction between these two professional groups. Coordinating activities across disciplinary borders is not an easy task. In the Cancer Foundation IL-2 trial it was even more difficult because of the paucity of earlier contact between clinicians and laboratory researchers and by the incommensurability of the medical and scientific understandings of malignant disease.[29] The clinicians' "cancer" and the scientists' "cancer" were measured and evaluated according to different methods that could not be entirely reduced to a common approach. Such incommensurability was usually not a problem for individual physicians or scientists who worked at the Cancer Foundation. Most of these professionals stayed within the limits of a single professional outlook. The rare medical oncologists (such as Pierre or Jacques) who simultaneously took care of cancer patients and conducted laboratory research adapted themselves to the oscillation between distinct frames of reference. They used the scientists' language when discussing scientific results and the clinicians' language in the clinic, and often boldly disregarded potential discrepancies between the two. Thus when Pierre discussed the pediatric IL-2 therapy in a clinical framework, he explained that in fact very little was known about the physiological effects of IL-2 treatment in young children, but that treatment was worth trying because "it may work." By contrast, when speaking with immunologists he presented a detailed evaluation of the effects of IL-2 on different subpopulations of lymphocytes in pediatric patients and interpreted these changes (such as the increase in NK activity) as directly related to the antitumor activity of the molecule.[30] Incommensurability is, however, problematic in intergroup relationships, and it may hamper attempts to stabilize interactions. The IL-2 trial brought to the fore the problem of compatibility between the clinicians' and the immunologists' professional outlooks. That problem was solved through placing "tumor-killing cytotoxic lymphocytes"—a "boundary object" that linked the domain of the clinicians with that of the immunologists—in the very center of the Cancer Foundation's IL-2 trial. That boundary object in turn facilitated the development of an intermediary zone that articulated the preoccupations of clinicians and scientists through investigations of the (potential) role of tumor-killing cytotoxic (LAK, TIL, NK) cells in cancer therapy.[31]

The problem of relations across professional and disciplinary boundaries and of interactions between heterogeneous professional groups is central to the understanding of the growth of modern medicine and the biomedical sciences. Susan Leigh Star and James Greisemer have proposed that the concept of boundary objects, derived from interactionist sociology, may help us to understand how "work can be done across different viewpoints and goals."[32] According to Star and Greisemer, boundary objects are concrete or conceptual objects that are robust enough to maintain unity but plastic enough to be manipulated in different "social worlds." They are weakly structured in the common use and become strongly structured in individual-site use. This property transforms them into negotiable entities that specify the content of professional agreements and may become a privileged site of interprofessional debates. Boundary objects, like the boundary stones from which they metaphorically borrow their name, simultaneously delimit and link particular territories: the domains of professional expertise. They also facilitate the development of intermediary zones: specific sites of interaction between professional cultures (in science and medicine, disciplines, specialties, professional segments).[33] Such boundary objects often have a double function. On the cognitive level they make possible the interaction of distinct professional cultures and thus permit the construction of a given segment of knowledge and the establishment of a given set of practices, while on the social level they facilitate the development of intergroup alliances and therefore advance specific social interests.[34]

The Cancer Foundation's IL-2 trial was based on the assumption that IL-2 activated a given subpopulation of cytotoxic lymphocytes (at first believed to be mainly, but not necessarily exclusively, LAK cells). These cytotoxic lymphocytes were, in turn, responsible for the observed reduction of volume of malignant tumors in IL-2-treated patients. The tumor-killing lymphocytes (cytotoxic T cells, NK cells, LAK cells) central to the proposed physiological mechanism of IL-2 antitumor activity were from the very beginning boundary objects. There was a near-universal agreement among specialists that some categories of activated white blood cells were capable of killing malignant cells in the test tube under well-controlled experimental conditions, and that several distinct white cell populations possessed such a capacity.[35] The causal link between the activation of specific subpopulations of "killer cells" and the elimination of tumors in laboratory animals was, however, more difficult to demonstrate, while the assumption that "killer cells" might play an important role in the elimination of malignancies in humans was based on indirect arguments. Thus the observation that, in some cases at least, the cytotoxic cells of a cancer patient were able to kill the patient's own tumor cells in a test tube was seen as indirect proof of the physiological role of these cells. Later investigations indicated, however, that cells of most spontaneously arising human tumors could not be killed by such cytotoxic lymphocytes.[36]

In their early research proposals and research reports Cancer Foundation investigators argued that their IL-2 trial aimed at the same time to improve IL-2 therapy and to better understand relations between the activation of immune mechanisms by IL-2 and the antitumor effects of the molecule. Clinical trials that test the efficacy of a new therapy often combine practical aims and cognitive goals (such as a better understanding of a given pathology or of the physiological effects of a given treatment).[37] The addition of cognitive goals to a design of a clinical trial may enhance the investigators' interest in that trial, bring supplementary professional rewards, and reduce the chances of a disappointing outcome. The trial organizers may claim, for example, that although the tested treatment did not work, they learned much during a given clinical trial, and that therefore the trial advanced the goal of the development of an efficient therapy. Cognitive goals were not, however, seen as ancillary to the Cancer Foundation's IL-2 trial; they were at the very center of the trial's structure. The correlations between the activation of white blood cells by interleukin and the clinical results of IL-2 therapy had not yet been found, the leaders of the Cancer Foundation trial explained, because the organizers of other clinical trials of IL-2 (as a rule, clinicians) were interested in rapidly obtaining practical results, not in immunological research. The Foundation's trial was different. It was developed by immunologists and clinicians who did not perceive immunological investigations as an appendix to clinical studies, but as an indispensable part of the trial's design and execution. The unique structure of the Cancer Foundation's trial thus greatly increased, its organizers believed, their chances of displaying the correlations between the stimulation of immune mechanisms in IL-2-treated patients and the antitumor effects of the molecule.

Nevertheless, the argument that immunologists' participation was central in the trial was fragile. The therapeutic goals of the IL-2 trial belonged entirely to the clinicians' jurisdiction, and the therapeutic protocols of treatment with IL-2 were closely modeled on standard chemotherapeutic protocols developed by medical oncologists. Once the conviction that LAK cells were an indispensable element of IL-2 therapy disappeared (an event that preceded the enrollment of the first adult patients in the Cancer Foundation's trial), it was possible to argue that clinical trials of IL-2 could have been conducted by medical oncologists alone. The Cancer Foundation IL-2 trial was, however, initiated and directed by immunologists. Moreover, one of its goals was to display successful collaboration between the laboratory and the clinic. The hypothetical tumor-destroying white blood cells were therefore essential for linking the distinct domains of the clinician and the immunologist and for legitimating the importance of the "scientific arm" of the IL-2 trial.

The term "cytotoxic cells" had a different meaning in immunological and in medical contexts. Immunologists viewed cytotoxic cells as a complex biological entity whose definition was embedded in a large body of specialized knowledge in cellular immunology. Immunologists were interested in the morphology and physiology of cells responsible for LAK and TIL activity, the distinction between LAK cells and NK cells (for example, LAK cells as a stage of development or, alternatively, a physiological variant of NK cells), or in the differences between the less specialized LAK/NK cells and the more specialized cyto-toxic T cells. They also developed a distinct set of standardized practices to study cytotoxic cells, and showed limited interest in other methods of assessing the antitumor activities of white blood cells. Thus, when in one meeting of the IL-2 group investigators from an-other hospital presented a method of coculture of tumor cells and lymphoid cells, aimed at measuring the inhibition of tumor cell growth by white blood cells (this effect was different from cell killing, usually studied in the immunology laboratory), their method evoked little in-terest among the immunologists. It did, in contrast, interest the clini-cians. The clinicians viewed cytotoxic cells as an undifferentiated en-tity with hypothetical antitumor activity in the patient, but they did not follow in detail the morphological details or the physiological mechanism(s) of that activity. Distinctions between subpopulations of tumor-killing lymphocytes interested the clinicians only insofar as such distinctions could be employed to find correlations between the results of biological tests and the clinical status of patients. Such cor-relations, moreover, are not necessarily causal, because a reliable marker of a response for a given therapy is not always directly related to a physiological mechanism that makes the therapy efficient. Persons who worked in the intermediary zone had an intermediate definition of the role of cytotoxic lymphocytes: they were interested in detailed morphological and functional studies of subpopulations of lympho-cytes of IL-2-treated patients, but they saw these studies as a means of finding correlations with the clinic, not as an independent goal. However, when the three groups met during the IL-2 group working sessions, the participants constantly employed terms such as "cyto-toxic T cells," "LAK cells," "TILs," or "NK cells," and it was auto-matically assumed that everyone in the room attributed the same meaning to these terms.[38] Cytotoxic cells were therefore boundary ob-jects, loosely structured in the common use by participants in the IL-2 trial, and strongly structured in their individual use by distinct pro-fessional communities.

The central role of immunologists in the Cancer Foundation's IL-2 trial, its organizers believed, would be automatically legitimated by the unveiling of the predicted correlation between biological tests (which defined the "cytotoxic lymphocytes" of immunologists) and the reduction of tumor volume (which defined the putative "tumor-killing by cytotoxic cells" of clinicians). The discovery of correlations between clinical results of IL-2 therapy and patterns of activation of subpopulations of lymphocytes would automatically align the goals of clinicians and immunologists. The interest of oncologists in cellular immunology would then be justified by their efforts to improve the treatment of their patients, while the participation of immunologists in the trial would be viewed as a direct response to the clinicians' demands.[39] Moreover, it was reasonable to assume that common goals such as selection and monitoring of IL-2-treated patients might lead to the development of common investigation methods and laboratory practices, while the sharing of instruments, reagents, and techniques might in turn reinforce links between the communities that shared these instruments and methods.

Efforts to uncover stable and reproducible correlations (even negative ones) between laboratory findings and clinical data were, however, unsuccessful. The central role of the immunology laboratory in the Cancer Foundation's IL-2 trial could not be justified in terms of an important contribution by immunological investigations to the improvement of the clinical results of IL-2 therapy. Their difficulty in demonstrating the direct participation of a specific subgroup of cytotoxic lymphocytes in the elimination of malignant tumors in IL-2-treated patients was shared by all the advocates of immunotherapy of cancer. In the absence of direct proof of the contribution of the putative IL-2-activated cytotoxic cells to eliminating cancer in humans, the argument was turned on its head, and specialists proposed that the therapeutic success of IL-2/LAK treatment might be seen as evidence of the anticancer activity of IL-2-activated human lymphocytes.[40] Interleukin therapy has a modest practical value but a great theoretical value: "it is now clearly established that IL-2 does not act directly on malignant cells but its antitumor activity is mediated through cells that possess a 'killer activity' and/or that, when stimulated by IL-2, secrete a 'cascade' of cytokines that reach the cancer cells,"[41] a "proof of a principle" that "demonstrates that immunotherapy of cancer is a highly promising research avenue."[42] The IL-2 project at the Cancer Foundation was destined, however, to develop not new avenues for fundamental and preclinical research but a new therapy and new relationships between biologists and oncologists. The participants in the IL-2 trial therefore developed alternative ways to legitimate and consolidate the relationship between laboratory and clinic. It is possible to classify these alternative approaches into three interrelated categories: material techniques—the development of new practices in the laboratory and the clinic; discursive techniques—the presentation of results and the attribution of meaning; and social techniques—the development of social links and of institutional structures.[43]

Articulating the Domains of Physicians and Scientists

Material Techniques

The first stages of the Cancer Foundation IL-2 trial were centered on the putative role of LAK cells (that is, IL-2-activated peripheral blood lymphocytes—PBLs) in destroying tumors. The idea that LAK cells (or rather, lymphocytes that displayed an "LAK function") played a role in the antitumor activity of IL-2 was not completely abandoned, but in the later stages of the trial researchers focused mainly on tumor infiltrating lymphocytes. The switch from LAK to TIL as the "star cytotoxic cell" of the IL-2 trial was not, however, merely a replacement of one category of candidate "tumor destroying cells" with another.[44] It was also a change from an activity (preparation of LAK) that depended mainly on the immunologists' skills (and on the technical skills of cytapheresis experts) to an activity that could not happen without the contribution of clinicians. A candidate for TIL therapy needed to have an accessible and operable tumor (in melanoma, usually a subcutaneous metastatic nodule) that could be removed by surgeons and then put in culture with IL-2 to prepare autologous TILs, or, alternatively, to possess a preexisting "stock" of TILs prepared from the patient's primary tumor and then frozen, to be used if the patient developed metastatic disease. Efficient coordination between the clinician who took care of the patient and the specialist who prepared the cells was then necessary to determine the right moment (if any) to inject TILs and IL-2 (for example, doctors were opposed to the treatment of patients who had rapidly growing tumors or to the therapy of stable patients who they believed "should be left in peace"). In the absence of such coordination, the opportunity to start a TIL culture might be missed, or the effort invested in the preparation of a given patient's TILs might be wasted. TIL therapy was thus a collective effort that involved aligning the efforts of several distinct professional groups.[45] It might therefore have been more efficient than "standard" IL-2 therapy in consolidating contacts between the laboratory and the clinic.

The role of the immunology laboratory in the planning and execution of the Cancer Foundation's IL-2 trial was legitimated first by the central role of LAK cells in the therapy proposed by Rosenberg. Later the growing body of evidence that LAK cells were not indispensable for the therapeutic effects of IL-2, in addition to the high costs of producing LAK cells, led to a decision to focus the clinical trial of the French IL-2 on the study of the therapeutic effects of IL-2 alone. LAK therapy was "rescued," however, through the claim that the addition of LAK cells increased the percentage of complete regressions of tumors in renal cell carcinoma.[46] Cancer Foundation researchers had an additional argument to promote LAK therapy: the proposal that a depletion of adherent cells would allow the production of more active and more efficient LAK cells. This last argument also opened the way for cooperation between the clinicians and the laboratory. "Standard" LAK cells (and later also "standard" TILs) could become semiroutine products, crafted by competent technicians. The development of "super LAK" was, however, a research-linked activity.

The proposal that depleting adherent cells prior to stimulating PBLs with IL-2 would improve the clinical results of IL-2/LAK therapy was based on several assumptions: that LAK cells played an important role in IL-2's antitumor effects, that higher LAK activity was correlated with improved antitumor effects, and that results observed in the test tube—such as an increase in LAK activity in the absence of adherent cells (or monocytes)—were relevant to clinical situations.[47] Leaders of the Cancer Foundation's IL-2 trial decided that instead of trying to prove all the hypotheses that sustained their proposal to apply "super LAK" to cancer therapy—a near-impossible task—it would be easier to start with a clinical experiment, that is, to eliminate monocytes from the white blood cells obtained through cytapheresis, to stimulate these cells with IL-2, to inject the LAK cells prepared with the new method into patients, and to look for improved therapeutic effects. They had no difficulty in convincing cancer charities and the French producer of IL-2 that it was worthwhile to finance preclinical and clinical experimentation on this subject. They also consulted with a manufacturer of cytapheresis machines to consider the possibility of making a technical modification in the cytapheresis apparatus in order to allow an automatic separation of adherent cells during the process of preparation of the patients' white blood cells. The argument "it may be worth trying" is frequently employed in oncology, a specialty based to a large extent on a trial-and-error approach. The preparation, then clinical application of "super LAK" pointed in addition to concrete ways to articulate the preoccupations of distinct professional groups: immunologists, blood bank specialists, producers of blood separation equipment, and clinicians.

In the meantime, however, LAK therapy generated powerful resistance in the Foundation's hospital. Obtaining white blood cells was not possible without the contribution of an unrelated professional group, the blood bank experts. François finally convinced them to perform the cytaphereses necessary for LAK preparation, but their participation in the trial was far from enthusiastic. Later the addition of one more step in the already complicated cytapheresis process—the separation of monocytes using a chemical substance (polymyristic ester, or PME)—further complicated the blood bank specialists' task. In December 1988 one of these specialists came to an IL-2 group meeting to complain that after a PME treatment the patient's blood was "full of lumps." Pierre and Georges proposed an alternative hypothesis—the lumps had been induced not by PME, but by an insufficient amount of heparin (the substance added to blood to prevent clotting) in the collected blood, and thus indirectly blamed the blood bank staff for their problems with cytaphereses. The blood bank specialist disagreed and left the meeting murmuring, "I don't understand a thing."

The injection of LAK cells also increased the work load of intensive care nurses. The reluctance of these nurses to survey LAK-treated patients increased when several of these patients suffered severe, life-threatening complications from LAK therapy. The difficulty of persuading professional groups external to the IL-2 trial to participate in the preparation and the administration of LAK probably contributed to the rapid abandonment of that therapy.

By contrast, TIL therapy did not generate major resistance. The expansion in the test tube of the small amount of tumor infiltrating lymphocytes (usually harvested from a single tumor) into the 10^{11} interleukin-2-activated cells that were injected into a patient was a long and tedious process that consumed expensive reagents (culture media) and equipment (culture flasks or plastic bags, other tissue culture materials). The main burden of labor (and of expenses) was, however, carried by the laboratory—in the Cancer Foundation's IL-2 trial, by the hematology laboratory. Madeleine and her collaborators were interested in TIL culture and were willing to work hard to prepare these cells. The culture of TILs seldom involved additional work for surgeons, because TILs were frequently prepared from tumors that had been removed surgically for unrelated medical reasons. Moreover, the injection of TILs did not as a rule provoke severe side effects, and the patients did not need additional nursing care. During the first two injections of TILs, physicians and nurses who had previously witnessed the dramatic effects of LAK injection were, Madeleine reported, so surprised not to observe any visible reaction (fever, chills) that she—jokingly of course—added that next time she would accelerate the pace of injection of TILs "to make the patient shiver a little; otherwise the clinicians will never believe that we are injecting an active product."

TILs and LAK cells linked the domains of clinicians and immunologists because both groups assumed that a direct relationship would be found between the capacity of IL-2-activated lymphocytes to destroy malignant cells in the test tube (measured by immunologists) and the reduction of tumor volume in patients injected with TILs or LAK cells (measured by oncologists). The same assumption guided efforts to correlate the results of biological tests of IL-2-treated patients with the clinical results of IL-2 therapy. Clinicians and immunologists supposed that they would find a correlation between a specific pattern of activation of cytotoxic lymphocytes and clinical results of IL-2 therapy. The search for one or more "winning pictures," that is, patterns of activation of white blood cells that would be associated with a clinical response to IL-2, was stimulated by the observation that one of the first patients treated by the French IL-2, and first "miracle" of that trial, Ms. R., developed an unusual pattern of lymphocyte activation.[48] Later the organizers of the trial looked systematically for an "R. profile" of activation of white blood cells, hoping to uncover reliable signs of clinical success. The search for patterns of activation of lymphocytes able to predict clinical success of IL-2 therapy could be likened to "clinical inference"—the doctor's search for diagnostic or predictive clinical signs.[49] However, whereas clinical inference is usually viewed as reflecting the tacit knowledge of a skilled medical practitioner (the "art of medicine"), the search for a "good" pattern of activation of lymphocytes by IL-2 was grounded in presuppositions originating in fundamental immunological studies and was directly related to efforts to quantify the effects of IL-2 treatment.[50]

The organizers of the IL-2 trial believed that the combination of biological studies and clinical observations would probably lead to a successful triangulation, that is, mutual reinforcement of the results of laboratory research and of observations made at the bedside.[51]

Their belief was based on the hypothesis that phenomena measured by different methods in the laboratory and the clinic reflected the same fundamental mechanism, because the therapeutic effects of IL-2 in cancer patients should be ascribed to the activation of tumor-killing lymphocytes by interleukin. If that hypothesis was correct, progress in the understanding of the biological pattern of response to IL-2 should improve the understanding of individual patients' clinical reactions, while a better definition of patients' pathophysiological reactions should further understanding of the mechanism(s) of IL-2's physiological activity. Successful triangulation might lead to a mutual validation of clinical and laboratory findings (and thus to the expansion of biological and medical knowledge) but also to the development of individualized treatments tailored to the "biological" and "clinical" profiles of each patient (and thus to the development of efficient cancer therapy).

The organizers of the Cancer Foundation's IL-2 trial started with the hypothesis that at least rough data, such as the extent of "lymphocytic rebound" (the increase in the number of circulating lymphocytes in IL-2-treated patients) or the global level of LAK activity, would be somehow related to clinical response. They assumed that patients who showed a stronger cellular reaction to IL-2 should also show a stronger therapeutic response. It was hoped, moreover, that these rough data would be refined later. They found, however, that even a rough measurement of individual response to IL-2 could not be reliably related to clinical response. The next step was to neglect the rough data and to concentrate on selected "target populations" of lymphocytes, potentially responsible for IL-2's antitumor activity (for example, cytotoxic T lymphocytes, NK cells, LAK cells). That approach also failed to reveal correlations between the results of biological tests and the regression of tumors. Finally, in the spring of 1990 the Foundation investigators replaced evaluations of the size of biological response with evaluations of its persistence.[52] The proposal that patients who were "doing well" were those who had relatively high cytotoxic responses at day 0 of a new cycle of IL-2 treatment (that is, after a rest period), if confirmed, could limit the unnecessary suffering of those treated, save labor and money, and, perhaps most important, vindicate the immunological hypothesis of IL-2 activity. However, the persistence of biological response also failed to become a reliable predictive measurement.

In the years 1988–1990 the difficulty of finding regular correlations between laboratory data and clinical findings did not lead to the abandonment of the search for such correlations or to a challenge to the validity of the theoretical assumptions guiding the search. Madeleine and her coworkers continued to follow the distribution of lymphocyte subpopulations in the blood of every patient enrolled in the IL-2 trial and to evaluate the cytotoxic activity of each patient's white blood cells, and they viewed this activity as an important one. For example, in the winter of 1989–90, after the IL-2 group became aware of the difficulties in correlating "biological" and "clinical" results, Madeleine threatened that if the blood samples did not arrive in time she would stop doing biological tests altogether. These studies, however, were seen, in principle at least, as a research activity that should not affect clinical decisions. François clearly stated in the spring of 1989 that the relationship between the results of biological tests and the clinical status of a given patient should be viewed as "unproved." "Unproved," however, could also be interpreted as "not yet proved." Georges, Madeleine, and François often included debates on the results of biological tests in their evaluation of patients. The estimation of a response to the IL-2 therapy, everybody agreed, should be based on measurements of the reduction in tumor volume. But it was not always easy to decide rapidly if the patient's tumor(s) had shrunk as a result of IL-2 treatment. The disappearance of subcutaneous metastases of melanoma could be easily observed by the clinicians (and often by the patients themselves). In other malignancies, however, the physicians had to wait for the results of X rays or a CAT scan, and these results were occasionally difficult to obtain or to interpret. In the meantime, the organizers of the IL-2 trial had easy access to the results of the biological tests of interleukin-treated patients. They tacitly agreed on several parameters of good biological response such as a high "rebound" of lymphocytes following IL-2 injection, an increase in the percentage of NK cells and/or cytotoxic T cells, an increase in LAK activity as measured with standard targets (tumor cell lines Raji, K-562, and Daudi). They were therefore able to affirm that a given patient had an excellent biological response, while another patient's response was rather weak.

The biological tests generated an impressive amount of quantitative data (tables, graphics) that were collectively commented upon during the meetings of the IL-2 group. These data, visible boundary objects, led to animated debates among members of heterogeneous professional communities. The organizers of the IL-2 trial had an ambivalent attitude toward the results of biological tests. They called for caution in the interpretation of the biological results, and François explained that "we have many results; what we need are more answers." On the other hand, the leaders of the group frequently made comments such as "Mr. T. seems to respond to the therapy, but we do not have his biological results yet"; "It's a pity that Mr. B. developed a cardiac arrhythmia and his doctors had to interrupt his treatment. His anti-K-562 response was excellent"; or "The biological response of that child is gradually disappearing; she should perhaps be boosted with a few injections of IL-2." François, Pierre, and Madeleine were preoccupied by the problem of the "exhaustion" of biological response (that is, the gradual decrease in activation levels of white blood cells in patients who had initially experienced a high biological response to IL-2) and frequently discussed the ways to prevent that phenomenon, indirectly implying that "exhaustion" of biological response to IL-2 would have a negative influence on the therapeutic effects of that molecule.

A constant flow of contradictory messages can be confusing, and indeed the intern Annette ended up confused. She probably lacked the experience necessary for the distinction between "potential" and "real" indicators for the clinic and understood the remarks about "beautiful biological response" as unproblematic descriptions of clinically relevant data. At some point she wondered out loud at a meeting of the IL-2 group, "If the cytotoxic activity of Mr. T. is so good, why is his tumor growing so fast?" François's answer was, "In this group, observation precedes interpretation" (in other words, "Don't speculate; it is not your business"). On another occasion she asked if the results of the biological tests of a given patient were good, adding that if they were not so good, she would recommend interrupting the patient's IL-2 therapy. She was immediately scolded by François, who stressed that "the decision to interrupt the IL-2 treatment belongs exclusively to the clinician. We are not going to take this decision in your place." Speculations about the contribution of biological tests to the global evaluation of the patient's status could be made, François's reaction implied, only if the tests retained their "fuzzy" (or boundary) character and were not transformed into firm recommendations for the clinician.[53]

The immune hypothesis of IL-2 antitumor activity was watered down during the IL-2 trial. The first research proposals written for the Cancer Foundation's IL-2 trial (1986 and 1987) insisted on the role of interleukin-2 in the generation of LAK activity. Later, however (1989 and 1990), therapeutic protocols and articles written by Cancer Foundation researchers started with a standard description of the effects of IL-2: "First described as a growth factor for lymphocytes, IL-2 has in fact pleiotropic activities: it supports the proliferation of all T cell subsets as well as NK and B lymphocytes. IL-2 activates the lytic potential of T and NK lymphocytes as well as monocytes. It also induces the synthesis and the release of other cytokines such as interferon gamma, IL-6, and TNF; finally, IL-2 acts on cells other than lymphocytes or monocytes such as polymorphonuclear cells by activating their oxygen burst or inhibiting chemotaxis." This description of IL-2 activity was broad enough to account for a large spectrum of physiological effects produced by the molecule. It included, however, only activities that could have been linked to specific or nonspecific functions of the immune system. Other physiological activities of the interleukin-2 molecule, such as an increase in the permeability of blood vessels (a property that, the American producers of IL-2 later believed, could be used to enhance the efficacy of chemotherapeutic drugs) or effects on blood pressure (among the 24 melanoma patients treated with French IL-2 at the Cancer Foundation in 1989 and 1990, 13 developed severe hypotension), were not included in the standard description of IL-2 activity.

Immunological data were presented in reports and publications of Cancer Foundation researchers as "immunological monitoring of patients receiving IL-2," "analysis of immune modifications induced by an IL-2 preparation," or "alternation of immune parameters by IL-2"—that is, as a broadly oriented collection of data about the immunological status of IL-2-treated patients. The results of attempts to correlate "lymphocyte activation" (a very general term) with "tumor responses" were often described in negative terms: "neither the increase of total lymphocytes nor that of CD3(+) (= cytotoxic T cell marker), CD56(+) (= NK marker), or CD25(+) (= IL-2 receptor) evaluated at day 8 of the first cycle could differentiate the group of responding versus nonresponding patients. Similarly, no difference was observed between the two groups of patients when the same analysis was performed at day 8 of the second IL-2 cycle." Cancer Foundation investigators nevertheless made two claims concerning correlations between laboratory results and clinical observations: "*In most cases* the ratio of CD56(+) and CD25(+) cells was higher at day 0 of the second cycle in patients with objective response than in patients with stable or progressive disease. In addition, both the peak values (at day 8 of the first cycle) and the baseline values (at day 0 of the second cycle) of the cytotoxic activities on K-562 target cells were higher *in most patients* with PR than in patients with stable disease or progressive disease" (emphasis added).[54] These assertions, however, were weakened by the low number of patients enrolled in that clinical trial (among the 24 patients enrolled, 6 were described as displaying an "objective response") and by the vagueness of the term "most."[55] The first article published by Cancer Foundation researchers and clinicians (the phase I trial of the French IL-2) explained that the major contribution of the IL-2 trial was to find "the conditions that allowed optimal stimulation of the immune system." This explanation took for granted that a stimulation of the immune system was indeed a desirable goal for the clinician. The next article on the same subject (phase II of the French IL-2 trial) stated more modestly that "immunological data *suggest* a *possible* role of maintaining a high cytotoxic activity" (emphasis added).[56]

The obstacles to the routinizing of cell-based therapies (LAK and TILs), combined with the difficulty of correlating the results of biological tests with clinical findings, might have led at least some members of the IL-2 group to question the role of immunologists in the IL-2 trial.[57] This did not happen, however. Interactions between clinicians and scientists continued to flourish, thanks to the existence of an intermediary zone articulated around shared practices (culture of LAK cells and TILs, quantification of levels of IL-2 receptors in the serum, measurement of the cytotoxic activity of white blood cells, studies of the distribution of cell surface markers in lymphocyte populations). In addition, other research projects (for example, studies of mixed lymphocyte reaction, investigations of the immunological functions of lymphocytes, kinetics of lymphokines in the serum, characterization of cell populations using molecular biology techniques) that employed patient-derived biological materials consolidated links between the immunology laboratory and the clinicians and contributed to the legitimation of the important role of immunologists in the IL-2 trial. Consequently, the researchers who worked in the immunology lab gained access to new materials (patient-derived cells and sera) and to a new subject of study (the biological effects of IL-2 in humans) and were able to enlarge the scope of their investigations.

The organizers of the Cancer Foundation's IL-2 trial believed that they would be able to align the interests of immunologists, clinicians, and industrialists and center them on a single object: interleukin-activated white blood cells that played an active role in the destruction of tumors (LAK cells, later viewed as an IL-2-activated NK cell). Gradually the proposed triangular alignment was transformed into several bilateral interactions. Industrialists cooperated with medical oncologists, who increasingly viewed IL-2 as a new anticancer drug that enriched their therapeutic arsenal. Industrialists also collaborated with immunologists, who studied the properties of IL-2 and employed the molecule as a tool to study cellular interactions during immune responses. Finally, the Cancer Foundation's IL-2 trial favored the development of close contacts between clinicians and immunologists. Although the putative boundary object—the tumor-destroying cytotoxic cells—had lost many of its "boundary" properties during the IL-2 trial, interactions between clinicians and scientists continued to flourish thanks to the maintenance of shared practices that linked the preoccupations of immunologists and of clinicians, thanks to the circulation of biological materials from IL-2-treated patients and the development of trial-related immunological research, and thanks to discursive and social techniques that consolidated the links between the laboratory and the clinic.

Social and Discursive Techniques

The organizers of the Cancer Foundation's IL-2 trial belonged to distinct professional cultures (or "social worlds"), but the collective conduct of that trial obliged them to accomplish numerous tasks together. Clinicians and scientists collaborated in writing grant proposals and discussed the shared management of funds—a new development at the Cancer Foundation. Later in the trial, they also met regularly in an official structure—the IL-2 group. Persons external to the IL-2 group readily perceived its regular and uneventful functioning as a visible sign of successful collaboration between physicians and scientists. Clinicians and immunologists who participated in the Cancer Foundation IL-2 trial also organized together several scientific meetings dedicated to different aspects of IL-2 therapy and IL-2 activity on cells. The shared preparation of these meetings—a truly collaborative endeavor—reinforced the ties between Cancer Foundation scientists and clinicians, while their conduct displayed these ties.

In addition, the Cancer Foundation's IL-2 trial was, from its very beginnings, an important political enterprise. It played an important role in interactions between the Cancer Foundation and cancer charities, other French cancer treatment centers, the biotechnology industry, the French government, and the media. The IL-2 trial became officially known outside the Cancer Foundation through a public act that associated most of these political aspects: a press conference (sponsored by the Cancer Foundation and by INSERM) that announced an official agreement between a cancer treatment hospital, a research laboratory funded by the French government, and a major French pharmaceutical firm. The statement read at the press conference stressed the exemplary character of the agreement, which would bring together for the first time French industrialists, clinicians, and biomedical researchers.

The official support of the French government for the IL-2 trial did not in itself guarantee the success of the trial. The IL-2 trial was open to criticisms from oncologists who were opposed to that therapeutic method and/or to the intervention of scientists in the jurisdiction of cancer therapy, of health administrators concerned about the cost-effectiveness ratio of new cancer treatments, and of colleagues/competitors interested in the domain of cancer biotherapy and worried that the Foundation investigators would monopolize the attention of the lay public and politicians. The leaders of the Foundation's IL-2 trial were engaged in a permanent effort to defend their clinical experiment and to present the IL-2 trial as a highly promising enterprise. The French Ministry of Health's creation of a special budget for clinical trials of biotherapies of cancer, the development of a "biotherapy unit" headed by François in the Cancer Foundation, and indirectly the creation of a clinical biology division, also headed by François, testify to the success of the public demonstration of the promise of "cancer biotherapy."[58]

Discursive techniques are often closely related to social techniques. Agreement on terms was a precondition for writing common grant proposals, organizing joint meetings, or negotiating with industrialists, hospital administrators, and government officials. The Cancer Foundation's IL-2 trial started with meetings to discuss the general framework of the trial. An important proportion of these preparatory discussions was dedicated to the search for trial-related research projects. The Cancer Foundation's IL-2 trial, François argued, should not become a mere repetition of clinical studies made in U.S. hospitals. The trial could potentially develop original scientific and therapeutic approaches thanks to close collaboration between a leading clinical department and a leading immunology laboratory, and thanks to the willingness of the French producer of IL-2 to take an active part in preclinical and clinical studies of that molecule. The aspiration to develop original IL-2 trial-related research at the Cancer Foundation was first concretized through a proposal to elaborate an animal model of human malignancy—"nude mice" grafted with a human tumor. Such an experimental approach, the organizers of the IL-2 trial believed, might permit the study of the sensitivity of a patient-derived tumor (grafted into a "nude mouse") to IL-2 therapy and, at the same time, might facilitate investigations of the mechanisms of IL-2/LAK activity in "near-life" conditions.[59] It would therefore successfully connect the preoccupations of clinicians, immunologists, and industrialists. For technical reasons, the "nude mouse" model was never developed at the Cancer Foundation, and the only animal studies conducted during the IL-2 trial were the investigations of the toxicity of IL-2 in mice, performed by Jacques and Marie. But the debates on animal models that might be employed to study LAK activity—together with more technical discussions on the culture and testing of LAK cells—played an important role in acclimating the participants, during preparatory meetings, to shared terms and techniques.

The people who participated in preparatory meetings of the IL-2 trial, it was implicitly assumed, had no major disagreements about the validity of IL-2/LAK therapy. The absence of disagreement did not necessarily mean that all the participants had carefully read all the papers published by Rosenberg's group and agreed with their conclusions. Some of the participants were perhaps more interested in other aspects of the trial, such as the opportunity to work in the laboratory or to experiment with innovative cancer therapies. Their participation in the preparatory group was interpreted, however, as an agreement with the fundamental assumptions underlying the IL-2 trial, namely that cancer could be cured by adoptive immunotherapy and that LAK cells (or cells possessing LAK activity) played an important role in such a cure. Consequently, the participants did not discuss the principles of adoptive immunotherapy and its relevance to the treatment of malignancies in humans, but rather the best ways to cultivate LAK cells, to increase LAK activity, and to develop animal models that might allow better studies of that activity. LAK cells could become efficient boundary objects because discussions about these cells were centered on laboratory techniques (methods of cell culture, measurement of the percentage of lysis of target cells, quantification of surface markers) that could be viewed as shared by the participants insofar as there was no disagreement on their principle and meaning. Thus clinicians were not expected to test LAK activity themselves, but it was assumed that they viewed these tests as the unproblematic quantification of a biological parameter, akin to, say, a measurement of hemoglobin levels or a platelet count. Squabbles over minor technical details increased the participants' interest in the experimental system employed during the IL-2 trial, and may have indirectly reinforced agreement over the general principles underlying the trial. The consensus over the meaning of shared concepts was consolidated by writing texts together. The participants in the Cancer Foundation's IL-2 trial wrote research proposals, signed agreements with the French and American producers of IL-2, prepared therapeutic protocols, and wrote research reports, abstracts for scientific meetings, scientific papers, and general reviews. They elaborated standardized or semistandardized explanations of the meaning of key terms such as (successively) "adoptive immunotherapy," "immunotherapy," and "IL-2 therapy" or "cytotoxic cells." These carefully worded explanations reflected carefully elaborated compromises that facilitated smooth interaction among participants.

The Cancer Foundation's IL-2 trial was guided by the assumption that the antitumor effects of interleukin-2 were mediated through the activation of cytotoxic cells able to kill malignant cells. But the precise meaning of the term "cytotoxic cells" depended on the context in which it was used. An early project to establish an appropriate therapeutic protocol for treatment of neuroblastoma by IL-2 and LAK mentioned "activated lymphoid killer cells" and "activated cytotoxic effectors," both rather imprecise terms.[60] A protocol proposed for the clinical trial of French IL-2 in adults explained that "interleukin-2 may induce the proliferation of all the subclasses of T lymphocytes, of NK cells, and of LAK cells and the differentiation of cytotoxic lymphocytes"—a definition of "IL-2 activated cells" that included de facto every known category of cell-killing white blood cells.[61] A research report written in 1989 mentioned "LAK cells" when discussing activities measured in the test tube, and a less restrictive category of "IL-2 activated peripheral blood lymphocytes" when discussing cells injected in patients. One neuroblastoma protocol defined a particularly large category of cells, the "IL-2-activated mononuclear cells"; another mentioned NK cells, T cytotoxic lymphocytes, and LAK cells. Articles published by participants in the Cancer Foundation IL-2 trial in the years 1989–1991 discussed the "stimulation by IL-2 of natural killer cells," the "increase in the cytotoxic activities of natural killer cells," and "enhancement of the LAK function" (all observed in the test tube). They also proposed loose definitions such as "the stimulation, by IL-2, of PBL (peripheral blood leukocytes) population."

All the imprecise expressions employed by the Cancer Foundation investigators nevertheless reflected their faithfulness to an interpretive framework which explained the antitumor effects of IL-2 through the activation of cellular immune mechanisms, and which assumed that a stimulation of immune mechanisms would be beneficial to cancer patients. The researchers were not concerned with the possibility that IL-2 therapy might have negative effects on tumor growth. Some patients showed accelerated tumor growth during or immediately after IL-2 therapy. Such rapid tumor growth was invariably interpreted as reflecting the intrinsic properties of a given tumor, an interpretation facilitated by the fact that most of these patients suffered from melanoma, a tumor that has an erratic and sometimes very rapid rhythm of growth. The assumption that a reduction in tumor volume in IL-2-treated patients was related to the interleukin therapy, while accelerated growth was unrelated to that therapy, was not unquestionable. IL-2 treatment induced numerous physiological effects, some of which, it was not entirely illogical to suppose, might have unfavorably affected the trajectory of a malignant disease. More specifically, "immunological enhancement"—the potential increase in the rapidity of tumor growth by immune mechanism(s)—was, Graham Currie explained in 1974, feared by all tumor immunologists.[62] Cancer Foundation researchers repeatedly affirmed that IL-2 had multiple (and not entirely understood) effects on immune system components, an affirmation that could have been interpreted as allowing for the possibility that in some cases IL-2 might also stimulate tumor growth. However—as far as I know—such a possibility was never raised by the organizers of the Cancer Foundation's IL-2 trial, not even in order to be immediately refuted, say, on statistical grounds.

Articles summarizing the results of the Cancer Foundation's IL-2 trial included in their introductory and concluding paragraphs indeterminate explanations, vague proposals of mechanisms, and fuzzy terms. But the core of these papers contained precise quantitative data. The presence of numerous tables and graphs summarizing the reac-

tions of the human organism to injections of high doses of recombinant IL-2 might have allowed clinicians to benefit from the prestige
of being associated with advanced scientific research. Data on the biological reactions of IL-2-treated patients were obtained with advanced immunological techniques, seldom employed by oncologists.
Articles that combined—as the Cancer Foundation's publications
did—detailed clinical data with detailed immunological data thus contributed, one may argue, to a process of bilateral "connotation" or
transposition of "elements of style."[63] In the absence of regular correlations between laboratory findings and tumor regression in patients, a true triangulation—that is, the consolidation of laboratory
data by clinical data and of clinical data by laboratory results—was
difficult to achieve. The systematic alignment of immunological and
clinical data in articles that reported the Cancer Foundation's IL-2 trial
results (and the similar alignment of talks on the activation of immune
mechanisms by IL-2 and on the therapeutic effects of that molecule in
scientific meetings) implicitly indicated the existence of a relationship
between the results obtained in the laboratory and in the clinic. It
associated the clinicians with an "immunological style" and the immunologists with a "clinical style." Such effects could be beneficial to
both professional groups: association with the "immunological style"
conveyed an impression of being at the "cutting edge of biomedical
research"; association with the "clinical style," a message of being
"useful to society."

To sum up, the central role of immunologists in the Cancer Foundation's IL-2 trial, the organizers of that trial explained at first, held
a promise of important scientific discoveries. Such discoveries, however, failed to materialize. In the years 1988–1990 the clinical and
scientific results of the Foundation's IL-2 trial were no better (and no
worse) than the results of other clinical trials of that molecule. Thereafter the presentation of the Foundation trial as a success was based
on two elements: the successful transfer of a new cancer therapy from
the United States to France, and the development of exemplary collaboration between oncologists and immunologists at the Cancer
Foundation. The scientists and the clinicians who co-organized the
Foundation's IL-2 trial were very proud of their ability to make their
collaboration work. Their success was even more remarkable if one
recalls the initial handicap of that trial—the relative dearth of interactions between laboratory and clinic in French oncology, and the
near-total absence of cooperative traditions at the Cancer Foundation.

An interview with François published in a popular French magazine in 1988 ended with the question (possibly inspired by François himself): "Isn't it rare to see such close collaboration between a laboratory scientist like you and an oncologist?" "For me, it's the first time things have happened this way," François answered, "and I find it absolutely extraordinary. The research laboratory has now entered into the clinic. And that's just a beginning. Over the next few years, we are going to do wonderful things with interleukins."

Rough Edges of a Smooth Collaboration: The IL-2 Trial and the Treatment of Terminal Cancer

The development and stabilization of links between the participants in the Cancer Foundation IL-2 trial was a complicated and energy-consuming endeavor. One of its most problematic aspects was the consolidation of ties with "traditional" clinical oncologists. The Cancer Foundation IL-2 trial started as a collaboration between the immunology laboratory and the French producer of IL-2. During the early stages of the trial the "clinic" side of the experiment was represented by Madeleine, Daniel, Jacques, and Pierre, that is, by atypical and relatively marginal clinicians who were not at all or only partly involved in patient care and who developed a strong interest in immunological research. The head of the medical oncology department at the Foundation's hospital agreed to conduct clinical tests of IL-2 in his ward, but according to François and Pierre, at first he viewed IL-2 therapy as an additional and not very promising drug treatment for advanced cancer. In the fall of 1988, the observation of "miracles" during phase I clinical trials of French IL-2 in adults led to a conversion of several medical oncologists and to their enthusiastic endorsement of the new therapeutic method, enthusiasm concretized through the establishment of the IL-2 group. Later, however, the "miracles" became rare, and the "true" (that is, full-time) clinicians (represented in the IL-2 group by Georges and by the interns Annette and Sandra) occasionally reverted to their previous, reserved attitude toward the IL-2 therapy.

Several examples may illustrate the clinicians' skepticism. In May 1989 Madeleine insisted on the necessity of convincing patients to stay in hospital until Monday (their treatment cycle usually ended Friday evening) to allow a systematic collection of blood for biological tests at day 8 of IL-2 therapy. Georges disagreed. He strongly resisted Madeleine's argument that the blood tests were "for the patient's own good." "Many patients," he explained, "especially those who are knowledgeable about their therapy, will never accept such an argument." At the same time Georges returned perplexed from a meeting organized by the American producer of IL-2, disturbed by the numerous contradictions between the clinical results reported. François tried to dissipate Georges's negative impressions and affirmed that "soon we will have more precise knowledge. There are more than a thousand patients in clinical trials of IL-2 worldwide." "Yes," Georges answered, "but without randomization." In September 1989 François summarized the first results of IL-2 therapy in adults and explained that out of 18 treated patients, 5 should be classified as partial responses, and thus "one may say that our results are within the average response range." Georges's reaction (as usual, pronounced softly and directed to François) was, "The only thing we can say now is that we cannot say much." Discussing a patient who had gastrointestinal bleeding following LAK injection (December 1989), Annette explained that the patient "is not ready to start again soon," while Georges added, following a suggestion that the patient had seemed to respond to LAK treatment earlier, that he had no intention of trying to convince a patient suffering from severe complications of interleukin/LAK therapy to return to the clinical trial.

The medical oncologists' skepticism had, I believe, a simple explanation: clinicians were directly confronted with the sufferings of terminal cancer patients and with the iatrogenic consequences of IL-2 treatment. Patients' subjective experience was usually carefully excluded from IL-2 group meetings. Patients were represented by numbers and graphs, while their clinical status was usually briefly mentioned in information given furtively and *en passant* by Georges, sometimes when the IL-2 meeting had already officially ended: "Ms. C. is regressing, Mr. B. is regrowing, Mr. K. had cardiovascular complications." But patients' experience was not entirely excluded from the IL-2 group meetings and from other professional interactions during the IL-2 trial. Terminal cancer cropped up, sometimes in unexpected places. In tables summarizing the data on LAK activity, the initials of certain patients were adorned with the letters *DCD* (for *décédé*, "deceased"), carefully written in calligraphy characters by Chantal. In the spring of 1987 Chantal and Dominique brought to the hematology laboratory a gift from the clinicians: three liters of ascitic fluid (fluid secreted into the peritoneal cavity) taken from a patient suffering from advanced, disseminated melanoma. The ascitic fluid, the clinicians believed, contained lymphocytes that might have been used for a TIL culture. The view—and the weight—of the ascitic fluid flasks could not be easily dissociated from thoughts about how that patient (38 years old and terminally ill) felt with several liters of fluid in his abdomen.[64]

The clinicians attempted to create a distance between the subjective experience of terminal cancer and the objective running of the IL-2 trial. Pierre explained that the results of a consolidation trial in ABMT "were very stimulating intellectually, but very difficult to support emotionally," because the patients underwent harsh treatment that could at best bring them a small gain in survival. Georges usually gave short, detached information about the patients' clinical status, but occasionally he demonstrated his feelings. When the members of the IL-2 group advanced multiple theoretical explanations to account for severe iatrogenic complications of LAK treatment, Georges exploded: "You should go to the ward and see the patient yourself. It is easy to discuss around a table in a conference room." Annette's attitude was different. She sometimes seemed to play the role of the naive (or falsely naive) beginner who repeatedly breached an unwritten etiquette—one that recommended elimination of the subjective experience of patients from a forum dedicated to objective, scientific evaluations.[65] She complained about the difficulty of caring for very sick, often mentally confused and frightened patients, and occasionally made comments on the futility of treating some of them. For example, she noted that a young patient suffering from disseminated, progressive melanoma and who "is not exactly one of the trial's big successes" should be left alone and allowed to die in his house. My impression was that the participants in the IL-2 group were relieved when Annette was replaced by the placid Sandra, who gave short, factual information about patients, without emotional undertones.

The fragility of the "objectivization" shield that covered the patients' suffering was perhaps best revealed in the cases in which the patient was himself a doctor. The need to treat a colleague put a particular strain on the participants in the IL-2 trial. One such case occurred early in the trial. Dr. A., a physician and biomedical researcher who worked in a prestigious French research institute, suffered from disseminated cancer with extended pulmonary metastases. He closely followed new developments in cancer therapy and knew several of the participants in the IL-2 project, among them François and Daniel. Dr. A. asked in the spring of 1987 to be treated with IL-2. François was very angered by the request. He and Madeleine thought that Dr. A.'s physician—one of the Foundation's leading medical oncologists—had committed a serious breach in professional ethics when he told his patient about the project to start IL-2/LAK therapy at the Foundation's hospital. The strong emotional reaction of the trial's organizers (and the equally strong rejection of the possibility that Dr. A. would be among the first persons treated by IL-2/LAK at the Cancer Foundation) probably reflected their identification with the patient (a colleague, of roughly the same age) but also a fear of contaminating the scientific sphere of the IL-2 trial with emotional elements. In addition, François explained, if the therapy failed because, say, the production of LAK was unsuccessful, the patient would immediately know that his status was hopeless, "and what will we tell him then?" François and Madeleine, hinting at their colleague's professional preoccupations, also evoked the possibility (viewed by them as particularly threatening) that "he might like to come here to cultivate his LAK cells himself." Finally the organizers of the IL-2 decided that only a doctor would be allowed to negotiate the participation of his or her patient in a clinical trial. The patient should never be permitted to enter directly into contact with researchers "because we need to protect the privileged doctor-patient relationship." Similarly, Dr. M., an oncologist and a friend of the head of the medical oncology division at the Cancer Foundation, who had been enrolled as an "out of protocol" patient at the request of the head of the medical oncology division, was seen as a double nuisance because of his privileged relationship with a hierarchical superior and his precise understanding of the trial's goals and his own clinical status. Discussing the case of Dr. M. (and invoking other cases too), Madeleine and François noted half-seriously that one should add to the long list of criteria that prevented inclusion in the IL-2 trial (nonmeasurable or nonevaluable tumor, brain metastases, recent chemotherapy, poor health status) an exclusion clause for physicians and their immediate families.[66]

The attempts to objectivize patients enrolled in the IL-2 trial did not reflect a desire among the trial's organizers to appear "cold," "unfeeling," or "science-centered." Just the opposite is true; participants in the IL-2 trial often insisted on the importance of paying close attention to the individual needs of patients. The clinicians, however, sometimes had difficulty separating the "experimental subject" from the individual patient. Their difficulty was illustrated by their attitude toward patients who suffered from severe neurological disturbances during IL-2 therapy (about one-third of those treated at the Cancer Foundation). Neurological problems were perceived as stemming from a purely mechanical cause: IL-2 therapy provoked a capillary leak syndrome, and the pressure of the release of liquid from blood vessels in the brain often led to mental confusion. The mechanical explanation of neurological problems of IL-2-treated patients was confirmed, the specialists explained, by the observation that when the intravenous drip of interleukin was discontinued, the neurological complications rapidly disappeared. The mentally confused IL-2-treated patient was therefore viewed exclusively as a "medicalized body," submitted to the general laws of anatomy and physiology, and the mechanical explanation of IL-2-induced neurological troubles radically dissociated the delirium of an IL-2-treated patient from the patient him- or herself. But Cancer Foundation clinicians were not at ease with such a dissociation, and they repeatedly raised the possibility that neurological troubles might be related to the psychological predispositions of the individual patient. For example, Georges explained that it was necessary to interrupt a given patient's therapy because of the severity of her neurological problems, then added: "She always did have rather peculiar behavior, didn't she?" One patient was described by the interns as suffering from a "preexisting schizoid state, made evident by IL-2 therapy," another as a "schizoid personality, exacerbated by IL-2 therapy." Indeed, although—as far as I know—the neurological problems observed during IL-2 therapy continued to be explained exclusively in terms of the mechanical pressure of fluids on the brain, beginning in 1989 psychiatric antecedents became one of the exclusion criteria in therapeutic protocols proposed by the American producer of IL-2.[67]

Coping with Difficulties

The Cancer Foundation was a potentially fragile enterprise. The low efficacy of the new therapy, coupled with its high cost—in terms of both money and patients' suffering—made it vulnerable to external criticism but also to internal dissent. The latter danger was very real. The heterogeneous origins of the organizers of the IL-2 trial increased the risks of tensions and conflict. Such tensions might threaten the cohesion of the group and undermine successful collaboration between the laboratory and the clinic. Foundation researchers used various devices to limit external criticism and internal tensions: the fragmentation and the routinization of tasks, the exclusion of singular and unexpected events, flexible definitions of success and failure, and, finally, black humor, self-directed irony, and cynicism. These devices increased the efficacy of the clinical experiment—and the IL-2 trial was indeed an efficient enterprise. As an external observer, I was often quick to notice conflicts, controversies, or deviations from routine, and my study of the Cancer Foundation IL-2 trial is rich in descriptions of such events. But difficulties and deviations from routine were noticeable (and interesting for the observer) precisely because of their exceptional character.

The routinization of tasks facilitated the smooth execution of the trial. Such routinization was mediated by therapeutic protocols. Protocols not only held a central place in negotiations among clinicians, scientists, and industrialists; they also determined the broad lines of the distribution of tasks and responsibilities during the clinical experiment. The protocols used during the IL-2 trial were not written "from scratch" but were modeled on earlier protocols. Cancer Foundation investigators were inspired by North American protocols of IL-2/LAK treatment, in particular those elaborated by Rosenberg and his collaborators. They were also inspired by more general models; the criteria for the inclusion of patients in the IL-2 trial, the definition of toxic and tolerable doses of interleukin during phase I trials, the codifications of the measurement of tumor volume and of the evaluation of the patient's clinical status, the list of routine tests necessary to trace the patient's reaction to therapy—all were modeled on chemotherapy protocols. The close resemblance between therapeutic protocols that tested the effects of IL-2 treatment and those that tested the effects of anticancer drugs facilitated the "naturalization" of IL-2 by medical oncologists. Moreover, therapeutic protocols structured the daily activities of staff members who treated the patients enrolled in the trial (doctors, nurses, auxiliary staff). One may assume that a protocol based on the repetition of routine or semiroutine tasks will be perceived by the (often overworked) staff of an oncology ward as less difficult and less stress-generating than a protocol that proposes numerous new tasks and new professional obligations.

The writing of therapeutic protocols also determined the questions that might be asked by the trial and the way to ask these questions, defined the framework of the trial, and neutralized questions about its aims. Decisions concerning the utility of a trial and the definition of its goals should in principle precede the stage of protocol writing. In practice, as is shown by the negotiations over the protocol of consolidation, by IL-2, of autologous bone marrow graft (ABMT), negotiations over the technical details of a protocol may partly replace debates over the necessity or urgency of a given clinical experiment. Clinicians may have a vague idea that a certain therapeutic hypothesis is worth testing. However, when an individual or a group of individuals (colleagues, competitors, industrialists) proposes a concrete clinical experiment, the debate may switch immediately to the "how" questions, and skip the "if" questions altogether. The conviction that certain therapeutic approaches should be tested may be consolidated through discussions about practical details. Even the very first, completely unofficial drafts of the ABMT consolidation protocols already contained numerous technical aspects: inclusion criteria, drug doses, follow-up of patients, laboratory tests. Ultimately Pierre and his colleagues agreed to a therapeutic protocol whose aims were very different from those of their original project. Some of the technical details defining the day-to-day tasks of the physician, the nurse, the laboratory worker (doses of drugs, routine follow-up of patients, ways of coping with drug-induced complications) were, however, similar in both projects. The consolidation trial was presumably based on agreement with the general (and imprecise) idea that it might be interesting to study the effects of IL-2 in children who received ABMT, and the willingness of clinicians to take responsibility for accomplishing a certain number of trial-related routine and semiroutine tasks. The new, radically modified form of the consolidation trial could still be perceived as acceptable by pediatric oncologists because it was well adapted to their "habitus."[68]

Protocols shaped the daily conduct of the IL-2 trial. A therapeutic protocol, however, describes predictable events. It is not devised to deal with the atypical, the unusual, the accidental, the unique. Exceptional events during a clinical trial may be classified as inexplicable accidents that do not carry any particular meaning and should be quickly forgotten or, alternatively, as incidents that reveal a hidden pattern and should be integrated into the collective record of a given clinical experiment. Many of the side effects of IL-2 (fever, rash, diarrhea, hypotension, weight gain, anemia, weakness, infections, disorientation) were seen by the Cancer Foundation's clinicians as normal (that is, expected), because they had been reported by other doctors and included in previous descriptions of the physiological effects of IL-2. But several patients treated with IL-2 at the Cancer Foundation developed unexpected pathological symptoms. Mr. F. developed an echytomatic purpura (a severe, sometimes gangrenous inflammation of the skin; the intern's description was: "large portions of his skin peeled off"); Mr. B. developed a vasculitis and huge parrotidis (inflammation of the salivary glands; "he really looked like a hamster," the intern added); and one of the patients treated with IL-2 and LAK developed life-threatening bleeding from the digestive tract. These cases were perceived by the participants in the Cancer Foundation IL-2 trial as true accidents, devoid of special meaning. They were not mentioned after the patient got better and were not included in a written description of the trial's results.[69] Another unusual complication, a dysfunction of the thyroid (hypothyroidism), was, however, tentatively classified as a "sign" rather than as "noise." During the phase I trial of the French IL-2, hypothyroidism occurred in two patients: Ms. R., the "star patient" of that phase; and Mr. T., who initially reacted to IL-2 therapy with a spectacular regression of his tumors. When François and Georges observed the second coincidence of hypothyroidism and rapid regression of tumors, they speculated that there might be a causal association. No other coincidences of hypothyroidism and tumor regression were found, however, and Mr. T.'s tumors grew back rapidly (Ms. R. remained stable). Hypothyroidism was classified as a "rare secondary effect" of IL-2 therapy.[70]

Classification of unusual events as "normal" or "true accidents" was but one discursive technique that helped to deflect trial-related tensions. Thus, a loose definition of what constituted an acceptable cost of IL-2 treatment allowed the Cancer Foundation researchers to justify the choices they made.[71] When researchers at another leading French cancer treatment center proposed to individualize IL-2/LAK therapy by cloning LAK cells of a given patient, then inject the patient with the most active clones only, François and Pierre explained that such a method, even if successful, was too expensive to be introduced into the clinic. In contrast, an innovation proposed by the Foundation investigators—the preparation of LAK from the nonadherent fraction of white blood cells—could, they claimed, be easily routinized and mechanized, and thus made inexpensive if necessary. On the other hand, François repeatedly affirmed that he was not excessively concerned about the cost of LAK or TIL therapies. Any efficient therapy for otherwise incurable cancers would be financed somehow, because no politician would be able to ignore public pressure in favor of it.[72]

The broadening of the definition of the trial's success, or rather, the restriction of the definition of failure, helped to reduce the participants' frustrations and the critiques of external observers. For example, the term "clinical response" had different interpretations in different circumstances. Reactions to anticancer drugs are usually classified under three main headings: progressive disease (PD)—continuation of the tumor's growth; complete response (CR)—complete disappearance of measurable disease signs; and partial response (PR)—the reduction of at least 40 percent of tumor volume. But Cancer Foundation researchers introduced in their publications other categories of reaction to IL-2 therapy: stable disease (SD), minor response (MR; a measurable response that did not achieve a 40 percent reduction in the tumor), and objective response (OR; an evaluable positive response that did not fit the rigid criteria of PR). Such terms allowed the clinicians to single out patients who appeared to respond to the IL-2 treatment, although these reactions could not be fitted into previously existing, stringent categories.

The fluid definition of the expression "to be in the protocol" (that is, to be included in evaluation of clinical results of a trial) also helped to limit the number of patients classified as IL-2 trial failures. Severe side effects prevented many from completing their therapeutic cycle. Such patients could not be included in, say, official applications for a marketing permit. The Foundation researchers maintained, however, that a patient who responded to a shorter cycle of IL-2 therapy could be considered a confirmed therapeutic success.[73] Thus one of the patients treated during the phase II trial, Ms. C., was never able to complete a full five-day treatment cycle. Nevertheless, she was viewed as the most successful case in phase II of the IL-2 trial because she had a permanent, near-complete regression of her tumor. On the other hand, patients who did not respond to a partial dose of IL-2 could be viewed as patients who had an unknown status, not as failures of therapy. During July 1989, when very few patients were responding to the therapy, François reacted to Madeleine's and Annette's pessimistic evaluation of the current results by pointing to the fact that many of the patients had been obliged to interrupt their treatment in the middle, and therefore "you should count how many among these patients really *were* in the protocol."

Black humor helped the researchers to cope with the uncertainties of clinical experimentation and with fears of terminal disease and death.[74] When a gross abdominal mass was discovered in Mr. R., a melanoma patient scheduled to be treated with TILs, Madeleine affirmed that she was "relieved." Now she was sure, she explained, that the patient's disease was severe enough to demonstrate the (expected) dramatic effects of TIL therapy. When Georges explained that Mr. B., one of the first patients treated with TILs, would be evaluated clinically in a week or so, Madeleine's reaction was, "Well, his tumor will have enough time to regrow." After the "out of protocol" patient Dr. M. refused to donate blood for biological tests Madeleine stated that she could not find his name in her laboratory notebooks and added, "That's it. Dr. M. has definitively disappeared," while other participants inquired when a patient would finally reach the status of "the late Dr. M."

Self-directed irony helped researchers to acknowledge some of the limits of the IL-2 trial without undermining its positive evaluation. Thus the organizers' frequent affirmation, "We are the best, aren't we?" conveyed the message "Well, in fact we know we are not *that* great" but also reflected a real pride in trial-related achievements. When François announced that he was going to participate in a radio program, he added, "I am going, as usual, to sing the praises of IL-2."[75] Cancer Foundation investigators also liked to joke about the way the IL-2 trial's results should be presented. Listing the clinical reports during a "good week" (nearly all the patients enrolled in the trial seemed to react to IL-2 therapy), François noted, "We have now four responses out of four for this protocol. This is the right moment to stop." Another time, admiring the "clear" X-ray plates of Ms. C., the only "miracle" of the phase II trial, Georges explained that he was going to show them in a scientific meeting, adding, "I will explain, of course, that these photographs were selected entirely by chance from a big pile of patients' results."

Another discursive device, cynicism, helped the researchers to cope with the multiple, sometimes contradictory, aims of the clinical experiment. The IL-2 trial was a multifunctional enterprise, and the real-life complexity of clinical research in oncology was quite different from the unidimensional, stereotyped images that depicted cancer researchers as selfless seekers of truth, preoccupied exclusively with the fate of present and/or future patients.[76] These flattering images undoubtedly affected the investigators' self-image, all the more so because many who joined the trial were indeed motivated by the excitement of immunological research, the desire to "do something" to help patients suffering from advanced cancer, or both. On the other hand, the Foundation researchers also sought to use the IL-2 trial to forward their social goals, but they were aware that such aspirations, if made explicit, might be perceived as a corruption of the purity of medical research by ambition for glory, power, or money. Cynicism was used to deflect such accusations.

Cynical remarks exaggerated the "impure" aims of the IL-2 trial in a self-mocking way, in order to neutralize them. Thus during one of the preparatory meetings, someone declared that an ethics committee should be constituted rapidly at the Cancer Foundation; "otherwise we will not be able to publish our results in the *New England Journal of Medicine.*" Pierre spoke semiseriously about the IL-2 trial as "my thing," a device that would allow him to have his name first on clinical articles and would open the way for professional promotion. "We should go ahead with the 'super LAK' project," François affirmed in the fall of 1988, "because even if it does not work, we can still make a lot of noise about it." Daniel explained that the true goal of the LAK project was to study the stimulation of human cells in the test tube. "And the clinic?" I asked. "Well, everybody knows that the clinic is only an excuse," he answered. The message conveyed by such comments was that the organizers were well aware of the web of personal and collective interests underlying the trial, but at the same time they viewed these issues as nonessential, secondary, just a good subject for a joke.[77] The cynical declarations thus provided a rhetorical bridge over the gap between the real and official images of the IL-2 trial, and allowed the participants to come to terms, though in an indirect and distorted way, with the trial's multifunctionality.

Material, social, and discursive techniques, shared objects and concepts, control over resources and persons, and the development of a specific "intermediary zone" facilitated the development of efficient links between the heterogeneous professional groups participating in the Cancer Foundation's IL-2 trial, shaped the routine and semiroutine tasks of participants, helped to deflect criticism, and limited trial-related tensions. Together these techniques allowed the work to be done and contributed to the (relatively) smooth functioning of a complex, multilayered enterprise.

CHAPTER SIX

A Science-Laden Pathology between Bench and Bedside

The early career of a given medical innovation—that is, the probability that this innovation will not be quickly rejected or shelved and will reach the stage of extended clinical testing—is strongly affected by the degree of compatibility between the innovation and a specific medical culture.[1] The idea that new therapies will be successful if they can find an "ecological niche" and "fit into" a well-defined culture should not be understood, however, as contrasting an infinitely flexible "innovation" with a totally rigid "environment." The IL-2 story illustrates just the opposite circumstance: the rich and complex interaction between a new medical practice (here, the introduction of IL-2 to cancer therapy) and its "environment"—other practices, knowledge claims, and organizational devices (here, the culture of clinical experimentation in oncology). Such interaction simultaneously modifies the innovation and its "neighbors."[2] In addition, as the study of the IL-2 trial at the Cancer Foundation shows, local elements and contingent events often shape new developments in science and medicine.

On the other hand, medical innovations need to find their place in a "full world"—full, that is, with existing practices and knowledge claims that constrain and guide the choices of doctors and scientists. Scientists and engineers are sometimes impatient with historical investigations. Thus, the immunologist Peter Medawar has asserted that scientists do not need to be concerned with history, because present science integrates past learning, and therefore "comprehends history within itself," while the engineer and inventor Charles F. Kettering of General Motors (who gave his name to the Sloan-Kettering Cancer Treatment Center in New York) explained that "you never get anywhere looking in your rear-view mirror" and proposed to focus on the future instead, "because we are going to spend the rest of our lives there."[3] But both Medawar and Kettering disregarded the powerful restraints imposed on the present and the future by decisions made in the past. Some technological choices, historians of technology explain, became irreversible, and this irreversibility sets limits on subsequent developments.[4] Medicine, and in particular technology-dependent hospital medicine, is a "highly prestructured activity in which early choices delineate the space of further choices."[5] The development of the culture of clinical experimentation in oncology in the 1950s and 1960s was affected by specific events such as the concentration of cancer patients in specialized institutions, the faith in "miracle drugs" following the development of antibiotics, the influx of public funds into biomedical research, the increased role of research-oriented cancer charities, and the development of close links between government-sponsored research and industry. Here I discuss an additional element that, I propose, favored the growth of the culture of clinical experimentation in oncology: the development of (orthodox) cancer therapy as an area of medical intervention that is strongly "science-laden" and weakly affected by "life-style" considerations.

Hospital-based "high-tech" scientific medicine is usually described as a single type of practice, opposed to other models of medical intervention: nonorthodox ("parallel") medicine, behaviorist medicine, folk medicine. This division points to an important difference between the reductionist approach, which views human diseases as the dysfunction of specific molecular, cellular, or organic mechanisms, and other medical practices. It may, however, obscure the existence of important distinctions within the entity "scientific medicine."[6] Thus, the strength of the links between distinct areas of medical intervention and laboratory-derived knowledge varies. This variability is more perceptible in the area of therapy than in that of diagnosis and classification of diseases. The development of diagnostic devices is usually directly related to the state of medical knowledge in a given area. New understanding of diseases (such as the bacterial theory of causation of disease) led to elaboration of new diagnostic tools (bacteriological and serological tests), and conversely, new diagnostic devices (such as the electrocardiogram or CAT scan) changed the definition of pathological states and occasionally led to the establishment of new disease entities. In contrast, therapy maintains more complicated relationships with medical science. "Knowledge about diseases" is not always successfully translated into curative practices, while efficient therapy may stem from poorly understood clinical experience.[7]

It is possible to construct a spectrum of medical activities that extends from strongly "science-laden" domains such as AIDS therapy, endocrinology, or medical genetics, in which important segments of therapeutic intervention depend directly on laboratory findings, to intermediate areas such as urology, rheumatology, or gastroenterology, in which some aspects of therapy are guided by laboratory-derived knowledge and others by clinical experience, to "clinical practice-laden" areas such as emergency medicine, therapy of chronic pain, geriatrics, or obstetrics, in which medical intervention is usually loosely connected to laboratory research.[8] Cancer therapy would be found near the "science-laden" end of such a scale. From the late nineteenth century on, cancer was seen as the disease of "deviant cells." The cell-centered view of cancer was strengthened in the twentieth century by the central role of cytology in cancer diagnosis and by the (partial) success of cancer therapies based on the principle of elimination of rapidly dividing cells—first radiation therapy and then chemotherapy. The definition of cancer as a cellular disease was conducive to the belief that the solution to the "cancer problem" is directly related to the understanding of the fundamental biological mechanisms regulating the proliferation of normal cells. This belief, together with the fact that malignant cells, easy to cultivate in a test tube, were a highly convenient research material for biologists, led to the development of close relationships between experimental studies of cancer and disciplines such as cell biology, cytology, biochemistry, genetics, and molecular biology. It also associated recent attempts at development of anticancer therapies with laboratory investigations.

Another important distinction can be made, however, between areas of medical intervention—the distinction between areas in which "life-style" considerations are perceived by (orthodox) medicine as affecting morbidity and outcome, and those in which life-style elements are viewed as unable to arrest a declared morbid process.[9] The degree of science-ladenness and the perceived importance of life-style elements are independent variables. Some areas of medical intervention—such as the therapy of chronic pain—are viewed by orthodox medicine as weakly science-laden (there are no clear-cut causal explanations and no efficient "scientific" therapies) and as strongly life-style-dependent (changes in the patient's behavior may directly affect morbid symptoms). In other areas of medical intervention, however, such as cardiology or diabetes therapy, strong reliance on laboratory-originated knowledge and practices is combined with life-style considerations. Our understanding of cardiac pathologies depends on complex measuring instruments and fundamental physiological and pharmacological studies, and that of diabetes on endocrinological research and tests that measure sugar in the blood. At the same time, patients suffering from cardiac disease or diabetes receive precise advice concerning diet and exercise and are instructed in techniques of self-monitoring and self-medication. These patients are simultaneously encouraged by their (orthodox) doctors to submit themselves to appropriate therapies (drugs, surgery) and to take responsibility for their own well-being through control of their behavior and changes in their life-style.

A diseased heart, blood vessel, pancreas, or liver is viewed as a poorly functioning but nevertheless integral part of the body. The perception of cancer is different. The disease is conceptualized as an external element, an aggregate of alien entities—the malignant cells—that have a life of their own, independent of the life of the individual who is harboring them. The inventor of IL-2/LAK therapy, Dr. Steven Rosenberg, articulated an extreme form of such a view of malignant disease. He presented his obstinate search for an immunotherapy of cancer as a personal crusade against evil, fueled by a hatred of the "cancer holocaust." Cancer, Rosenberg asserted, is a "hateful disease," a hidden enemy within the body that kills "by felony and in a treacherous way" and that "eats slowly the body of its victims and obliges them and their families to watch, impotent, the tumor's growth."[10] This image of an impotent body inexorably "devoured" by malignant cells may have stimulated Rosenberg's efforts to develop a therapeutic

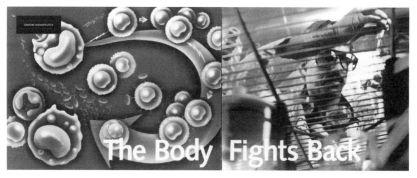

From *Chiron Annual Report, 1993:* "The Body Fights Back." (Courtesy Chiron/ Cetus Corporation.)

approach based on the activation of immune mechanisms, that is, on increasing the organism's capacity to fight a treacherous enemy.[11]

The perception of cancer cells as uncontrollable alien elements limits the ability of individuals diagnosed with cancer to find a meaning for their illness and to regain some degree of control over their lives. Many patients resist such a view of their illness and strive to escape the tyranny of the randomness of disease. As the historian of medicine Charles Rosenberg puts it, "Although most of us retain secure faith in reductionist medicine and its credentialed practitioners, we nevertheless seek an understanding that will allow us to predict our future and impose a morally coherent meaning on individual actions."[12] "Pathographies" (that is, autobiographical disease accounts) written by cancer patients or their family members often reflect, Anne Hunsaker Hawkins has found, a desire to relate illness to specific events in the patient's life, and to explain the disease trajectory as reflecting life-style changes. This desire is not fulfilled by mainstream medicine.[13] The great majority of cancer patients in industrialized countries are treated by (and put their faith in) doctors who do not believe that changes in life-style are able to arrest or reverse the progress of their disease. The only alteration in life-style that people suffering from cancer are asked to make is to become "exemplary patients," fully compliant with their treatment. Hence doctors' positive reinforcement of patients who do not "give up" and bravely "fight their disease"— that is, who are ready to undergo harsh and trying treatments, and occasionally to participate in clinical trials of new therapies. Hence also the faith in the "miracles of science" shared by many patients caught in a strongly science-laden and weakly life-style-dependent area of medical intervention. These patients may view adherence to a scientific credo as the only way to conceptualize their illness and regain control over their lives.

Karen Osney Browstein's bestselling pathography, *Brainstorm,* is a particularly vivid illustration of the process through which the "high-tech" and "science-laden" culture of oncology shapes a (perceived) cure of cancer.[14] The author, a New York journalist, suffered from recurring violent headaches. A visit to a neurologist revealed an excess of pressure in her brain, but a CAT scan and an additional (and dangerous) test, a pneumoencephalogram, were unable to reveal the cause of this pressure. Two hypotheses were then advanced: a pinealoma, a very rare tumor of the pineal gland; or an aqueductal stenosis, an abnormal (and equally rare) circulation defect. If the first hypothesis was correct, the doctor's recommendation was radiation therapy with a cobalt bomb (an experimental treatment, since the tumor is very rare); if the second hypothesis was correct, the specialist's advice was to do nothing, because the circulation defect is self-limiting. In the meantime the installation of a shunt reduced the fluid pressure in the brain, taking care of Ms. Browstein's symptoms. The few experts who could be consulted about the case disagreed about what to do next. Some advised waiting, others radiation therapy. Finally the author, impressed by the authoritative statement of one well-known expert— "my clinical intuition tells me that you have a tumor"—but also afraid to live with a possible "time bomb" in her brain, and pressed by family and friends to "do something," started a cobalt bomb therapy. The diagnostic uncertainty, however, enhanced her fears of the treatment and increased her negative reaction to its side effects (nausea, fatigue, hair loss). To overcome her depression, she entered psychotherapy. The therapist then convinced her that the negative reaction to the radiation therapy was in fact a denial of her tumor. He also attempted to cure her of a fear of the cobalt machine: "The technology, Mrs. Browstein. Think of the technology. Maybe your husband can help you to appreciate this. If your tumor recurs in two years there will be a laser therapy that may cure you. The tumor did not grow in your brain overnight; it took time. More time than it takes for technology to advance. Trust it. Trust the technology."[15] At the end of the radiation treatment the radiologist responsible for her therapy declared her cured of a malignant pinealoma. The paperback edition of *Brainstorm* is advertised as a "book about a brain tumor" and as a "medical success story."

Brainstorm is a story of the genesis and development of medical facts (diagnosis, then cure of a brain tumor) within a specific biomedical culture. The fuzziness of the initial pathological phenomenon— increased pressure in the brain—is gradually transformed into scientific and medical conviction and into a strong individual belief. This combined effect is produced by machines such as CAT scanners and cobalt bombs but above all by the authoritative declarations of experts and by the gradual transformation (here, also by a psychotherapist) of the patient's perception of her disease.[16] The case of the "brain tumor" described in *Brainstorm* is unusual, insofar as it involves not only a (frequent) therapeutic uncertainty but also a (much less frequent) diagnostic uncertainty. Gerda Lerner's pathography, *A Death of One's Own,* presents a more typical case in which the diagnosis (of an inoperable brain tumor in her husband) is accepted as an indisputable fact, the prognosis is viewed as being accurate in its general outline but not in important details (the trajectory of the patient's illness did not conform in many points to the expected one; he did not die three days but three weeks after a withdrawal of life-sustaining drugs), and the effects of the therapy remain unclear (Carl Lerner's doctor thought that an experimental chemotherapy slowed the progress of his disease, but the family disagreed).[17]

Although the story told in *A Death of One's Own* differs in many important details from the one told in *Brainstorm*, it is also fully embedded in the current culture of oncology—a "high-tech" specialty with a strong trialist ethos. Gerda Lerner's reasoning is expressed in scientific terms, and she shares the doctors' view of cancer as the inexorable progress of deviant cells that will kill her husband because there is no possibility of eliminating these cells by surgery or of destroying them with appropriate drugs. On the other hand, while most cancer pathographies either uncritically accept the medical point of view or, alternatively, radically reject it, Gerda Lerner's fine-tuned account of her husband's terminal illness points to the incommensurability between the biomedical view of cancer—fully accepted by all the participants in Carl Lerner's drama—and the concrete experience of the sick person and his family. Gerda Lerner does not attempt to accomplish an impossible synthesis between contradictory perceptions of cancer, and her book contains several versions of the same story. Her faithful record of the failure to construct a coherent narrative of her husband's illness and death nevertheless achieves a transcendence of a kind through her writing.

Similarly, when the poet Ted Rosenthal was diagnosed with leukemia, he at first felt that his imminent death gave him an extraordinary feeling of freedom to "do anything" he wanted with his life. Later, however, he became afraid because he was increasingly unable to align his subjective emotions and bodily sensations with the image of his disease projected by the scientific medicine, that is, with the results of laboratory tests. "My medical condition was such that it changed dramatically from moment to moment. I was never able to synchronize my feelings with the information . . . [from blood tests and bone marrow samples] and every bit of information had to alter my feelings about myself in terms of survival and where I stood in relation to the future and even that moment. I became frightened."[18]

The experiences of Gerda Lerner, Karen Osney Browstein, and Ted

Rosenthal are typical insofar as they reflect the (sometimes reluctant) adherence of most cancer patients and their families to the oncologists' concepts and practices. Proposals advanced by advocates of cancer immunotherapy may have facilitated such adherence, because they connected the oncologists' view of cancer as an alien entity to the more familiar idea of "stimulation of the defense mechanisms of the body."[19] The patients enrolled in the IL-2 trial at the Cancer Foundation, the doctors who conducted it, the industrialists who supplied interleukin and funding, the health administrators and cancer charities that supported this clinical experiment—all shared the conviction that a suc-

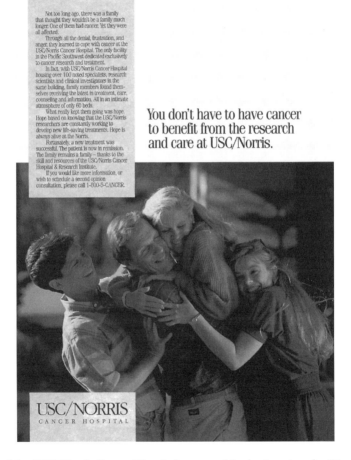

This ad for USC/Norris Cancer Hospital appeared in the *Los Angeles Times Magazine,* April 7, 1991. (Courtesy USC/Norris Hospital.)

cessful linking of an immunology laboratory with an oncology ward would increase the chances of developing a cure for a disseminated cancer. This conviction was rooted in the history of the perception of the disease "cancer" and in the history of the practices of biologists and oncologists, and was stabilized in the culture of clinical experimentation in oncology. It informed doctors' and scientists' decisions and favored the development of multiple material, social, and rhetorical connections between the laboratory and the clinics during the IL-2 trial. These connections, one may object, remained weak. Weak ties, however, may have a strength of their own.[20] Network theories stress the importance of developing long and stable links between actors.[21] In contrast, I propose that the indeterminacy of concepts and practices, the development of "hedges" (fuzzy practices) and intermediary zones, and the circulation of boundary objects contributed to stabilization of the alliance between biologists and oncologists through the development of loose but relatively stable ties. These ties affected trial-related practices but also helped make the IL-2 trial into a vehicle for organizational changes at the Cancer Foundation.

In its current form the culture of clinical experimentation in oncology reflects "the power of structures that already exist."[22] The long-standing alliance between the research laboratory and the oncology clinics is among the most powerful of these preexisting structures. But one should not confuse power and rigidity. The cooperation between basic biological research and the cancer clinic is unlikely to continue forever in its present form. Attitudes and practices may change, and perhaps they are already changing. Thus the discourse of the leaders of the U.S. National Cancer Institute was less optimistic in the early 1990s than in the 1970s and 1980s.[23] In the meantime, however, one may reasonably assume that as long as cancer is defined as a disease of "deviant cells," as long as there is no efficient treatment of cancer "at hand," and as long as the therapy of human malignancies is structured as a weakly life-style-dependent and strongly science-laden area of medical intervention, connections between the biology laboratory and the oncology ward will remain stable.

Notes

Introduction

1. Sandra Panem, *The Interferon Crusade* (Washington, D.C.: Brookings Institution, 1984).
2. Steven A. Rosenberg et al., "Observations on the systemic administration of autologous lymphokine-activated killer cells and recombinant interleukin-2 to patients with metastatic cancer," *New England Journal of Medicine,* 313 (1985), 1485–92.
3. "Cancer Patience," *Wall Street Journal,* December 16, 1985.
4. Eli Kedar and Eva Klein, "Cancer immunotherapy: Are the results discouraging? Can they be improved?" *Advances in Cancer Research,* 59 (1992), 245–322.
5. For example, a survey made in the early 1990s (and reported by the French minister of health, Philippe Douste-Blazy) revealed that only 30 percent of French cancer patients suffering from disease-related pain received efficient antipain treatment, and that half of the patients suffering from cancer-related pain received no pain medication; Franck Nouchi, "La douleur maltraitée," *Le Monde,* August 29, 1993. See also M. Zenz and A. Willweber-Strumpf, "Opiophobia and cancer pain in Europe," *Lancet,* 1993, pp. 1075–76. Similar observations have been made in the United States. A study conducted by the Eastern Cooperative Oncology Group revealed that 85 percent of the oncologists included in that study believed that cancer patients in the United States are undermedicated for disease-related pain, and two-thirds admitted that they did not prescribe enough pain killers to their cancer patients; Joel Greenberg, "Treatment of cancer patients found to be low priority," *Los Angeles Times,* May 27, 1991. In 1995 both French and American doctors claimed that they now pay more attention to cancer pain.
6. The results of the Cancer Foundation's IL-2 trial were published in rec-

ognized professional journals, but a "black" account might argue that these results merely confirmed findings published by other groups.

7. The contamination of blood and blood products, the trial of the directors of the French blood transfusion system revealed, resulted from strict adherence to managerial criteria. The directors of blood transfusion agencies decided to distribute contaminated products to patients in order to avoid financial losses; Anne-Marie Casteret, *L'affaire du sang* (Paris: La Découverte, 1992); Michel Setbon, *Les pouvoirs contre le Sida* (Paris: Le Seuil, 1993).

8. The proposition that societal structures are valid analytic units does not assume that these structures are stable and rigid entities. It does assume, however, differences in their plasticity and their degree of resistance to change.

9. Robert E. Kohler, *Partners in Science: Foundations and Natural Scientists, 1900–1945* (Chicago: University of Chicago Press, 1991), p. xiv.

10. Clifford Geertz, "Thick description: Towards an interpretative theory of culture," in *The Interpretation of Cultures* (New York: Basic Books, 1973), pp. 3–30.

11. Jacques Degain, "Les médicaments avant leur AMM. Une victoire pour les grands malades?" *Le quotidien du médecin,* October 14, 1991, pp. 4827–28.

12. George J. Annas, "Faith (healing) hope and charity at the FDA: The politics of AIDS drug trials," *Villanova Law Review,* 34 (1989), 771–797.

13. Some AIDS activists stress the complexity and ambiguities of the new situation, e.g., Cindy Patton, *Inventing AIDS* (London: Routledge, 1990).

14. Harold Edge and David J. Rothman, "New rules for new drugs: The challenge of AIDS to the regulatory process," *Milbank Quarterly,* 68, supp. 1 (1990), 111–142; Anne Christine d'Adesky, "Empowerment or co-optation," *The Nation,* February 11, 1991, 158–161; Daniel Defert, "La rhétorique des conférences," *Transcriptase,* 17 (1993), 2–3; Peter S. Arno and Karyn L. Freiden, *Against the Odds: The Story of AIDS, Drug Development, Politics, and Profits* (New York: Harper Perennial, 1992), pp. 225–235.

15. This sentence evokes Ludwik Fleck's pioneering study, *Genesis and Development of a Scientific Fact* (1935), trans. Fred Bradley and Thaddeus J. Trenn (Chicago: University of Chicago Press, 1979).

16. E.g., Bruce Nussbaum, *Good Intentions: How Big Business and the Medical Establishment Are Corrupting the Fight against AIDS, Alzheimer's, Cancer, and More* (New York: Penguin, 1990); Arno and Freiden, *Against the Odds.* Such schematic images are related to representations

of biomedical research in popular books such as Sinclair Lewis' *Arrowsmith* (1925). On the perpetuation of such stereotyped images by the media see, e.g., Joseph Turow, *Playing Doctor: Television Storytelling and Medical Power* (New York: Oxford University Press, 1989); Anne Karff, *Doctoring the Media: The Reporting of Health and Medicine* (London: Routledge, 1988); and, on schematic representations of scientific research, John C. Burnham, *How Superstition Won and Science Lost* (New Brunswick, N.J.: Rutgers University Press, 1987).

17. John S. James, *AIDS Treatment News* (Berkeley, Calif.: Celestial Arts, 1989), p. xxxv (emphasis added). For an analysis of the influence of AIDS activists in shaping clinical trials for new anti-AIDS drugs, see Steven Epstein, "The construction of lay expertise: AIDS activism and the forging of credibility in the reform of clinical trials," *Science, Technology and Human Values,* 20(4) (1995), 408–437.

18. Kathryn M. Hunter, *Doctor Stories: The Narrative Structure of Medical Knowledge* (Princeton: Princeton University Press, 1991), p. 47. One may add that the success of modern medicine may depend not merely on the ignorance of its epistemological paradoxes but also on their efficient utilization.

19. The AIDS epidemic brought to the fore the issue of cost-effective analysis of clinical trials of new therapies. See, e.g., A. D. Paltiel and E. H. Kaplan, "Modeling Zidovudine therapy: A cost-effectiveness analysis," *Journal of AIDS,* 4 (1991), 795–804; idem, "The epidemiological and economic consequences of an AIDS trial," ibid., 6 (1993), 179–190; Yves-Antoine Flory, "Analyse coût-bénéfice des essais thérapeutiques," *Transcriptase,* 18 (1993), 22–25.

20. Even in highly complex scientific or technological enterprises, small changes may sometimes have far-reaching consequences. See, e.g., Bruno Latour, *The Pasteurization of France,* trans. Alan Sheridan and John Law (Cambridge, Mass.: Harvard University Press, 1988). Beyond a certain point, however, technological choices become irreversible; Thomas Hughes, *Networks of Power: Electric Supply Systems in the United States, England, and Germany, 1880–1930* (Baltimore: Johns Hopkins University Press, 1983).

21. The classic philosophical study on this subject is Georges Canguilhem, *Le normal et le pathologique* (1943) (Paris: Presses Universitaires de France, 1966). See also Nancy Maul, "The practical art of medicine," *Journal of Medicine and Philosophy,* 6 (1981), 215–232; Ronald Munson, "Why medicine cannot be science," ibid., 6 (1981), 183–208; Christiane Sinding, *Le clinicien et le chercheur. Des grandes maladies de carence à la médecine moléculaire, 1880–1980* (Paris: Presses Universitaires de France, 1991).

22. Joseph Ben-David, "The professional role of physicians in bureaucratized medicine: A study in role conflict," *Human Relations,* 11 (1958), 255–274.

23. N. D. Jewson, "The disappearance of the sick-man from medical cosmology, 1770–1870," *Sociology,* 10(2) (1976), 225–244; Charles E. Rosenberg, "The therapeutic revolution: Medicine, meaning, and social change in nineteenth-century America," in *The Therapeutic Revolution: Essays in the Social History of American Medicine,* ed. M. J. Vogel and C. E. Rosenberg (Philadelphia: University of Pennsylvania Press, 1979), pp. 3–26; C. E. Rosenberg, *The Care of Strangers* (New York: Basic Books, 1987).

24. Erwin Ackerknecht, *Medicine at Paris Hospital* (Baltimore: Johns Hopkins Press, 1967); Stanley Reiser, *Medicine and the Reign of Technology* (Cambridge: Cambridge University Press, 1978).

25. Joseph Dietl, "Praktische Wahermungen," in *Unzusammen Werken* (Vienna, 1845).

26. Latour, *The Pasteurization of France;* Claire Salomon-Bayet, ed., *Pasteur et la révolution pasteurienne* (Paris: Payot, 1988); John Harley Warner, "Science in medicine," in *Historical Writings on American Science: Perspectives and Prospects,* ed. Sally Georgy Kohlsted and Margaret W. Rossiter (Baltimore: Johns Hopkins University Press, 1986), pp. 37–58; John Harley Warner, "Science, healing, and the physician's identity: A problem of professional character in nineteenth-century America," *Clio Medica,* 22 (1991), 65–88; Gerald L. Geison, *The Private Science of Louis Pasteur* (Princeton: Princeton University Press, 1995).

27. Vogel and Rosenberg, *The Therapeutic Revolution;* Christopher Lawrence, "Incommunicable knowledge: Science, technology, and the clinical art in Britain, 1850–1914," *Journal of Contemporary History,* 20 (1985), 503–520; John Harley Warner, *The Therapeutic Perspective: Medical Practice, Knowledge, and Identity in America* (Cambridge, Mass.: Harvard University Press, 1986).

28. Paul DeKruif, *The Microbe Hunters* (New York: Harcourt and Brace, 1926).

29. E.g., James S. Coleman, Elihu Katz, and Herbert Menzel, *Medical Innovation: A Diffusion Study* (Indianapolis: Bobbs-Merrill, 1966); Daniel M. Becker, Dan Satel, and Laurence Gardner, "Decision to adapt new medical technology: A case study of thrombolytic therapy," *Social Sciences and Medicine,* 21(3) (1985), 291–298; Edward B. Roberts, *Biomedical Innovation* (Cambridge, Mass.: MIT Press, 1981); F. Gremy, ed., *De la recherche biomédicale à la pratique des soins* (Paris: Editions INSERM, 1986); Renaldo N. Battista, "Innovation and diffusion of health-related technologies," *International Journal of Tech-*

nology Assessment in Health Care, 5 (1989), 227–243. Stuart Blume's *Insight and Industry: On the Dynamics of Technological Change in Medicine* (Cambridge, Mass.: MIT Press, 1991) is a notable exception.

30. E.g., Russel Maulitz, "Physician versus bacteriologist: The ideology of science in clinical medicine," in Vogel and Rosenberg, *The Therapeutic Revolution;* Lawrence, "Incommunicable knowledge"; Reiser, *Medicine and the Reign of Technology;* Rosenberg, *The Care of Strangers;* Bernike Pasveer, "The Knowledge of Shadows" (Ph.D. diss., University of Amsterdam, 1992).

31. For examples of the "linear" view, see, e.g., C. D. Dickinson, "The value for medical practice of basic and applied medical research," in *Social Researching: Politics, Problems and Practice,* ed. Colin Bell and Helen Roberts (London: Routledge & Kegan Paul, 1984), pp. 54–69; Lewis Thomas, "The future of medicine," in *New Prospects for Medicine,* ed. Jonathan M. Austy (New York: Oxford University Press, 1988), pp. 114–126.

32. See, e.g., Vogel and Rosenberg, *The Therapeutic Revolution;* John Pickstone, ed., *Medical Innovations in Historical Perspective* (London: Macmillan, 1992); Ilana Löwy, ed., *Medicine and Change: Historical and Sociological Studies of Medical Innovation* (London and Paris: John Libbey and INSERM, 1993).

33. Eliot Freidson, *Profession of Medicine: The Study of Sociology of Applied Knowledge* (New York: Dodd, Mead, 1970), pp. 223, 277, 288.

34. E. Freidson and Judith Lorber, "Producing medical knowledge," in *Medical Men and Their Work,* ed. E. Freidson and J. Lorber (New York: Aldine-Atherton, 1972), pp. 385–472.

35. Renée C. Fox, *Experiment Perilous: Physicians and Patients Facing the Unknown* (1959; reprint, Philadelphia: University of Pennsylvania Press, 1974); R. C. Fox and Judith Swazey, *The Courage to Fail: A Social View of Organ Transplantation and Dialysis* (Chicago: University of Chicago Press, 1974.)

36. Later Fox considerably changed her outlook, and her recent publications question medical knowledge and medical practices. See, e.g., R. C. Fox and J. Swazey, *Spare Parts* (Oxford: Oxford University Press, 1992); R. C. Fox, " 'An ignoble form of cannibalism': Reflections on the Pittsburgh protocol for procuring organs for non-heart-beating cadavers," *Kennedy Institute of Ethics Journal,* 3(2) (1993), 231–239.

37. Peter Wright and Andrew Treacher, *The Problem of Medical Knowledge: Examining the Social Construction of Medicine* (Edinburgh: Edinburgh University Press, 1982); David Armstrong, *The Political Anatomy of the Body* (Cambridge: Cambridge University Press, 1983); Malcolm Bury, "Social constructivism and the development of medical sociology," *Sociology of Health and Illness,* 8 (1986), 137–169; Mal-

colm Nicholson and Cathleen McLaughlin, "Social constructivism and medical sociology: A reply to M. Bury," ibid., 9 (1988), 107–126; idem, "Social constructivism and medical sociology: A study of the vascular theory of multiple sclerosis," ibid., 10 (1988), 107–126.

38. Peter Galison, *How Experiments End* (Chicago: University of Chicago Press, 1987), p. 2.

39. See, e.g., Isabelle Baszanger, "Deciphering chronic pain," *Sociology of Health and Illness*, 14 (1992), 181–215; Mark Berg, "The construction of medical disposals: Medical sociology and medical problem solving in clinical practice," ibid., pp. 151–180; Warwick Anderson, "The reasoning of the strongest: The polemics of skill and science in medical diagnosis," *Social Studies of Science*, 22 (1992), 653–684; Nicolas Dodier, *L'expertise médicale. Essai de sociologie sur l'exercice du jugement* (Paris: A. M. Métailié, 1993); Annemarie Mol, "What's new? Doppler and its others: An empirical philosophy of innovations," in Löwy, *Medicine and Change*, pp. 107–125.

40. Ilana Löwy, "The impact of medical practice on biomedical research: The case of lymphocyte antigen studies," *Minerva*, 25 (1987), 173–199; idem, "Variances in meaning in discovery accounts: The case of contemporary biology," *Historical Studies in Physical and Biological Sciences*, 21 (1990), 87–112.

41. Robert K. Merton, "Paradigm for the sociology of knowledge" (1945), reprinted in idem, *The Sociology of Science* (Chicago: University of Chicago Press, 1973), pp. 7–40.

42. Gerald M. Swatez, "Social organization of a university laboratory," *Minerva*, January 1970, 36–58; Robert S. Anderson, "The necessity of field methods in the study of scientific research," in *Science and Cultures*, ed. Everett Mendelsohn and Yehuda Elkana (Dordrecht: D. Reidel, 1981), pp. 213–244.

43. Thomas S. Kuhn, *The Structure of Scientific Revolutions* (Chicago: University of Chicago Press, 1962).

44. Harold Garfinkel, *Studies in Ethnomethodology* (Englewood Cliffs, N.J.: Prentice-Hall, 1966); Aaron Cicourel, *Method and Measurement in Sociology* (New York: Free Press, 1964); idem, *The Social Organization of Juvenile Justice* (New York: John Wiley and Sons, 1968).

45. Harry M. Collins, "The seven sexes: A study of a phenomenon of replication of experiments in physics," *Sociology*, 9(2) (1975), 205–224; H. M. Collins and Robert Harrison, "Building a TEA laser: The caprices of communication," *Social Studies of Science*, 5 (1975), 441–445; Bruno Latour and Steve Woolgar, *Laboratory Life: The Social Construction of Scientific Facts* (Beverly Hills: Sage, 1979); Karen Knorr-Cetina, *The Manufacture of Knowledge: An Essay on the Constructivist and Contextual Nature of Science* (Oxford: Pergamon Press, 1981);

Andrew Pickering, "Constraints on controversy: The case of magnetic monopole," *Social Studies of Science*, 11 (1981), 63–93; Michael Zenzen and Sal Restivo, "The mysterious morphology of immiscible liquids: A study of scientific practice," *Social Science Information*, 21 (1982), 447–473; S. Leigh Star, "Simplification in scientific work: An example from neurosciences research," *Social Studies of Science*, 13 (1983), 205–228; Michael Lynch, *Art and Artifact in Laboratory Science: A Study of Shop Work and Shop Talk in a Research Laboratory* (London: Routledge and Kegan Paul, 1985); Trevor J. Pinch, "Toward the analysis of scientific observations: The externality and evidential significance of observation reports in physics," *Social Studies of Science*, 15 (1985), 1–22.

46. Latour and Woolgar, *Laboratory Life*, p. 39.

47. H. M. Collins and Trevor Pinch, *Frames of Meaning: The Social Construction of Extraordinary Science* (London: Routledge & Kegan Paul, 1982); H. M. Collins, "Researching spoonbending: Concepts and practice of participatory fieldwork," in Bell and Roberts, *Social Researching*, pp. 54–69.

48. Robert M. Emerson, "Introduction," in *Contemporary Field Research* (Prospect Heights, Ill.: Waveland Press, 1983), pp. 1–35, esp. pp. 12–13.

49. Suziko Y. Fagarhaugh and Anselm Strauss, *Politics of Pain Management: Staff–Patients Interactions* (Menlo Park, Calif.: Addison-Wesley, 1977).

50. Barry Barnes and David Edge, *Science in Context: Readings in the Sociology of Science* (Cambridge, Mass.: MIT Press, 1982), p. 65.

51. Ilana Löwy, "The scientific roots of constructivist epistemologies: Hélène Metzger and Ludwik Fleck," in *Etudes sur/Studies on Hélène Metzger*, ed. Gad Freudenthal (Paris: Corpus, 1988), pp. 219–235; Gad Freudenthal and Ilana Löwy, "Ludwik Fleck's roles in society: A case study using Joseph Ben David's paradigm for the sociology of knowledge," *Social Studies of Science*, 18 (1988), 625–651; Ilana Löwy, *The Polish School of Philosophy of Medicine: From Tytus Chalubinski (1820–1889) to Ludwik Fleck (1896–1961)* (Dordrecht: Kluwer, 1990).

52. This opinion is shared by other historians and sociologists of science. As Ian Golinski put it: "sociologists and historians . . . might still profitably consider whether their visions of scientific practice can match the elegance and subtlety of Fleck's"; "The theory of practice and the practice of theory: Sociological approaches in the history of science," *Isis*, 81 (1990), 505.

53. Geertz, "Thick description."

54. Latour and Woolgar, *Laboratory Life*, p. 254.

55. For some students of science, all participants in a network (e.g., patients,

interleukin-2, tumors, immunologists, white blood cells, oncologists, cytapheresis machines) belong to a single category of "actants"; Michel Callon, "Some elements of a sociology of translation: Domestication of the scallops and fishermen of St. Brieuc Bay," in *Power, Action and Belief: A New Sociology of Knowledge?* ed. J. Law (London: Routledge and Kegan Paul, 1986), pp. 196–233; Bruno Latour, *Nous n'avons jamais été modernes* (Paris: La Découverte, 1991).

56. C. G. Moertel, "On lymphokines, cytokines, and breakthroughs," *Journal of the American Medical Association,* 256 (1986), 3141–42.

57. For a detailed account of the problems of witnessing in the clinics, see Charles L. Bosk, *All God's Mistakes: Genetic Counseling in a Pediatric Hospital* (Chicago: University of Chicago Press, 1992).

58. Following Abbott, I define *jurisdiction* as a link between a profession (or a professional segment) and its work; Andrew Abbott, *The System of Professions: An Essay on the Division of Expert Labor* (Chicago: University of Chicago Press, 1988). This meaning of the term *jurisdiction* is akin to the meaning of the term *ownership,* proposed by Joseph Gusfield; J. R. Gusfield, *The Culture of Public Problems: Drinking, Driving, and the Symbolic Order* (Chicago: University of Chicago Press, 1981).

59. Jean-Paul Gaudillière, "Biologie moléculaire et biologistes en France dans les années soixante" (Ph.D. diss., Université de Paris VII, 1991).

60. Scientists tend to report their experiments in the order in which they should have been done, not in chronological order. Sir Peter Medawar noted that this tendency is not viewed as dishonest, because scientists (unlike historians of science) are convinced that a faithful record of false trails and chance events during a scientific investigation is of anecdotal value only; Peter Medawar, *The Art of the Soluble* (Harmondsworth: Penguin, 1969), p. 169.

61. E. P. Thompson, "The moral economy of the English crowd in the eighteenth century," in *Customs in Common: Studies in Traditional Popular Culture* (New York: New Press, 1993), p. 187 (first published in *Past and Present,* 50 (1971), 76–136). Thompson's writings contributed to the development of more fine-grained analyses of interactions between economic and cultural developments.

62. E.g., Mario Biagolli, *Galileo, Courtier: The Practice of Science in the Culture of Absolutism* (Chicago: University of Chicago Press, 1993); Lorraine Daston, "Baconian facts, academic civility, and the prehistory of objectivity," *Annals of Scholarship,* 8 (1991), 337–363; Peter Dear, "From truth to disinterestedness in the seventeenth century," *Social Studies of Science,* 22 (1922), 619–631; Steven Pumphrey, " 'Ideas above his station': A social study of Hooke's curatorship of experiments," *History of Science,* 29 (1991), 1–44; Steven Shapin and Simon

Schaffer, *Leviathan and the Air Pump: Hobbes, Boyle, and the Exper-imental Life* (Princeton: Princeton University Press, 1985); S. Shapin, *A Social History of Truth: Civility and Science in Seventeenth-Century England* (Chicago: University of Chicago Press, 1994).

63. Notable exceptions are historical studies centered on use of instruments and tools. These studies often combine detailed accounts of bench (or bedside) practices with "larger pictures" that include economic consid-erations and industrial partners. See, e.g., Nicolas Rasmussen, "Making a machine instrumental: RCA and the wartime beginnings of biological electron microscopy," *Studies in the History and Philosophy of Science* (in press); Alberto Cambrosio and Peter Keating, "A matter of FACS: Constitution novel entities in immunology," *Medical Anthropology Quarterly,* 6(4) (1992), 362–384; Blume, *Insight and Industry.*

1. The Culture of Clinical Experimentation in Oncology

1. David Cantor has proposed that close linking of cancer research and cancer therapy served mainly the interest of the biomedical scientists; "Contracting cancer: The politics of commissioned histories," *Journal of the Social History of Medicine,* 5 (1992), 136. Cantor does not men-tion that clinicians too may benefit from an association with prestigious domains of biomedical research.

2. Richard A. Rettig, *Cancer Crusade: The History of the National Cancer Act of 1971* (Princeton: Princeton University Press, 1977); James Patterson, *The Dread Disease: Cancer and Modern American Culture* (Cambridge, Mass.: Harvard University Press, 1987), pp. 171–200.

3. Janny Scott, "Women's new push for health," *Los Angeles Times,* April 30, 1991. On the struggle of AIDS activists to ensure equal access to experimental treatments, see Harold Edgar and David J. Rothman, "New rules for new drugs: The challenge of AIDS to the regulatory process," *Milbank Quarterly,* 68 (1990), 111–142.

4. Lou Fintor, "Patient activism: Cancer groups become vocal and politi-cally active," *Journal of the National Cancer Institute,* 83(8) (1991), 528–529.

5. *Los Angeles Times,* April 23, 1991.

6. Patterson, *The Dread Disease;* Patrice Pinell, *Naissance d'un fléau. La lutte contre le cancer en France 1890–1940* (Paris: A. M. Métailié, 1992).

7. Ronald W. Raven, "The surgeon and oncology," *Clinical Oncology,* 10 (1984), 311–318; idem, "Radical and extended surgery for cancer," *On-cology: Proceedings of the Tenth International Cancer Congress,* 4 (1970), 197–203.

8. For example, in the years 1867–1876 Billroth operated upon 170 cancer

patients, 4.7 percent of whom were alive three years after the operation; Patterson, *The Dread Disease,* p. 29.

9. J. Bergonié, "Effets des rayons X dans le cancer du sein," *Journal de médecine de Bordeaux,* 13 (1904), 228; Pinell, *Naissance d'un fléau.*

10. Manuel Lederman, "The early history of radiotherapy: 1895–1939," *International Journal of Radiation Oncology, Biology and Physics,* 7 (1981), 639–648; Pinell, *Naissance d'un fléau,* chap. 2.

11. Lederman, "Early history of radiotherapy"; Pinell, *Naissance d'un fléau.*

12. Such centers were typically multidisciplinary institutions. The first such center in France, the Curie Institute, was a subdivision of the Pasteur Institute, which was seen as a model for the association between an advanced biomedical research institute and a hospital.

13. Michael B. Shimkin, *Contrary to Nature,* NIH Publication 76-720 (Bethesda, Md.: National Institutes of Health, 1979), pp. 271–295; Patrice Pinell, "Cancer policy and health system in France: Big medicine challenges the conception and organization of medical practice," *Social History of Medicine,* 4(1) (1991), 75–101.

14. C. G. Kardinal and J. W. Yabro, "A conceptual history of cancer," *Seminars in Oncology,* 6 (1979), 396–536; J. Ratner, *The Genesis of Cancer: A Study in the History of Ideas* (Baltimore: Johns Hopkins University Press, 1978).

15. Patrice Pinell and Sylvia Brossat, "The birth of cancer policies in France," *Sociology of Health and Illness,* 10(4) (1988), 576–607; Patterson, *The Dread Disease,* pp. 56–87; Pinell, *Naissance d'un fléau.*

16. Stephen P. Strickland, *Politics, Science, and Dread Disease: A Short History of United States Medical Research Policy* (Cambridge, Mass.: Harvard University Press, 1972); Donald Swain, "Rise of a research empire: NIH, 1930–1950," *Science,* 138 (1962), 1233–37; Pinell, "Cancer policy and health system in France."

17. Carl G. Cardinal, "Cancer chemotherapy: Historical aspects and future considerations," *Postgraduate Medicine,* 77(6) (1985), 165–174.

18. James B. Murphy, in "Reports of the Directors of the Laboratories," vol. 3, April 1914, pp. 259–261, Rockefeller Archives, North Tarrytown, N.Y.

19. E. B. Krumbhaar and H. D. Krumbhaar, "The blood and bone marrow in mustard gas poisoning: Changes produced in the bone marrow of fatal cases," *Journal of Medical Research,* 11 (1919–20), 497–507.

20. E.g., I. Berenblum, "Experimental inhibition of tumor induction by mustard gas and other compounds," *Journal of Pathology and Bacteriology,* 40 (1935), 549–558.

21. A. Gilman, "The initial clinical trial of nitrogen mustard," *American Journal of Surgery,* 105 (1963), 574–578; Jerzy Einhorn, "Nitrogen

mustard: The origins of chemotherapy for cancer," *International Journal of Radiation Oncology, Biology and Physics,* 11 (1985), 1375–78.

22. Helen Coley Nauts, Walker E. Swift, and Bradley E. Coley, "The treatment of malignant tumors by bacterial toxins developed by the late William B. Coley, M.D., reviewed in the light of modern research," *Cancer Research,* 6 (1946), 205–216.

23. M. J. Shear and F. C. Turner, "Chemical treatment of tumors: V. Isolation of hemorrhage-producing factor from *Serratia marcescens (Bacillus prodigiosus)* culture filtrate," *Journal of the National Cancer Institute,* 1 (1943), 81–97; G. Schwartzmann, "Phenomenon of local skin reactivity of *Serratia marcescens:* Immunological reactions between *Serratia marcescens* culture filtrate and Shear's polysaccharide," *Cancer Research,* 4 (1944), 191–196; A. M. Brues and M. J. Shear, "Chemical treatment of tumors: Reactions of four patients with advanced malignant tumors to injection of polysaccharide from *Serratia marcescens* filtrate," *Journal of the National Cancer Institute,* 5 (1944), 195–208; A. L. Hollman, "Reactions of patients and of tumors to the injection of *S. marcescens* polysaccharide in eight cases of malignant disease," in *Approaches to Tumor Chemotherapy,* ed. F. M. Moulton (Washington, D.C.: American Association for the Advancement of Science, 1947), pp. 273–276; R. Oakey, "Reactions of patients to injections of *S. marcescens* polysaccharide in nine further cases of malignant disease," ibid., p. 277.

24. Joan Austoker, *A History of the Imperial Cancer Research Fund, 1902–1986* (Oxford: Oxford University Press, 1988), pp. 181–182.

25. Jean-François Picard, "Poussée scientifique ou demande des médecins? La recherche médicale en France de l'Institut National d'Hygiène à l'INSERM," *Sciences sociales et médecine,* 10(4) (1992), 47–106.

26. C. Gordon Zubrod, Saul A. Schepartz, and Stephen K. Carter, "Historical background of the National Cancer Institute's Drug Development Trust," *National Cancer Institute's Monographs,* 45 (1977), 8. This paper explains that screening programs for anticancer drugs were influenced by the example of antibiotics.

27. Robert F. Bud, "Strategy in American cancer research after World War II: A case study," *Social Studies of Science,* 8 (1978), 425–459.

28. Ibid., p. 433.

29. C. G. Zubrod, "Origins and development of chemotherapy research at the National Cancer Institute," *Cancer Treatment Reports,* 68(1) (1984), 9; Bud, "Strategy in American cancer research," pp. 440–445.

30. Zubrod, Schepartz, and Carter, "Historical background," p. 8.

31. Zubrod, "Origins and development"; Zubrod, Schepartz, and Carter, "Historical background"; Carl G. Baker, "Cancer research program

strategy and planning: The use of contracts for program implementation," *Journal of the National Cancer Institute*, 59, supp. (1977), 651–
669.

32. Kenneth M. Endicott, "The chemotherapy program," *Journal of the National Cancer Institute*, 19 (1957), 283.

33. C. G. Zubrod, "Historic milestones in curative chemotherapy," *Seminars in Oncology*, 6(4) (1979), 500; Bud, "Strategy in American cancer research," p. 442; Austoker, *History of Imperial Cancer Research Fund*, p. 181.

34. The growth of cancer chemotherapy at the NCI may be compared to the development of chemical physiology in England in the early twentieth century; Steve Sturdy, "Chemical physiology and clinical medicine: Academics and the scientisation of medical practice in England," in *Medicine and Change: Historical and Sociological Studies of Medical Innovation*, ed. Ilana Löwy (London and Paris: John Libbey/INSERM, 1993), pp. 371–393.

35. S. Farber et al., "Temporary remission in acute leukemia in children produced by folic acid antagonist, 4-aminoptenyl-glutamic acid (aminopterin)," *New England Journal of Medicine*, 238 (1948), 787–793.

36. Eugene A. Stead (chair), Report of the Advisory Panel on Biomedical Research and Medical Technology, *Development of Medical Technology: Opportunities for Assessment* (Washington, D.C.: U.S. Congress, Office of Technology Assessment, 1976), pp. 74–75.

37. Zubrod, "Origins and development."

38. In 1945 the ACS replaced the ASCC. The reorganization of the major U.S. cancer charity—orchestrated by the philanthropists Albert and Mary Lasker—resulted in a dramatic increase in its ability to mobilize resources and political support; Strickland, *Politics, Science, and Dread Disease*.

39. Endicott, "The chemotherapy program"; Zubrod, "Origins and development"; Zubrod, Schepartz, and Carter, "Historical background"; Zubrod, "Historic milestones in curative chemotherapy."

40. Zubrod, "Origins and development," p. 11.

41. Endicott, "The chemotherapy program"; Zubrod, "Origins and development"; Zubrod, Schepartz, and Carter, "Historical background."

42. The sums allocated to chemotherapy studies were small, however, in comparison to funds allocated in the 1950s for, e.g., research in high-energy physics.

43. Zubrod, Schepartz, and Carter, "Historical background," p. 12.

44. Zubrod, "Origins and development," p. 12; Endicott, "The chemotherapy program," p. 292.

45. The production of "standard" inbred organisms that are in fact engineered tools played an important role in biological research; see Robert

E. Kohler, "Systems of production: Drosophila, Neurospora, and bio-chemical genetics," *Historical Studies in the Biological and the Physical Sciences,* 21 (1991), 87–127; idem, *Lords of the Fly: Drosophila Genetics and the Experimental Life* (Chicago: University of Chicago Press, 1994).

46. Zubrod, Schepartz, and Carter, "Historical background," p. 10; Endicott, "The chemotherapy program," p. 280.

47. Harry M. Marks, "Notes from the underground: The social organization of therapeutic research," in *Grand Rounds: One Hundred Years of Internal Medicine,* ed. Russell C. Maulitz and Diana E. Long (Philadelphia: University of Pennsylvania Press, 1987), pp. 297–335.

48. Ian Robinson, "Clinical trials and the collective ethics: The case of hyperbaric oxygen therapy and the treatment of multiple sclerosis," in *Social Science Perspectives on Medical Ethics,* ed. George Weisz (Dordrecht: Kluwer Academic Publishers, 1990), pp. 19–41.

49. George Weisz, "Introduction," in *Social Science Perspectives,* pp. 3–17; Bernard S. Bloom, "Controlled studies in measuring the efficacy of medical care: A historical perspective," *International Journal of Technology Assessment in Health Care,* 2 (1986), 299–310; A. R. Feinstein and N. Kosso, "The changing emphasis in clinical research: III. Follow-up report for the years 1965–1969," *Archives of Internal Medicine,* 125 (1970), 885–891.

50. Robert H. Fletcher and Suzanne W. Fletcher, "Clinical research in general medical journals: A thirty-year perspective," *New England Journal of Medicine,* 301 (1979), 180–183; S. W. Fletcher, R. H. Fletcher, and M. Andrew Gerganti, "Clinical research trends in general medical journals, 1946–1976," in *Biomedical Innovation,* ed. Edward B. Roberts et al. (Cambridge, Mass.: MIT Press, 1981), fig. 17.3, pp. 292, 298.

51. Fletcher, Fletcher, and Gerganti, "Clinical research trends," p. 298; Bloom, "Controlled studies in measuring efficacy"; Feinstein and Kosso, "Changing emphasis in clinical research."

52. H. G. Mather et al., "Myocardial infarction: A comparison between home and hospital care for patients," *British Medical Journal,* 1976, pp. 925–929; J. D. Hill, R. J. Hampton, and J. R. Mitchell, "A randomized trial of home versus hospital management of patients with suspected myocardial infarction," *Lancet,* 1978, pp. 837–841.

53. Bryan Jennett, "Surgery to prevent stroke: High hopes and deep disappointments," *International Journal of Technology Assessment in Health Care,* 5 (1988), 443–457. The recent focus on cost-efficiency evaluation of new treatments may, however, change this trend.

54. The nineteenth-century controversies over the legitimation of medical practice which opposed bedside practice to abstract knowledge are discussed by, e.g., Morris J. Vogel and Charles E. Rosenberg, eds., *The*

Therapeutic Revolution: Essays in the Social History of American Medicine (Philadelphia: University of Pennsylvania Press, 1979); John Harley Warner, *The Therapeutic Perspective: Medical Practice, Knowledge, and Identity in America* (Cambridge, Mass.: Harvard University Press, 1986); Ilana Löwy, *The Polish School of Philosophy of Medicine* (Dordrecht: Kluwer Academic Publishers, 1990); Christopher Lawrence, "Incommunicable knowledge: Science technology and the clinical art in Britain, 1850–1914," *Journal of Contemporary History,* 20 (1985), 503–520.

55. William J. Mackillop and Pauline A. Johnston, "Ethical problems in clinical research: The need for empirical studies of clinical trial process," *Journal of Chronic Diseases,* 39(3) (1986), 177–188.

56. Samuel Hellman and Deborah S. Hellman, "Of mice but not men: Problems of the randomized clinical trial," *New England Journal of Medicine,* 324(22) (1991), 1585–89.

57. A. R. Feinstein, "The intellectual crisis in clinical science: Medaled models and muddled mettle," *Perspectives in Biology and Medicine,* 30(2) (1987), 215–230; idem, "An additional basic science for clinical medicine: II. The limitations of randomized trials," *Annals of Internal Medicine,* 99 (1983), 549. A proposal to create a specific clinical science through the "scientization" of clinical practice was advanced in the late nineteenth century by the Polish philosopher of medicine Wladyslaw Bieganski; Löwy, *The Polish School,* pp. 69–90.

58. Anne Fagot-Largeault, *L'homme bio-éthique. Pour une déontologie de la recherche sur le vivant* (Paris: Maloine, 1985), p. 51.

59. Robinson, "Clinical trials and the collective ethics," p. 25.

60. Evelleen Richards, "The politics of therapeutic evaluation: The vitamin C and cancer controversy," *Social Studies of Science,* 18 (1988), 653–701; idem, *Vitamin C and Cancer: Medicine or Politics?* (London: Macmillan, 1991); Toine Pieters, "Interferon and its first clinical trial: Looking behind the scenes," *Medical History,* 37 (1993), 270–295.

61. Trevor Pinch and W. Bijker, "The social construction of facts and artifacts," in *The Social Construction of Technological Systems,* ed. Trevor Pinch, T. B. Hughes, and W. Bijker (Cambridge, Mass.: MIT Press, 1987); Andrew Feenberg, *Critical Theory of Technology* (New York: Oxford University Press, 1991).

62. William Coleman, "Experimental strategies and statistical interference: The therapeutic trial in nineteenth-century Germany," in *The Probabilistic Revolution,* ed. Lorraine Daston, Michael Heidelberger, and Lorenz Kruger (Cambridge, Mass.: MIT Press, 1986); Warner, *The Therapeutic Perspective;* Theodore M. Porter, *The Rise of Statistical Thinking, 1820–1900* (Princeton: Princeton University Press, 1986),

pp. 157–162; G. Gigenerzener et al., *The Empire of Chance* (Cambridge: Cambridge University Press, 1989), pp. 129–131.

63. Marks, "Notes from the underground."

64. Picard, "Poussée scientifique ou demande des médecins?"

65. Medical Research Council, "Streptomycin treatment of pneumonary tuberculosis," *British Medical Journal,* 1948, pp. 769–782; idem, "The prevention of whooping cough by vaccination," ibid., 1951, pp. 1462–71.

66. H. M. Marks, "Historical perspectives on clinical trials," Working paper for the National Research Council Committee on AIDS Research, August 1, 1990.

67. H. M. Marks, "Ideas as social reforms: The ambiguous legacy of randomized clinical trials" (Manuscript, September 1984), p. 15; idem, "Historical perspectives," p. 9; idem, "Notes from the underground," p. 319. In the United States the importance of clinical trials was officially recognized through Congress' 1962 Drug Amendment and through the establishment in 1970 of regulatory standards of controlled trials by the FDA. Such standards do not exist in all Western countries. For example, France does not have published guidelines for performing clinical trials, and new drugs are evaluated by the procedure of *autorisation de mise sur le marché* (marketing permit), created in 1972; Luis Lasagna and Lars Werkö, "International differences in drug regulation philosophy," *International Journal of Technology Assessment in Health Care,* 2 (1986), 615–618; Lucien Steru and Pierre Simon, "French drug policy," ibid., pp. 637–642.

68. William F. Raub, "Management of multicenter controlled clinical trials," in *Issues in Research with Human Subjects,* NIH Publication 80-1858 (Bethesda, Md.: National Institutes of Health, 1980), pp. 55–62.

69. Marks, "Ideas as social reforms," p. 2.

70. Lawrence, "Incommunicable knowledge."

71. Marks, "Notes from the underground," pp. 301–305.

72. Theodore M. Porter, "Objectivity as standardization: The rhetoric of impersonality in measurements, statistics, and cost-benefit analysis," *Annals of Scholarship,* 9 (1992), 19–59; idem, *Trust in Numbers* (Princeton: Princeton University Press, 1995).

73. I am indebted to Harry Marks for attracting my attention to this alternative view.

74. Lack of consensus over what is viewed as a good outcome of a clinical trial may complicate the evaluation of therapies for acute infectious diseases too. See, e.g., William C. Summers, "Cholera and plague in India: The bacteriophage inquiry of 1927–1936," *Journal of History of Medicine and Allied Sciences,* 48 (1993), 275–301.

75. Marks, "Ideas as social reforms"; H. M. Marks, "Ideas as reforms: Therapeutic experiments and medical practice, 1900–1980" (Ph.D. diss., MIT, 1987), esp. chaps. 6 and 7. On the impact of preexisting ideas on the understanding of pathological phenomena see, e.g., Malcolm Nicholson and Cathleen McLaughlin, "Social constructivism and medical sociology: A study of the vascular theory of multiple sclerosis," *Sociology of Health and Illness*, 10(3) (1988), 234–261. For a late nineteenth-century reflection on the influence of physicians' preconceived ideas on "clinical facts," see Zygmunt Kramsztyk, "A clinical fact," in Löwy, *The Polish School*, pp. 155–159.

76. Andrew Abbott, *The System of Professions: An Essay on the Division of Expert Labor* (Chicago: University of Chicago Press, 1988), pp. 184–195.

77. Bud, "Strategy in American cancer research," pp. 442–446.

78. Shimkin, *Contrary to Nature*; Pinell, *Naissance d'un fléau*.

79. Paul Star, *The Social Transformation of American Medicine: The Rise of a Sovereign Profession and the Making of a Vast Industry* (New York: Basic Books, 1982); Rosemary Stevens, *In Sickness and in Wealth: American Hospitals in the Twentieth Century* (New York: Basic Books, 1989), pp. 17–50; Pinell, *Naissance d'un fléau*, pp. 201–230.

80. Endicott, "The chemotherapy program," p. 280.

81. Ibid., p. 285.

82. Harry F. Bisel, "Clinical aspects of the cancer chemotherapy program," *Current Research in Cancer Chemotherapy*, 5 (1956), 7.

83. Endicott, "The chemotherapy program," p. 283.

84. Ibid., p. 293.

85. Zubrod, "Historic milestones in curative chemotherapy," pp. 496–497.

86. M. C. Li, R. Hertz, and D. B. Spencer, "Effect of methotrexate upon choriocarcinoma and chorioadenoma," *Proceedings of the Society for Experimental Biology and Medicine*, 93 (1956), 361–366; M. C. Li, "Trophoblastic disease: Natural history, diagnosis and treatment," *Annals of Internal Medicine*, 74 (1971), 102–112.

87. R. Hertz, J. Lewis, and M. B. Lipsett, "Five years' experience with the chemotherapy of metastatic trophoblastic diseases in women," *American Journal of Obstetrics and Gynecology*, 86 (1963), 808–814.

88. Zubrod, "Origins and development," p. 14.

89. Ibid., p. 15.

90. Zubrod, Schepartz, and Carter, "Historical background," p. 11.

91. E. Frei and E. J. Freireich, "Progress and perspectives in the chemotherapy of acute leukemia," *Advances in Chemotherapy*, 2 (1965), 269–298; J. H. Burchenal, "Long-term remission in acute leukemia," in *Chemotherapy of Cancer*, ed. P. A. Plattner (Amsterdam: Elsevier, 1964), pp. 257–262.

92. V. T. De Vita and A. Serpik, "Combination chemotherapy in the treatment of advanced Hodgkin's disease," *Proceedings of the American Association for Cancer Research,* 8 (1967).

93. E.g., Thomas C. Chalmers, Jerome Block, and Stephanie Lee, "Controlled studies in clinical cancer research," *New England Journal of Medicine,* 278 (1972), 75–78.

94. Franz Ingelfinger, "The randomized clinical trial," *New England Journal of Medicine,* 278 (1972), 100–101; Edmund A. Gehan and Emil J. Freireich, "Non-randomized controls in clinical trials," ibid., 290 (1974), 198–203.

95. Zubrod, Schepartz, and Carter, "Historical background," p. 11.

96. David J. Rothman and Harold Edgar, "Scientific rigor and medical realities: Placebo trials in cancer and AIDS research," in *AIDS: The Making of a Chronic Disease,* ed. Elisabeth Fee and Daniel M. Fox (Berkeley: University of California Press, 1992), p. 196.

97. Joint Task Force, National Cancer Institute and U.S. Food and Drug Administration, *Anticancer Drugs: The NCI Development and FDA's Regulations* (Washington, D.C.: U.S. Department of Health and Human Services, 1982), pp. 101–102; quoted by Rothman and Edgar, "Scientific rigor and medical realities," p. 199.

98. Zubrod, "Origins and development," pp. 16–17.

99. A few "dissident" oncologists claimed, however, that the current biological models of malignancy, which view cancer exclusively as the proliferation of abnormal cells, do not provide adequate explanation of the totality of pathological events in advanced cancer. See, e.g., Jean-Claude Salomon, "Cancer classification," *Cancer Journal,* 1 (1987), 286–289.

100. Joint Task Force, NCI and FDA, *Anticancer Drugs,* pp. 198, 202.

101. On the historical role of measuring instruments in normalizing and instrumentalizing health and disease see Audry B. Davis, *Medicine and Its Technology: An Introduction to the History of Medical Instrumentation* (Westport, Conn.: Greenwood Press, 1981), pp. 185–241.

102. V. Ventafridda et al., eds., *Assessment of Quality of Life and Cancer Treatment* (Amsterdam: Excerpta Medica, 1986); J. J. Berenheim, "Evaluation de la qualité de vie en cours de traitement," *Bulletin du cancer,* 73 (1986), 614–619; Basil A. Stoll, "Saying no is difficult in cancer," in *Cost versus Benefit in Cancer Care,* ed. Stoll (Baltimore: Johns Hopkins University Press, 1988), p. 101.

103. Brigid L. Leventhal and Robert F. Wittes, *Research Methods in Clinical Oncology* (New York: Raven Press, 1988), pp. 4–22; Jane E. Smith, "Measuring response in incurable cancer," in *Cancer Treatment: End Point Evaluation,* ed. Basil A. Stoll (London: John Wiley & Sons, 1983), pp. 23–41.

104. B. J. Kennedy et al., "Training program in medical oncology," *Annals of Internal Medicine,* 78 (1973), 127–130.

105. Henry J. Aaron and William B. Schwartz, *The Painful Prescription: Rationing Hospital Care* (Washington, D.C.: Brookings Institution, 1984), p. 48.

106. Pinell, *Naissance d'un fléau,* pp. 69–75.

107. Barrie R. Cassileth, "The evolution of oncology as a sociomedical phenomenon," in *The Cancer Patient: Social and Medical Aspects of Care,* ed. Cassileth (Philadelphia: Lea & Febiger, 1979), pp. 3–15. The NCI budget increased from $91 million in 1960, to $200 million in 1970, to $1.02 billion in 1979.

108. Charles E. Rosenberg, "Looking forward, thinking backward: The roots of the hospital crisis," *Transactions & Studies of the College of Physicians of Philadelphia,* 5th ser., 12 (1990), 127–150.

109. Albert S. Braverman, "Medical oncology in the 1990s," *Lancet,* 1991, pp. 901–902. It was not unusual for a leading U.S. teaching hospital to participate in more than a hundred collaborative trials of cancer therapies.

   Kathryn M. Taylor and Merrijoy Kelner, "Informed consent: The physician's perspective," *Social Sciences and Medicine,* 24 (1987), 135–143; K. Antman, L. E. Schipper, and E. Frei, "The crisis in clinical cancer research: Third-party insurance and investigational therapy," *New England Journal of Medicine,* 319 (1988), 46–48; W. C. Scott et al., "Special report of the American Medical Association Council on Scientific Affairs: Viability of cancer clinical research: Patient accrual, coverage and reimbursement," *Journal of the National Cancer Institute,* 83 (1991), 225–259; Daniel Belanger, Malcolm Moore, and Ian Tannock, "How American oncologists treat breast cancer: An assessment of influence of clinical trials," *Journal of Clinical Oncology,* 9 (1991), 7–16. The term "clinical trials of cancer therapies" employed in these articles refers both to highly visible trials of new and promising anticancer drugs, usually conducted in leading cancer centers, and to the much less visible "routine" trials that aim at the reevaluation or the improvement of existing anticancer treatments and are often conducted by "rank-and-file" oncologists.

110. Some French oncologists saw training in a U.S. cancer treatment center as a decisive event that stimulated their interest in clinical research. See, e.g., Claude Jasmin, *Parce que je crois au lendemain* (Paris: Editions Robert Laffont, 1983), pp. 70–79.

111. In addition, in 1981 there were in Britain more than a dozen senior oncology registrars in training. (Senior registrars occupy an accredited post in medical oncology and aspire to a consultant position after four years of training, which includes both laboratory and clinical research

experience.) In 1981 there were, however, no vacant positions for consultants in medical oncology; J. S. Tobias, P. G. Harper, and M. H. N. Tattersall, "Who should treat cancer?" *Lancet,* 1981, pp. 885–886. In the same year there were about 1,700 board certified medical oncologists in the United States; Aaron and Schwartz, *The Painful Prescription,* pp. 48, 51.

112. Gareth J. G. Rees, "What is best for the patient? A European view," in Stoll, *Cost versus Benefit,* p. 34.

113. Tobias, Harper, and Tattersall, "Who should treat cancer?"; editorial, "Who should treat cancer?" *Lancet,* 1981, pp. 674–675; M. J. Peckham, "Clinical oncology: The future of radiotherapy and medical oncology," ibid., pp. 886–887.

114. Editorial, "Who should treat cancer?" p. 674.

115. David Radstone, "The physician's attitude in Britain," in Stoll, *Cost versus Benefit,* pp. 49–56.

116. Pierre Denoix, *Clefs pour la cancérologie* (Paris: Seghers, 1974), pp. 175–185; Pinell, *Naissance d'un fléau,* pp. 201–216. After the Second World War a significant proportion of French radiologists elected to practice in private hospitals and clinics. For this reason, nearly half of French cancer patients were treated in private or semiprivate institutions.

117. In 1990, reorganization of the medical curriculum in France led to official recognition of the subspecialty oncology through the creation of a *diplôme d'études supérieures complémentaires* in that field.

118. At first their number was very small—seventeen on January 1, 1992; Conseil National de l'Ordre des Médecins, Paris, December 1992.

119. Jean Bernard and Michel Boiron, "Current status: treatment of acute leukemia," *Seminars in Hematology,* 7 (1970), 427–440; Georges Mathé, ed., *Advances in the Cure of Acute (Blastic) Leukemias* (Berlin: Springer-Verlag, 1970). Bernard presents a 1947 French attempt to cure leukemia by multiple transfusions as the first step toward the cure of that disease; Jean Bernard, *L'enfant, le sang et l'espoir* (Paris: Buchet/Chastel, 1984), pp. 23–24. This episode is not mentioned in non-French histories of the search for a cure for leukemia.

120. Denoix, *Clefs pour la cancérologie,* pp. 186–197. The EORTC was directed by the Belgian Henry Tagnon and was supported by an NCI grant and by European cancer charities.

121. Maurice Tubiana, *La lumière dans l'ombre* (Paris: Editions Odile Jacob, 1991), pp. 389–390, 508–515.

122. Yves Cachin, *La lutte contre le cancer en France. Perspectives—propositions* (Paris: La Documentation Française, 1985), pp. 11–17. The central place of hematology and of immunology reflects some of the peculiarities of the French biomedical sciences. Jean-Paul Gaudillière,

"Biologie moléculaire et biologistes dans les années soixante. La naissance d'une discipline" (Ph.D. diss., Université de Paris VII, 1991).

123. For example, Jean Bernard, *L'espérance ou le nouvel état de la médecine* (Paris: Buchet/Chastel, 1978); Bernard, *L'enfant, le sang et l'espoir*; Jasmin, *Parce que je crois au lendemain*; Georges Mathé, *Dossier cancer* (Paris: Stock, 1976); Maurice Tubiana, *Le refus du réel* (Paris: Robert Laffont, 1977); idem, *La lumière dans l'ombre.* These books belong to the French tradition of doctors' writings and display the literary and philosophical ambitions of their authors.

124. Bernard, *L'espérance,* p. 209; Jasmin, *Parce que je crois au lendemain,* p. 173. Literary skills have been an important asset for a professional career at the upper levels of the French medical establishment; Pierre Bourdieu, *Homo Academicus* (Paris: Editions de Minuit, 1989).

125. Leventhal and Wittes, *Research Methods in Clinical Oncology,* pp. 40–54; Mortimer B. Lipsett, "On the nature of ethics of phase I clinical trials of cancer chemotherapies," *Journal of the American Medical Association,* 248 (1982), 941–942. See also E. M. Smith and J. C. Bailar, "Progress against cancer?" *New England Journal of Medicine,* 314 (1986), 1226–32; Braverman, "Medical oncology in the 1990s"; Aman U. Buzdar, "What is the best for the patient? A United States view," in Stoll, *Cost versus Benefit,* pp. 19–26. Advanced cancer, other specialists emphasize, is highly distressing, and an experimental therapy may offer hope of alleviating the patient's suffering; Barrie R. Cassileth et al., "Survival and quality of life among patients receiving an unproven as compared with conventional therapy," *New England Journal of Medicine,* 324 (1991), 1180–85; Irvin H. Krakoff, "The hospice movement and its relationships to active treatment," in *Cancer Treatment and Research in Humanistic Perspective,* ed. Steven C. Gross and Solomon Garb (New York: Springer, 1985), pp. 155–160.

126. Brian A. Stoll, "What is overtreatment in cancer?" in Stoll, *Cost versus Benefit,* pp. 7–17; idem, "Quality of life as objective in cancer treatment," in Stoll, *Cancer Treatment,* pp. 113–138; John A. Beal, "Mercy for the terminally ill cancer patient," *Journal of the American Medical Association,* 249 (1983), 2883; J. V. Watson, "What does 'response' in cancer really mean?" *British Medical Journal,* 1981, pp. 34–37; Smith and Bailara, "Progress against cancer?"; Braverman, "Medical oncology in the 1990s."

127. Joseph Lellouch and Daniel Schwartz, "L'essai thérapeutique. Ethique individuelle ou éthique collective?" *Revue de l'Institut International de Statistique,* 39 (1971), 127–136; Kenneth F. Schaffner, "Ethical problems in clinical trials," *Journal of Medicine and Philosophy,* 11 (1986), 297–316; F. Gifford, "The conflict between randomized clinical trials and the therapeutic obligation," *Journal of Medicine and Philosophy,*

11 (1986), 347–366. For the opinion that no such conflict exists see, e.g., David J. Roy, "Editorial: Controlled clinical trials: An ethical imperative," *Journal of Chronic Diseases,* 39 (1986), 159–162.

128. Rothman and Edgar, "Scientific rigor and medical realities," p. 194.

129. Joint Task Force, NCI and FDA, *Anticancer Drugs,* pp. 101–102.

130. Aaron and Schwartz, *The Painful Prescription,* pp. 46–48; G. J. G. Rees, "Cost effectiveness in oncology," *Lancet,* 1985, pp. 1405–07. Aaron and Schwartz compared treatment of several pathologies—end-stage kidney disease, hemophilia, total parenteral nutrition, bone marrow transplantation, and cancer in the United States and Britain. They found that while in the cases of hemophilia therapy, bone marrow transplantation, and radiation therapy of cancer the rate of treatment was nearly identical in both countries, dialysis, transplantation, total parenteral nutrition, and chemotherapy of cancer were less often used in Britain.

131. William J. Mackillop, G. K. Ward, and Brian O'Sullivan, "The uses of expert surrogates to evaluate clinical trials in non-small cell lung cancer," *British Journal of Cancer,* 54 (1986), 661–667; William J. Mackillop et al., "Clinical trials in cancer: The role of surrogate patients in defining what constitutes an ethically acceptable clinical experiment," ibid., 59 (1989), 388–395; Michael J. Palmer et al., "Controversies in the management of non-small cell lung cancer: The results of expert surrogate study," *Radiotherapy and Oncology,* 19 (1990), 17–27; Daniel F. Hayes, "What would you do if this were your wife, sister, mother, self?" *Journal of Clinical Oncology,* 9 (1991), 1–3.

132. Aaron and Schwartz, *The Painful Prescription,* p. 50.

133. Eliot Friedson, *The Patient's View of Medical Practice* (New York: Russell Sage Foundation, 1961).

134. Aaron and Schwartz, *The Painful Prescription,* p. 49; Watson, "What does 'response' in cancer therapy really mean?" The restriction of competition among U.S. doctors through the introduction of HMOs and managed care may diminish the differences between the U.S. and British models of health care.

135. Stoll, "Quality of life as an objective in cancer treatment," in Stoll, *Cancer Treatment,* pp. 113–138; Robert Zittun, "Medical decision making in daily practice," in Ventafridda et al., *Assessment of Quality of Life and Cancer Treatment.*

136. Dennis H. Novack et al., "Changes in physicians' attitude towards telling the cancer patient," *Journal of the American Medical Association,* 241 (1979), 897–900; Barney G. Glazer and Anselm L. Strauss, *Awareness of Dying* (New York: Aldine Press, 1965); Emil J. Freireich, "Should the patient know?" *Journal of the American Medical Association,* 241 (1979), 928; Stanley Joel Reiser, "Words as scalpels: Trans-

mitting evidence in a clinical dialogue," *Annals of Internal Medicine,* 92 (1980), 837–842; Mary-Jo DelVecchio Good, "The practice of biomedicine and the discourse of hope: A preliminary investigation into the culture of American oncology," *Anthropologies of Medicine,* 7 (1991), 212–235; Deborah R. Gordon, "Culture, cancer and communication in Italy," ibid., pp. 137–156; Jutta Dornheim, "Images and interpretations of severe illness," ibid., pp. 157–173.

137. For the same reason dissimulation is difficult for European medical oncologists; Tubiana, *La lumière dans l'ombre,* pp. 479–480.

138. An extreme version of this point of view was presented by promoters of patient-financed, for-profit cancer research, who explained that cancer patients who know that they face imminent death have but one rational choice, namely to seek (and pay for) new, experimental therapies; Frederick E. Porter, "Bioethics," *Journal of Biological Response Modifiers,* 6 (1987), 369–374; Robert K. Oldham, "The cure for cancer," ibid., 4 (1985), 111–116.

139. Radstone, "The physician's attitude in Britain"; Stoll, "Saying no is difficult in cancer," pp. 97–111.

140. Stoll, "Quality of life as objective in cancer treatment," p. 113.

141. Aaron and Schwartz, *The Painful Prescription,* pp. 49, 52–56.

142. Paul J. DiMaggio and Walter W. Powell, "The iron cage revisited: Institutional isomorphism and collective rationality in organizational fields," *American Sociological Review,* 48 (1983), 147; Stuart Blume, *Insight and Industry: On the Dynamics of Technological Change in Medicine* (Cambridge, Mass.: MIT Press, 1991).

143. Hospitals, Mary L. Fennell has argued, "can increase their range of services not because there is a particular need for a service or facility within the patient population, but because they will be defined as fit only if they can offer everything other hospitals in the area offer"; "The effects of environmental characteristics on the structure of hospital clusters," *Administrative Science Quarterly,* 25(3) (1980), 505.

144. Abbott, *The System of Professions,* pp. 184–195.

145. Harold Y. Vanderpool, "The ethics of clinical experimentation with anticancer drugs," in Gross and Garb, *Cancer Treatment and Research,* pp. 36–37; Melvin J. Krant, Joseph L. Cohen, and Charles Rosenbaum, "Moral dilemmas in clinical cancer experimentation," *Medical and Pediatric Oncology,* 3 (1977), 141–147. Stoll, "Saying no is difficult in cancer," pp. 101–102; N. Daniels, "Why saying no to the patients in the United States is so hard: Cost containment, justice and provider authority," *New England Journal of Medicine,* 314 (1986), 80–83.

146. Richards, *Vitamin C and Cancer;* Ilana Löwy, "Innovation and legitimation strategies: The story of the New York Cancer Institute," in Löwy, *Medicine and Change,* pp. 337–358. All the innovations dis-

cussed—both those labeled "successful" and those labeled "unsuccessful"—had low clinical efficacy.

147. Glazer and Strauss, *Awareness of Dying,* pp. 180–181.

148. Similar mechanisms may facilitate international diffusion of clinical trials.

149. Daniels, "Why saying no to patients is so hard," p. 82.

150. Cachin, *La lutte contre le cancer en France,* pp. 13–15; Antman, Schipper, and Frei, "The crisis in clinical cancer research"; Scott et al., "Special report of American Medical Association Council on Scientific Affairs." On the other hand, health administrators may fear that the
introduction of new and expensive experimental therapies may indirectly increase health care costs by raising the level of what will be seen
as an acceptable cost of "last-ditch" cancer treatments; Françoise La-
lande, "Cytokines et interferons. Aspects économiques et coût de la
santé," *Médecine et sciences,* 7 (1991), 715–718.

151. Renée C. Fox, *Experiment Perilous: Physicians and Patients Facing the
Unknown* (1959; reprint, Philadelphia: University of Pennsylvania
Press, 1974); Stoll, "What is overtreatment in cancer?" p. 7; idem,
"Quality of life as objective in cancer treatment," p. 135; Vanderpool,
"The ethics of clinical experimentation," p. 26.

152. John H. Glick, "Palliative chemotherapy: Risk/benefit ratio," in *Clinical
Care of the Cancer Patient,* ed. Barrie R. Cassileth and Peter E. Cassileth
(Philadelphia: Lea & Febiger, 1982), p. 60.

153. Jay Katz, *The Silent World of Doctor and Patient* (New York: Free
Press, 1984), pp. 171–173.

154. Vanderpool, "The ethics of clinical experimentation," p. 33; Elisabeth
A. Eisenhauer and William J. Mackillop, "Focus on clinical trials," in
Stoll, *Cost versus Benefit,* p. 61; Krant, Cohen, and Rosenbaum,
"Moral dilemmas in clinical cancer experimentation," p. 142.

155. J. Yabro, "Quo Vadis?" *Seminars in Oncology,* 12 (1985), 199–200;
quoted in Leventhal and Wittes, *Research Methods in Clinical Oncology,* p. 2.

156. Patterson, *The Dread Disease;* Pinell, *Naissance d'un fléau.*

157. Daniel S. Greenberg, "A sober anniversary of the 'War on Cancer,' "
Lancet, 1991, pp. 1582–83; Gershom Zajicek, "Progress against cancer: Are we winning the war?" *Cancer Journal,* 3 (1990), 2; Eliot
Marshall, "Breast cancer: Stalemate in the war on cancer," *Science,* 254
(1991), 1719–20.

158. Gavin Mooney, "Introduction," in Stoll, *Cost versus Benefit,* p. 3.

159. Stoll, "Saying no is difficult in cancer," pp. 101–103; Glazer and Strauss,
Awareness of Dying, p. 190; Vanderpool, "The ethics of clinical experimentation," p. 37; Robert Flamant, "Questions éthiques particulières
aux essais thérapeutiques de phase I réalisés chez les malades cancér-
eux," *Concours médical,* 32, supp. (October 3, 1987), 3020–22. Cancer

patients are often motivated to enroll in a clinical trial by an inseparable mixture of fear of disease, trust in their doctor, and hope for a cure; D. T. Pennmann et al., "Informed consent for investigational chemotherapy: Patients' and physicians' perceptions," *Journal of Clinical Oncology,* 2 (1984), 849–855.

160. Carl G. Kardinal and Bruce N. Strand, "Confrontation with cancer: Historical and existential aspects," in Gross and Garb, *Cancer Treatment and Research,* p. 173. French patients had similar reactions; Flamant, "Questions éthiques particulières," p. 3021.

161. Quoted by Rothman and Edgar, "Scientific rigor and medical realities," p. 195.

162. Ibid., p. 196.

163. Ibid., p. 198.

164. Kardinal and Strand, "Confrontation with cancer," p. 173.

165. Andrew Feenberg, "On being a human subject: Interest and obligation in the experimental treatment of incurable disease," *Philosophical Forum,* 23 (1992), 213–230.

166. Howard Brody, *Placebos and the Philosophy of Medicine* (Chicago: University of Chicago Press, 1980).

167. Feenberg, "On being a human subject." Recently, among other things under the pressure from AIDS activists, the access to clinical trials has been presented as a social good, and patients' advocates have stressed the right of different groups to equal access to experimental therapies; Eric Gagnon, "Médecine scientifique et médecine de l'individu. Les comités d'éthique et la légitimité de la recherche médicale," *Sciences sociales et santé,* 12(4) (1994), 5–34; Steven Epstein, "The construction of lay expertise: AIDS activism and the forging of credibility in the reform of clinical trials," *Science, Technology & Human Values,* 20(4) (1995), 408–437.

168. Stoll, "Saying no is difficult in cancer," p. 100; George Annas, "Faith (healing) hope and charity at the FDA: The politics of AIDS drug trials," *Villanova Law Review,* 34 (1989), 783; idem, "FDA's compassion for desperate drug companies," *Hastings Center Report,* January/February 1990, pp. 35–37. For a discussion of desperate experimental remedies in the American context, see Renée C. Fox and Judith Swazey, *Spare Parts* (New York: Oxford University Press, 1992).

169. Glazer and Strauss describe a cancer patient who, upon hearing that he would be given another dose of experimental chemotherapy, tried to put end to his life; *Awareness of Dying,* pp. 192–193.

170. Stoll, "What is overtreatment in cancer?" p. 16; Vanderpool, "The ethics of experimentation," p. 39; Glazer and Strauss, *Awareness of Dying,* p. 193.

171. Cassileth et al., "Survival and quality of life," p. 1184.

172. Richards, *Vitamin C and Cancer.* On the negative effects of cancer patients' excessive faith in unorthodox therapies, see also Anne Hunsaker Hawkins, *Reconstructing Illness: Studies in Pathography* (West Lafayette, Ind.: Purdue University Press, 1993), pp. 148–157.

173. Hawkins' *Reconstructing Illness* is centered on pathographies, patients' literary accounts of their illness experience. Many of these pathographies describe the experience of cancer, but the book does not discuss the patients' experience of participation in a clinical trial of a new anticancer drug, although this experience was described in some of the pathographies.

174. Kenneth A. Shapiro, *Dying and Living: One Man's Life with Cancer* (Austin: University of Texas Press, 1985); quotation p. 9.

175. Stewart Alsop, *Stay of Execution: A Sort of Memoir* (Philadelphia: J. B. Lippincott, 1973), pp. 83, 265.

176. Jack J. Lewis, "Acute myelogenic leukemia," in *When Doctors Get Sick,* ed. Harvey Mandell and Howard Spiro (London: Plenum Books, 1987), pp. 325–333; quotation p. 333.

177. Gerda Lerner, *A Death of One's Own* (New York: Simon and Schuster, 1978), pp. 168, 169.

178. Ibid., p. 208. This clinical trial took place in 1973, when there were still high hopes that the recent success of chemotherapy of childhood cancers would soon be extended to the cure of major cancers of the adult.

179. Ibid., p. 250. Dr. Goldman believed nevertheless that the chemotherapy did slow the progress of Carl Lerner's disease. Gerda Lerner disagreed.

180. Ibid., p. 168. See also Hawkins, *Reconstructing Illness,* pp. 123–124.

181. Ernest H. Rosenbaum, *Living with Cancer* (New York: Praeger, 1975), p. 21.

182. Gagnon, "Médecine scientifique et médecine de l'individu."

183. Zygmunt Baumann, *Mortality, Immortality and Other Life Strategies* (Cambridge: Polity Press, 1992).

184. Patterson, *The Dread Disease,* pp. 171–200.

185. The observation that tumor cells multiply rapidly was made in the second half of the nineteenth century; L. J. Rather, *The Genesis of Cancer: A Study in the History of Ideas* (Baltimore: Johns Hopkins University Press, 1978).

186. Patterson, *The Dread Disease,* p. 197.

2. Cancer Immunotherapy, 1894–1979

1. Steven A. Rosenberg, "Adoptive immunotherapy for cancer," *Scientific American,* May 1990, pp. 34–41.

2. William H. Woglom, "Immunity to transplanted tumors," *Cancer Review,* 4 (1929), 195.

3. Gustav J. V. Nossal, "The case history of Mr. T. I.: Terminal patient or still curable?" *Immunology Today,* 1 (1980), 5–9. Nossal made these observations in a keynote lecture delivered at the conference "Immunological Aspects of Experimental and Clinical Cancer," Tel Aviv, November 1979.

4. Robert K. Oldham and Richard V. Smalley, "Immunotherapy: The old and the new," *Journal of Biological Response Modifiers,* 2 (1983), 1–37; Ronald B. Herberman, "The evaluation of biological response modifiers for cancer therapy," in *New Directions in Cancer Treatment,* ed. Ian Magrath (Berlin: Springer Verlag, 1989).

5. S. Cohn, E. Pick, and J. J. Oppenheim, *The Biology of Lymphokines* (New York: Academic Press, 1979); Ronald B. Herberman, *Natural Cell-Mediated Immunity against Tumors* (New York: Academic Press, 1980).

6. J. L. Rather, *The Genesis of Cancer* (Baltimore: Johns Hopkins University Press, 1978).

7. The search for a "cancer bacillus" was abandoned in the early twentieth century. In contrast, the debate on the role of viruses in the origins of human cancer, which started in 1911 with the description of transmissible tumors of the fowl (Peyton Rous, "Transmission of a malignant new growth by means of cell-free filtrate," *Journal of the American Medical Association,* 56 [1911], 198), continues today. See also Jean-Paul Gaudillière, "NCI and the spreading genes: About the production of viruses, mice and cancer," *Sociology of Science Yearbook* (1993).

8. The history of immunology is summed up in Arthur M. Silverstein, *A History of Immunology* (San Diego: Academic Press, 1989); and Anne-Marie Moulin, *Le dernier langage de la médecine: Histoire de l'immunologie de Pasteur au Sida* (Paris: Presses Universitaires de France, 1991).

9. Elie (Ilyia) Metchnikoff, *L'immmunité dans les maladies infectieuses* (Paris: Mason, 1901); Paul Ehrlich, "Cronian lectures on immunity," *Proceedings of the Royal Society,* 66 (1900), 424.

10. G. Dean, "The types of immunity," in *Diphtheria,* ed. George H. Nuttal and George S. Graham (New York, 1907), p. 449.

11. Metchnikoff, *L'immmunité dans les maladies infectieuses,* pp. 283–284. The enhanced efficacy of phagocytes in immunized individuals was later explained by the increase in the efficiency of bacteria phagocytosis in the presence of specific antibacterial antibodies; J. Denis and J. Leclef, "Sur le mécanisme de l'immunité chez le lapin vacciné contre le streptocoque pyogène," *La Cellule,* 11 (1985), 177–211; Almroth Wright and S. Douglas, "An experimental investigation of the role of body fluids in connection with phagocytosis," *Proceedings of the Royal Society,* 72 (1903), 357.

12. Robert E. Kohler, "The enzyme theory and the origins of biochemistry," *Isis,* 64 (1973), 181–194.

13. Emile Duclaux, *Traité de microbiologie,* 4 vols. (Paris: Masson, 1898), vol. 1, pp. 727–730.

14. Maurice Nicolle, *Eléments de microbiologie générale* (Paris: Octave Doin, 1901), p. 296.

15. A. M. Silverstein, "The dynamics of conceptual change in twentieth-century immunology," *Cellular Immunology,* 132 (1991), 515–531.

16. Idem, "Introduction," in *Milestones in Immunology: A Historical Exploration,* ed. Debra Bibel (Berlin: Springer Verlag, 1988), pp. xiii–xv.

17. Rous, "Transmission of a malignant new growth."

18. James B. Murphy and P. Rous, "The behaviour of chicken sarcoma implanted in the developing embryo," *Journal of Experimental Medicine,* 15 (1912), 119–132.

19. J. B. Murphy, "Transplantability of malignant tumors to the embryos of foreign species," *Journal of the American Medical Association,* 59 (1912), 874–875; idem, "Transplantability of tissues to the embryo of foreign species," *Journal of Experimental Medicine,* 17 (1913), 482–492.

20. C. Da Fano, "Zellulare Analise der Geschulstimmunität Reaktionen," *Zeistschrift für Immunitätforscherung,* 5 (1910), 1; idem, "A cytological analysis of the reactions of animals to implanted carcinomata," *Fifth Scientific Report of the Imperial Cancer Research Fund,* 5 (1912), 57–78. For a history of early cancer research at the Imperial Cancer Research Fund see Joan Austoker, *A History of the Imperial Cancer Research Fund, 1902–1986* (Oxford: Oxford University Press, 1988), pp. 27–68.

21. J. B. Murphy, "Studies on tissue specificity: The ultimate fate of mammalian tissue implanted in chicken embryo," *Journal of Experimental Medicine,* 19 (1914), 181–186.

22. Idem, "Factors in resistance to heteroplastic tissue grafting: Studies on tissue specificity," ibid., pp. 513–522; idem, "Heteroplastic tissue grafting through Roentgen-ray lymphoid destruction," *Journal of the American Medical Association,* 62 (1914), 1459.

23. A large dose of X rays, Murphy found, decreased the number of circulating lymphocytes, while a low dose induced first a decrease in the number of these cells, then, several days later, a sharp increase; "Heteroplastic tissue grafting."

24. J. B. Murphy and John J. Morton, "The effects of X-rays on the resistance to cancer in mice," *Science,* 42 (1915), 842; idem, "The effects of X-rays on the rate of growth of spontaneous tumors in mice," *Journal of Experimental Medicine,* 22 (1915), 800–803. Murphy and Morton's claims that the stimulation of lymphocytes protected mice against grafts

of their own spontaneously arising tumors were not confirmed by other investigators.

25. Paul De Kruiff, *The Sweeping Wind* (New York: Harcourt, Brace & World, 1962).

26. Newspaper clippings from August 1915, J. B. Murphy's Papers, BM 956, American Philosophical Society, Philadelphia. On the attitude of the American press to cancer research at that time, see James Patterson, *The Dread Disease: Cancer and Modern American Culture* (Cambridge, Mass.: Harvard University Press, 1987), pp. 56–86.

27. J. B. Murphy, *The Lymphocyte in Resistance to Tissue Grafting, Malignant Disease, and Tuberculous Infection: An Experimental Study* (New York: Rockefeller Institute for Medical Research, 1926).

28. Simon Flexner, "Report to the corporation: October 1915," in "Reports of the Directors of the Laboratories," vol. 4, 1914–1915, p. 125, Rockefeller Archives, North Tarrytown, N.Y.

29. J. B. Murphy, in ibid., vol. 4, 1915–1916, pp. 226–227; vol. 5, 1917, p. 108; vol. 6, 1918, p. 54; vol. 9, 1921, p. 48; vol. 10, 1922, p. 101.

30. Simon Flexner, "Report to the corporation: October 1920," in ibid., vol. 8, 1920, p. 208.

31. Murphy, *Lymphocyte in Resistance to Tissue Grafting.* The explicit term "experimental study" probably aimed at differentiating Murphy's work from the numerous speculative or descriptive studies on similar subjects.

32. J. B. Murphy, "Certain etiological factors in the causation and transmission of malignant tumors," *American Naturalist,* 60 (1926), 227–236.

33. Clarence C. Little, "James Baumgardner Murphy," *Biographical Memoirs of the National Academy of Sciences,* 34 (1960), 183–203.

34. Ilana Löwy, "Variance of meaning in discovery accounts: The case of modern biology," *Historical Studies in the Physical and Biological Sciences,* 21 (1990), 87–121.

35. This resistance was called "natural" because it occurred without previous contact with the tumor.

36. Paul Ehrlich, "Experimentelle Carcinomstudien an Mäusen," *Arbeit aus der Königlischen Institut für experimental Therapie,* 1 (1906), 77.

37. Ernest F. Bashford, James A. Murray, and William Cramer, "The natural and induced resistance of mice to the growth of cancer," *Third Scientific Report of the Imperial Cancer Research Fund,* 3 (1908), 315.

38. L. Michaelis, "Versuche zur Einzeilung einer Krabsimmunität bei Mäusen," *Zeitschrift für Krebsforscherung,* 5 (1907), 163.

39. E. F. Bashford, J. A. Murray, and Magnus Haaland, "Resistance and susceptibility to inoculated cancer," *Third Scientific Report of the Imperial Cancer Research Fund,* 3 (1908), 358; E. F. Bashford and B. G. R.

Russell, "Further evidence on the homogeneity of the resistance to implantation of malignant new growths," *Proceedings of the Royal Society,* ser. B, 82 (1910), 298.

40. W. H. Woglom, *The Study of Experimental Cancer: A Review* (New York: Columbia University Press, 1913), pp. 130–137. From the point of view of current scientific knowledge one may attribute the inconsistency of experimental results reported by Woglom to the fluidity of the term "race" and to the variability of experimental tumors used by different investigators.

41. Alexis Carrel, "Remote results of the retransplantation of the kidneys and the spleen," *Journal of Experimental Medicine,* 12 (1910), 146.

42. Peyton Rous, "An experimental comparison of the transplanted tumor and transplanted normal tissue capable of growth," ibid., pp. 344–369.

43. Idem, "Resistance to tumor-producing agent as distinct from resistance to the implanted tumor cells," ibid., 18 (1913), 416.

44. Woglom, *The Study of Experimental Cancer.*

45. Patricia Peck Gossel, "A need for standard methods: The case of American bacteriology," in *The Right Tools for the Job: A Work in Twentieth-Century Life Sciences,* ed. Adele E. Clarke and Joan F. Fujimura (Princeton: Princeton University Press, 1992), pp. 287–311.

46. Although researchers occasionally exchanged animals and tumors, such exchanges became more systematic only in the 1930s; J.-P. Gaudillière, "Le cancer entre infection et hérédité. Gènes, virus et souris au National Cancer Institute," *Revue d'histoire des sciences,* 47(1) (1994), 57–89.

47. Austoker, *History of Imperial Cancer Research Fund.*

48. Katsusaburo Yamagiwa and Koichi Ichikawa, "Experimental study of the pathogenesis of carcinoma," *Journal of Cancer Research,* 3 (1918), 1–29.

49. J. B. Murphy and Ernest Sturm, "Primary lung tumors in mice following cutaneous application of coal tar," *Journal of Experimental Medicine,* 42 (1925), 693–700.

50. Woglom, "Immunity to transplantable tumors," p. 131.

51. Acquired resistance was observed when a tumor's recipient was injected with living cells from another individual belonging to the same species. Although it was highly reproducible in the laboratory, Woglom strongly doubted that it was relevant to the cure of naturally occurring malignant growths.

52. The whole domain of studies of grafted tissue and tumor transplantation almost completely disappeared in the 1920s and 1930s; Silverstein, *A History of Immunology,* pp. 275–304.

53. Woglom, "Immunity to transplantable tumors," p. 192.

54. E. E. Tyzzer, "Tumor immunity," *Journal of Cancer Research,* 1 (1916), 125; C. C. Little and E. E. Tyzzer, "Further experimental studies of the

susceptibility of transplantable tumor, carcinoma of the Japanese waltzing mouse," *Journal of Medical Research*, 3 (1916), 393–427.

55. C. C. Little and B. W. Johnson, "The inheritance of susceptibility to
implant of splenic tissue in mice: Japanese waltzing mice, albinos and
their F1 generation hybrids," *Proceedings of the Society for Experimental Biology and Medicine,* 19 (1922), 163–167; C. C. Little, "The
genetics of tissue transplantation in mammals," *Journal of Cancer Research,* 8 (1924), 75–95.

56. George D. Snell, "Methods for the study of histocompatibility genes,"
Journal of Genetics, 49 (1948), 87. The organization of the Jackson
Memorial Laboratory is the subject of Karen Rader's Ph.D. dissertation,
"Making Mice: C. C. Little, the Jackson Laboratory, and the standardization of *Mus musculus* for research" (University of Indiana). Rader
kindly made excerpts from this work available to me before its com-
pletion.

57. The development of an inbred line of mice made possible the selection
of "high-tumor" strains, that is, strains in which a high proportion of
the animals developed spontaneous cancer. These lines became an important research tool for experimental oncologists from the 1930s on;
Rader, "Making Mice"; Gaudillière, "Le cancer entre infection et hérédité."

58. Johannes Clemmensen, *The Influence of X-Radiation on the Development of Immunity to Heterologous Transplantation of Tumors* (London: Humphrey Milford, Oxford University Press, 1938), p. 17.

59. M. K. Barrett, "The influence of genetic constitution upon the induction
of resistance to transplantable tumors," *Journal of the National Cancer
Institute,* 1 (1940), 387–393.

60. J. B. Murphy, "An analysis of trends in cancer research," *Journal of the
American Medical Association,* 120 (1942), 107–111.

61. R. R. Spencer, "Tumor immunity," *Journal of the National Cancer Institute,* 2 (1942), 317–322.

62. Theodore S. Hauschka, "Immunologic aspects of cancer: A review,"
Cancer Research, 12 (1952), 615–633.

63. Chester M. Southam, "Relationships of immunology to cancer: A review," ibid., 20 (1960), 271–291.

64. Helen Coley Nauts, *Bibliography of Reports concerning the Clinical or
Experimental Use of Coley's Toxins (Streptococcus pyogenes and Serratia marcescens), 1893–1991* (New York: Cancer Research Institute,
1991); idem, "Coley's toxins—the first century," Paper delivered at a
meeting of the International Clinical Hyperthermia Society, Rome, May
1989.

65. Jules Bordet, *Annales de l'Institut Pasteur,* 12 (1899), 688.

66. Bashford and Russell, "Further evidence on homogeneity of resistance,"

p. 298; Robert A. Lambert, "A note on the specificity of cytokines," *Journal of Experimental Medicine,* 19 (1914), 277–282.

67. Woglom, The *Study of Experimental Cancer.*

68. Silverstein, *A History of Immunology,* pp. 262–270; Moulin, *Le dernier langage de la médecine,* pp. 239–240.

69. Chester M. Southam, "Applications of immunology to clinical cancer: Past attempts and future possibilities," *Cancer Research,* 21 (1961), 1302–16; Graham A. Currie, "Immunotherapy of human cancer: Prospect and retrospect," in *Cancer and the Immune Response* (Baltimore: Williams and Wilkins, 1974), pp. 71–96.

70. J. Hericourt and C. Richet, "Physiologie pathologique de la sérothérapie dans le traitement du cancer," *Comptes rendus des séances hebdomadaires de l'Académie des Sciences,* 121 (1895), 567.

71. M. N. Berkeley, "Results of three years of observation on a new form of cancer treatments," *American Journal of Obstetrics,* 69 (1914), 1060–63; G. A. Lindstrom, "Experimental studies of myelotoxic sera: Therapeutic attempts in myeloid leukemia," *Acta Medica Scandinavica,* 22, supp. (1927), 169–177; A. B. Vial and W. Callahan, "The effects of some tagged antibodies on human melanoblastoma," *Cancer,* 10 (1957), 999–1003.

72. E. von Leyden and F. Blumenthal, "Attempt to immunize humans by inoculation of their own cancer," *Deutsche Medizinische Wochenschrift,* 28 (1914), 637–638.

73. Southam, "Applications of immunology to clinical cancer," pp. 1305–08; A. F. Coca, G. M. Dorrance, and M. G. Lebredo, " 'Vaccination' in cancer: II. A report of the results of the vaccination therapy as applied in 79 cases of human cancer," *Zeitschrift für Immunitätsforscherung und Experimental Therapie,* 13(1) (1912), 543; J. W. Vaughan, "Cancer vaccine and anti-cancer globulins as an aid in the surgical treatment of malignancy," *Journal of the American Medical Association,* 63 (1914), 1258–1265; J. B. Graham, "The effects of vaccine on cancer patients," *Surgery, Gynecology and Obstetrics,* 109 (1959), 131–138.

74. William B. Coley, "The treatment of inoperable sarcoma with the mixed toxins of erysipelas and *Bacillus prodigiosus:* Immediate and final results in 160 cases," *Journal of the American Medical Association,* 31 (1898), 389–395, 456–465.

75. Idem, "Treatment of inoperable sarcoma by bacterial toxins (the mixed toxins of the *Streptococcus erysipelas* and the *Bacillus prodigiosus*)," *Proceedings of the Royal Society of Medicine and Surgery,* 3d ser., 1909, pp. 46–48.

76. S. P. Beebe and M. Tracey, "The treatment of experimental tumors with bacterial toxins," *Journal of the American Medical Association,* 49 (1907), 1493–98.

77. Coley's daughter, Helen Coley Nauts, who later became the main advocate for this therapy, attributed the difficulties of obtaining reproducible clinical results with Coley's toxins to the variability of commercial preparation of the toxins and to their inadequate use by physicians; H. Coley Nauts, Walker E. Swift, and Bradley L. Coley, "The treatment of malignant tumors by bacterial toxins as developed by the late William B. Coley, M.D., reviewed in the light of modern research," *Cancer Research,* 6 (1946), 205–216. I am indebted to Helen Coley Nauts for information about her own activities and those of her father.

78. C. Gordon Zubrod, "Origins and development of chemotherapy research at the National Cancer Institute," *Cancer Treatment Reports,* 68(1) (1984), 9–19.

79. Robert F. Bud, "Strategy in American cancer research after World War II: A case study," *Social Studies of Science,* 8 (1978), 425–459.

80. E. Vidal, "La sérothérapie des tumeurs malignes," in *Travaux de la deuxième conférence internationale pour l'étude du cancer* (Paris: Doin, 1911), pp. 293–342; Southam, "Applications of immunology to clinical cancer," pp. 1306, 1313.

81. Chester Southam, "Homotransplantation of human cell-lines," *Bulletin of the New York Academy of Medicine,* 34(6) (1958), 416–423; C. Southam and Alice Moore, "Induced immunity to cancer cell homografts in man," *Annals of the New York Academy of Science,* 73(3) (1958), 635–651.

82. In 1966 the regents of the State University of New York found Southam guilty of "unprofessional conduct" during these clinical trials and suspended his medical license for one year; Elinor Langer, "Human experimentation: New York verdict affirms patient's rights," *Science,* 151 (1966), 663–666.

83. Ibid., p. 663.

84. Peter B. Medawar, "The immunology of transplantation," in *The Harvey Lectures, 1956–57* (New York: Academic Press, 1958).

85. Woglom, "Immunity to transplantable tumors," p. 130. Today immunologists believe that some malignant cells may lose the "identity markers" that allow their recognition as foreign by the recipient's immune mechanisms.

86. Edward F. Scanlon et al., "Fatal homotransplanted melanoma," *Cancer,* 18 (1965), 782–789.

87. Zubrod, "Origins and development."

88. Patterson, *The Dread Disease,* pp. 245–254.

89. Murphy, "Certain etiological factors in causation and transmission of tumors."

90. Robert A. Good, "Runestones in immunology: Inscription of journeys in discovery and analysis," *Journal of Immunology,* 117 (1976), 1417.

91. Jack W. Milder, "Introduction," in proceedings of the symposium "The Possible Role of Immunology in Cancer," Rye, New York, March 16–18, 1961, *Cancer Research,* 21 (1961), 1169.

92. A. M. Moulin and A. M. Silverstein, "The history of immunophysiology," in *Immunophysiology: The Role of Cells and Cytokines in Immunity and Inflammation,* ed. Joost J. Oppenheim and Ethan M. Shevach (Oxford: Oxford University Press, 1990).

93. Michael M. Mastrangelo, David Berd, and Robert E. Bellet, "Review of immunotherapeutic studies in cancer patients," in *Immunocancerology in Solid Tumors,* ed. Marcel Martin and Luis Dionne (New York: Stratton Intercontinental Medical Books, 1976), pp. 155–177; William D. Terry, "Present status and future directions for cancer immunotherapy," in *Cancer Immunotherapy and Its Immunological Basis,* ed. Y. Yamama, M. Kitagawa, and I. Azuma (Tokyo: Japan Scientific Societies Press, 1977), pp. 239–246.

94. Lloyd J. Old, Donald A. Clarke, and Baruj Benacerraf, "Effects of Bacillus Calmette-Guerin infection on transplanted tumors in the mouse," *Nature,* 184 (1959), 291.

95. Murphy, *Lymphocyte in Resistance to Tissue Grafting.*

96. Georges Mathé et al., "Transfusions et greffes de moelle osseuse homologue chez des humains irradiés à haute dose accidentellement," *Revue française des études cliniques et biologiques,* 4 (1958), 3.

97. Georges Mathé et al., "Active immunotherapy for acute immunoblastic leukemia," *Lancet,* 1969, p. 697.

98. Georges Mathé et al., "Attempts at immunotherapy of 100 acute leukemia patients: Some factors influencing results," in *Investigation and Stimulation of Immunity in Cancer Patients,* ed. G. Mathé and R. Weiner (New York: Springer Verlag, 1974), pp. 434–448; Georges Mathé et al., "Immunothérapie active de la leucémie aiguë et du lymphosarcome léucemique. Une étude de 200 cas conduite pendant 10 ans," *Nouvelle presse médicale,* 4 (1975), 1337.

99. Georges Mathé, "Introduction," in Mathé and Weiner, *Investigation and Stimulation of Immunity,* pp. 1–3.

100. Patterson, *The Dread Disease,* pp. 56–87; Patrice Pinell, "Fléau moderne et médecine d'avenir. La cancérologie française entre les deux guerres," *Actes de la recherche en sciences sociales,* 68 (1987), 45–76.

101. Barrie R. Cassileth, "The evolution of oncology as a sociomedical phenomenon," in *The Cancer Patient: Social and Medical Aspects of Care,* ed. Cassileth (Philadelphia: Lea & Febiger, 1979), pp. 1–15; Michael B. Shimkin, *Oncology* (Austin, Texas: Silvergirl, 1986), pp. 2–5.

102. Mathé, "Introduction," in Mathé and Weiner, *Investigation and Stimulation of Immunity,* p. 3.

103. Jordan U. Gutterman et al., "Active immunotherapy with BCG for re-

current malignant melanoma," *Lancet,* 1974, p. 128; D. L. Morton et al., "BCG therapy of malignant melanoma: Summary of seven years of experience," *Annals of Surgery,* 10 (1974), 635.

104. See, e.g., Evan M. Hersh, Jordan U. Gutterman, and Giora Mavligit, eds., *Immunotherapy of Cancer in Man: Scientific Basis and Current Status* (Springfield, Ill.: Charles C. Thomas, 1973); Mathé and Weiner, *Investigation and Stimulation of Immunity;* Gilles Lamoreux, Raymond Turcotte, and Vincent Portelance, eds., *BCG in Cancer Immunotherapy* (New York: Grune and Stratton, 1976); Martin and Dionne, *Immunocancerology in Solid Tumors;* R. Lee Clark, Robert C. Hickey, and Evan M. Hersh, eds., *Immunotherapy of Human Cancer* (New York: Raven Press, 1978); W. D. Terry and D. Windhorst, eds., *Immunotherapy of Cancer: Present Status of Trials in Man* (New York: Raven Press, 1978); Albert L. LoBuglio, ed., *Clinical Immunotherapy* (New York and Basel: Marcel Dekker, 1980).

105. Dorothy Windhorst, "International registry of tumor immunotherapy: The contribution of an information service to a new specialty," in Terry and Windhorst, *Immunotherapy of Cancer.*

106. From 1973 on, the list of members of the scientific council of the Cancer Research Institute reads like a *Who's Who* of leading specialists in tumor immunology. The budget of the institute was $15,000 in 1953, $150,000 in 1965, $900,000 in 1975, $3.4 million in 1987, and $5.1 million in 1991; Cancer Research Institute, *Annual Reports.* (Dollar amounts are not corrected for inflation.)

107. In the 1950s the New York Cancer Research Institute financed a series of experimental and clinical investigations of the antitumor effects of Coley's toxins. These investigations confirmed that the preparation did indeed have antitumor properties in laboratory animals and in selected patients, but they did not lead to isolation of active compounds or elucidation of the toxins' supposed mechanisms of antitumor activity; H. F. Havas, M. E. Groesbeck, and A. J. Donnelley, "Mixed bacterial toxins in the treatment of tumors," *Cancer Research,* 18 (1958), 141–148; H. F. Havas, A. J. Donnelley, and Stanley I. Levine, "Mixed bacterial toxins in the treatment of tumors: III. The effect of tumor removal on the toxicity and mortality rates in mice," ibid., 20 (1960), 393–396; Rita S. Axelrod et al., "Effect of mixed bacterial vaccine on the immune response of patients with non-small-cell lung cancer and refractory malignancies," *Cancer,* 61 (1988), 2219–30; H. F. Havas et al., "The effect of a bacterial vaccine on tumors and the immune response of ICR/Ha mice," *Journal of Biological Response Modifiers,* 9 (1990), 194–204.

108. Nauts strongly recommends the method of preparation of toxins developed by Beebe and Tracy in 1907; S. P. Beebe and M. Tracy, "The

treatment of experimental tumors with bacterial toxins," *Journal of the American Medical Association,* 49 (1907), 1493–98.

109. What attracted Chinese doctors was precisely the simplicity of the method and the absence of a necessity to develop links with the laboratory; H. Coley Nauts, "Bacteria and cancer: Antagonisms and benefits," *Cancer Surveys,* 8 (1989), 713–723.

110. David Wilson, *Body and Antibody: A Report on New Immunology* (New York: Alfred A. Knopf, 1972); Harold M. Schmeck, *Immunology: The Many-Edged Sword* (New York: George Braziller, 1974); Ronald J. Glasser, *The Body Is the Hero* (New York: Random House, 1976). In the United States, books about medical science are often written by journalists; in France, leading cancer specialists often popularize their own and their colleagues' achievements. See Jean Bernard, *L'espérance ou le nouvel état de la médecine* (Paris: Buchet/Chastel, 1978); idem, *L'enfant, le sang et l'espoir* (Paris: Buchet/Chastel, 1984); Claude Jasmin, *Parce que je crois au lendemain* (Paris: Editions Robert Laffont, 1983); Georges Mathé, *Dossier cancer* (Paris: Stock, 1976); Maurice Tubiana, *Le refus du réel* (Paris: Editions Robert Laffont, 1977); M. Tubiana, *La lumière dans l'ombre* (Paris: Editions Odile Jacob, 1983).

111. Bernard Glemser, *Man against Cancer* (New York: Funk & Wagnalls, 1969), p. 207. The official image of Mathé's investigations was different. Thus in 1978, during the presentation of the Heath Memorial Award to Mathé, Robert C. Hickey stressed the importance of ethical considerations in the laureate's studies; "Introduction of Heath Memorial Award recipient, Professor Georges Mathé," in Clark, Hickey, and Hersh, *Immunotherapy of Human Cancer,* pp. 7–8.

112. Clark, Hickey, and Hersh, *Immunotherapy of Human Cancer,* p. ix.

113. June Goodfield, *The Siege of Cancer* (New York: Random House, 1975), p. 113.

114. "Concord trial: A preliminary report," *British Medical Journal,* 1971, pp. 189–194.

115. Georges Mathé, "Immunotherapy in the treatment of acute lymphoid leukemia," *Hospital Practice,* 6 (1971), 43–51; idem, "Round table," in Lamoreux, Turcotte, and Portelance, *BCG in Cancer Immunotherapy,* p. 383; Terry, "Present status and future directions for cancer immunotherapy"; William D. Terry and Steven Rosenberg, eds., *Immunotherapy of Human Cancer* (New York: Excerpta Medica, 1983).

116. Michael J. Mastrangelo et al., "Regression of pulmonary metastatic disease associated with intralesional BCG therapy of dermal melanoma metastases," *Cancer,* 36 (1975), 1305; Lucien Israel, *Conquering Cancer* (New York: Random House, 1978), p. 121. A critic of immunotherapy warned, however, that dramatic reduction in the size of pul-

monary metastases in melanoma following a BCG treatment may reflect the disappearance of lymphocytes that infiltrate melanoma nodes, which may be induced by immunotherapy to migrate elsewhere, not the disappearance of tumor cells; J. L. Bernheim, "Immunotherapy of a solid tumor (melanoma) with BCG: A comment on the risks of enhancement," in Mathé and Weiner, *Investigation and Stimulation of Immunity*, pp. 473–475.

117. Lamoreux, Turcotte, and Portelance, *BCG in Cancer Immunotherapy;* Martin and Dionne, *Immunology in Solid Tumors;* Terry and Windhorst, *Immunotherapy of Cancer;* LoBuglio, *Clinical Immunotherapy.*

118. Michael J. Mastrangelo, David Berd, and R. E. Bellet, "Limitations, obstacles, and controversies in the optimal development of immunotherapy," in Clark, Hickey, and Hersh, *Immunotherapy of Human Cancer,* p. 384.

119. Clark, Hickey, and Hersh, *Immunotherapy of Human Cancer,* pp. ix–x.

120. Gerald L. Bartlett, "Milestones in tumor immunology," *Seminars in Oncology,* 6(4) (1979), 515–535.

121. William D. Terry, "Concluding remarks," in Terry and Windhorst, *Immunotherapy of Cancer,* p. 669.

122. J. A. Habeshaw, "Tumor immunology: Is man the odd mouse out?" *Immunology Today,* 1 (1980), 4–5.

123. On the development of clinical trials of chemotherapies in the 1950s see C. Gordon Zubrod, Saul A. Schepartz, and Stephen K. Carter, "Historical background of the National Cancer Institute's Drug Development Trust," *National Cancer Institute's Monographs,* 45 (1977), 7–11; Zubrod, "Origins and development."

124. David W. Weiss, "Animal models of cancer immunotherapy: Some considerations," in Clark, Hickey, and Hersh, *Immunotherapy of Human Cancer,* p. 101.

125. Currie, "Immunotherapy of human cancer," p. 81.

126. Weiss, "Animal models of cancer immunotherapy," p. 105. EL4 cells are an established line of human malignant cells derived from leukemic cells that, like the great majority of established human cell lines, had long lost many of its original properties. On the difficulties of working with established tumoral lines see Michael Gold, *A Conspiracy of Cells* (Albany: State University of New York Press, 1986).

127. Currie, "Immunotherapy of human cancer," p. 89. The lack of obligatory correlation between strong immune response and cure was already noted in the late nineteenth century, when investigators observed that high titers of antityphoid antibodies did not prevent death from this disease.

128. Weiss, "Animal models of cancer immunotherapy," pp. 102–103.

129. Harold B. Hewitt, "Second point: Animal tumors and their relevance

to human tumor immunology," *Journal of Biological Response Modifiers*, 2 (1983), 210, 216. On the Laetrile controversy see Neil M. Elison, David P. Byar, and Guy R. Newell, "Special report on Laetrile: The NCI Laetrile review," *New England Journal of Medicine*, 299 (1978), 549–552; Gerald E. Markle and James C. Petersen, *Politics, Science, and Cancer: The Laetrile Phenomenon* (Boulder: Westview Press, 1980); Robert L. Schwartz, "Judicial deflection of scientific questions: Pushing the Laetrile controversy towards medical closure," in *Scientific Controversies: Case Studies in the Resolution and Closure of Disputes in Science and Technology*, ed. H. Tristram Engelhardt and Arthur L. Kaplan (Cambridge: Cambridge University Press, 1987), pp. 355–379.

130. Hewitt, "Second point," p. 216.
131. Currie, "Immunotherapy of human cancer," p. 94.

3. Cancer Immunotherapy and Mass Production of Biological Agents, 1980–1990

1. Robert A. Good, "Runestones in immunology: Inscription of journeys of discovery and analysis," *Journal of Immunology*, 111 (1976), 1417–29; *New Initiatives in Immunology: NIAID Study Group Report*, NIH Publication no. 81-2215 (Bethesda, Md.: National Institutes of Health, 1981); Pauline M. Mazumdar, "Working out of the theory," in *Immunology, 1930–1980: Essays on the History of Immunology*, ed. Mazumdar (Toronto: Wall & Thompson, 1989), pp. 1–12.

2. K. W. Baldwin, S. K. Carter, and Georges Mathé, "A new journal, *Cancer Immunology and Immunotherapy*," *Cancer Immunology and Immunotherapy*, 1 (1976), 1–2.

3. William H. West et al., "Natural cytotoxic reactivity of human lymphocytes with myeloid cell line," *Journal of Immunology*, 118 (1977), 359; Ronald B. Herberman, ed., *Natural Cell-Mediated Immunity against Tumors* (New York: Academic Press, 1980).

4. Harold B. Hewitt, "Second point: Animal tumor models and their relevance to human tumor immunology," *Journal of Biological Response Modifiers*, 2 (1983), 210–216.

5. Arthur M. Silverstein, *A History of Immunology* (New York: Academic Press, 1989), pp. 87–123.

6. Ilana Löwy, "The impact of medical practice on biomedical research: The case of human leukocyte antigen studies," *Minerva*, 25 (1987), 171–200.

7. S. Cohn, E. Pick, and J. J. Oppenheim, *The Biology of Lymphokines* (New York: Academic Press, 1979); Anne-Marie Moulin and Arthur Silverstein, "The history of immunophysiology," in *Immunophysiology: The Role of Cells and Cytokines in Immunity and Inflammation*, ed.

Joost J. Oppenheim and Ethan M. Shevach (Oxford: Oxford University Press, 1990).

8. On the first clinical trials of interferon see Toine Pieters, "Interferon and its first clinical trial: Looking behind the scenes," *Medical History,* 37 (1993), 270–295.

9. David Tyrrel, "Historical background," in *Interferon and Cancer,* ed. K. Sikora (New York and London: Plenum Press, 1983), pp. 11–15; Mike Edelhardt with Jean Lindemann, *Interferon: The New Hope for Cancer* (Reading, Mass.: Addison-Wesley, 1980).

10. Nicholas Wade, "Special Virus Cancer Program: Travails of a biological moonshot," *Science,* 174 (1971), 1036; C. G. Baker, "Cancer Research Program strategy and planning," *Journal of the National Cancer Institute,* 59 (1977), 651.

11. The application of interferon to cancer therapy was studied in detail by Sandra Panem and Toine Pieters: Sandra Panem, *The Interferon Crusade* (Washington, D.C.: Brookings Institution, 1984); Toine Pieters, "A comparative study of the development of two biologicals: The interferons," Paper presented at the workshop "Les biologistes entre l'état et l'industrie," December 3, 1993, Paris. My short presentation of the history of interferon as an anticancer drug follows the chronology established in these accounts.

12. I. Gresser, I. J. Coppey, and C. Burali, "Interferon and murine leukemia: IV. Effects of interferon preparations on the lymphoid leukemia of AKR mice," *Journal of the National Cancer Institute,* 43 (1969), 1083–89; Panem, *The Interferon Crusade,* pp. 50–55.

13. H. Koren, C. Brandt, and J. Laszlo, "Modulation of natural killer (NK) activity induced by human lymphoblastoid interferon," *Proceedings of the 13th Annual International Cancer Congress* (Seattle: n.p., 1982), p. 377. The activation of NK by interferon was, however, more consistent in the test tube than in laboratory animals.

14. I. Gresser, C. Maury, and D. Brouty-Boye, "Mechanism of the antitumor effect of interferon in mice," *Nature,* 239 (1972), 167–168; Ion Gresser, "Commentary: On the varied biological effects of interferon," *Cellular Immunology,* 34 (1977), 406–415.

15. K. Cantell and S. Hirvonen, "Preparation of human leukocyte interferon for clinical use," *Texas Reports in Biology and Medicine,* 35 (1977), 138–144.

16. H. Strander et al., "Interferon treatment of osteogenic sarcoma: A clinical trial," in *Conference on Modulation of Host Immune Resistance in the Prevention or Treatment of Neoplasms* (Washington, D.C.: U.S. Government Printing Office, 1974), pp. 28, 377; Tyrrel, "Historical background," pp. 12–13. Strander and his collaborators later affirmed that interferon induced regression of the tumor in myeloma patients; H. Mellested et al., "Interferon therapy in myelomatosis," *Lancet,* 1979,

pp. 245–247. Strander's early studies are seldom quoted in "official" histories of the introduction of interferons to cancer therapy, such as Kenneth A. Foon, "Biological response modifiers: The new immunotherapy," *Cancer Research,* 49 (1989), 1621–39.

17. Panem, *The Interferon Crusade,* pp. 16–18. Oncologists continue to use historical controls, as in the clinical trials of interleukin-2 conducted in the 1980s.

18. Richard A. Retting, *Cancer Crusade: The Story of the National Cancer Act of 1971* (Princeton: Princeton University Press, 1977); Robert Teitelman, *Gene Dreams: Wall Street, Academia, and the Rise of Biotechnology* (New York: Basic Books, 1989), pp. 27–35; Panem, *The Interferon Crusade,* pp. 18–19.

19. Enrico Mihich and Alexander Fefer, *Biological Response Modifiers: Subcommittee Report,* NIH Publication no. 83-2606 (Bethesda, Md.: National Institutes of Health, 1983), pp. 234–235.

20. Edward Shorter, *The Health Century* (Garden City, N.Y.: Doubleday, 1987), p. 241. The narrative model employed there is a "classical" one: the dramatic story of a new life-saving drug, at first not available in sufficient quantity. This plot was popular in literary works as early as Shaw's 1909 play, *The Doctor's Dilemma,* and it enjoyed even more use after the Second World War in popular accounts of the discovery of penicillin.

21. Mihich and Fefer, *Biological Response Modifiers,* p. 236.

22. Edelhardt, *Interferon.*

23. The program was directed by Robert Oldham, who had become familiar with cancer immunotherapy during a postdoctoral fellowship (funded by the New York Cancer Research Institute) in Georges Mathé's laboratory in Paris; *Annual Report of the New York Cancer Institute,* 1976, p. 8.

24. Saul A. Schepartz, "Historical overview of the National Cancer Institute Fermentation Program," *Recent Results in Cancer Research,* 63 (1978), 30–32; idem, "History of the National Cancer Institute and the Plant Screening Program," *Cancer Treatment Reports,* 60(8) (1976), 975–978; C. Gordon Zubrod, "Origins and development of chemotherapy research at the National Cancer Institute," ibid., 68(1) (1984), 9–19.

25. Mihich and Fefer, *Biological Response Modifiers,* pp. 245–246.

26. William D. Terry, "Concluding remarks," in *Immunotherapy of Cancer: Present Status of Trials in Men,* ed. W. D. Terry and D. Windhorst (New York: Raven Press, 1978), pp. 669–671; Albert LoBuglio, "Introduction," in *Clinical Immunotherapy,* ed. LoBuglio (New York and Basel: Marcel Dekker, 1980), pp. 2–4.

27. Robert K. Oldham and Richard V. Smalley, "Immunotherapy: The old and the new," *Journal of Biological Response Modifiers,* 2 (1983), 3, 6.

28. John W. Hadden, "Immunomodulators in the immunotherapy of cancer

and other diseases," *Trends in Pharmaceutical Sciences,* May 1982, p. 191.

29. "Dossier: Interferons—du singulier au pluriel," *Biofutur,* March 1982, pp. 9–16.

30. Panem, *The Interferon Crusade,* pp. 61–67.

31. Charles Weissman, "The cloning of interferon and other mistakes," in *Interferon 3,* ed. Ion Gresser (New York: Academic Press, 1981), p. 101.

32. "Enquête sur l'interferon," *Biofutur,* March 1983, pp. 5–22; Martin Kenney, *Biotechnology: The University Industrial Complex* (New Haven: Yale University Press, 1986), p. 198.

33. Usually only a few pharmaceutical firms are engaged in competition over the development of a new drug. A compound destined to cure a major disease for which no known therapy exists can reach the market much faster thanks to specific regulations that expedite its commercializaton (in the United States, the FDA "fast track"; in Europe, specific regulations for experimental drugs). Such a product can therefore rapidly bring profits to its producers. The reduction of the interval between the development and the commercialization of a new drug is particularly important for small venture-capital startups such as the new biotechnology firms that appeared in the late 1970s. These firms centered their efforts on a limited number of products and, unlike bigger and more diversified companies, could not afford to go for long periods without making a profit; Panem, *The Interferon Crusade,* p. 68; Teitelman, *Gene Dreams,* p. 145.

34. Mihich and Fefer, *Biological Response Modifiers,* p. 5.

35. Panem, *The Interferon Crusade,* p. 30. The suppression of medical evidence in the name of progress in medical knowledge is not a new phenomenon. An early episode of this type occurred in the early days of bacteriology. In 1886 a child, Joseph Rouyer, died following treatment with the newly developed rabies vaccine. The child's physician suspected that the death was induced by the vaccine, and the child's family threatened to sue the vaccine's discoverer, Louis Pasteur. Pasteur's friends and collaborators, Emile Roux and Pierre Bruardel, feared that a trial would "ruin the positive image of vaccination and set back the new science of bacteriology fifty years." They went to great lengths and possibly falsified post-mortem evidence and laboratory results in order to mask the possibility that the rabies vaccine could be dangerous; Adrien Loir, *A l'ombre de Pasteur. Souvenirs personnels* (Paris: Editions du Mouvement Sanitaire, 1937), p. 85; Maurice Valery-Radot, *Pasteur. Un génie au service de l'homme* (Paris: Editions Pierre-Marcel Favre, 1985), pp. 297–304.

36. Hairy cell leukemia, however, also responds to splenoctomy, to chemotherapy with pentostatin, and to a new drug, the 2-chlorodeoxy-

adenosine (2CdA). Interferon enlarged the range of therapeutic choices in hairy cell leukemia but did not provide a therapy for an otherwise incurable disease; R. I. Jahiel and M. Krim, "Interferons, clinical trials and effects on hematologic neoplasms," in *Biological Response and Cancer Therapy*, ed. J. W. Chiao (New York and Basel: Marcel Dekker, 1988), pp. 197–266; D. A. Carson et al., "Programmed cell death and adenine denucleotide metabolism in human lymphocytes," *Advances in Enzyme Regulation*, 27 (1988), 395–404.

37. In France four patients treated with cell-secreted interferon in 1982 died of cardiac arrest. Consequently, the French government ordered a temporary halt to clinical trials of interferon in France; "Interferon. Situation des essais cliniques en France," *Biofutur*, March 1983, p. 14.

38. Stephen K. Carter, "The clinical trial evaluation for interferon and other biological response modifiers—not an easy task," *Journal of Biological Response Modifiers*, 1 (1982), 102–105.

39. K. Sikora, "The cancer problem," in Sikora, *Interferon and Cancer*, pp. 7–8; Tabitha M. Powledge, "Interferon on trial," *Biotechnology*, March 1984, p. 218; James E. Talmage, Isaiah J. Fidler, and R. K. Oldham, *Screening for Immunological Response Modifiers: Method and Rationale* (Boston and Dordrecht: Martinus Nijhoff, 1985), pp. 180–181; Karl Fent and Gerhard Zbinden, "The toxicity of interferon and interleukin," *Trends in Pharmacological Sciences*, 8 (March 1987), 100–108.

40. Robert Weinberger and Frank Raucher, "New developments in cancer research," *Annual Report of the American Cancer Society*, 1983, p. 8.

41. Carter quoted in Shorter, *The Health Century*, p. 250. The New York–based Bristol-Myers Company was one of the main pharmaceutical companies involved in interferon production and marketing. In 1980 it acquired a worldwide license to use and sell interferon manufactured using Genentech Corporation technology. In 1981 it also acquired a worldwide license to use and sell interferon purchased from Interferon Sciences; "Enquête sur l'interferon," *Biofutur*, March 1983, pp. 5–22.

42. "Editorial: Topical BCG for recurrent superficial bladder cancer," *Lancet*, 1991, pp. 821–822.

43. Hélène Therre, "Le marché américain de monokines, cytokines et autres facteurs de croissance," *Biofutur*, January 1990, pp. 46–47; editorial, *Biotechnology News*, 9 (1990), 4–8; Betty Dodet, "Cytokines in the clinics: Choose your weapon," *European Cytokine Network*, 5 (1994), 369–376.

44. Oldham and Smalley, "Immunotherapy," pp. 25, 27. The claim that the "old" immunotherapy did not induce regression of solid tumors was not exact. In some cases investigators claimed that treatment with bac-

terial vaccines led to the regression of established, metastatic solid tumors such as lymphoma and melanoma; Michael J. Mastrangelo, David Berd, and Robert E. Bellet, "Review of immunotherapeutic studies on cancer patients," in *Immunology in Solid Tumors,* ed. Marcel Martin and Luis Dionne (New York: Stratton Intercontinental Medical Books, 1976), pp. 155–177; Lucien Israel, *Conquering Cancer* (New York: Random House, 1978). Although these reports were anecdotal, BCG was repeatedly found to induce shrinking of skin tumors and to inhibit superficial bladder cancer. Still earlier there had been numerous reports (complete with "before" and "after" photos) that Coley's toxins induced regression of solid tumors.

45. Jahiel and Krim, "Interferons."
46. Ronald B. Herberman, "The evaluation of biological response modifiers for cancer therapy," in *New Directions in Cancer Treatment,* ed. Ian Magrath (Berlin: Springer Verlag, 1989), p. 283.
47. Ibid., p. 286.
48. Foon, "Biological response modifiers," p. 1621.
49. J. W. Clark and D. L. Longo, "Biological response modifiers in cancer therapy," in Magrath, *New Directions in Cancer Treatment,* p. 301.
50. Panem, *The Interferon Crusade,* p. 103.
51. D. A. Morgan, F. W. Ruscetti, and R. Gallo, "Selective *in vitro* growth of lymphocytes from normal human bone marrow," *Science,* 193 (1976), 1007–08.
52. Didier Fradzelli and Willem Roskam, "Interleukine-2 humaine," *Biofutur,* September 1983, p. 340.
53. Steven A. Rosenberg and John M. Barry, *The Transformed Cell* (New York: G. P. Putnam's Sons, 1992), pp. 44–48.
54. S. A. Rosenberg, "Adoptive immunotherapy of cancer," *Scientific American,* May 1990, pp. 34–41; Rosenberg and Barry, *The Transformed Cell,* pp. 63–64.
55. William D. Terry and S. A. Rosenberg, eds., *Immunotherapy of Human Cancer* (New York: Elsevier North Holland, 1982).
56. S. A. Rosenberg, "Adoptive immunotherapy of cancer using lymphokine-activated killer cells and recombinant interleukin-2," in *Important Advances in Oncology,* ed. V. T. DeVita, S. Hellman, and S. A. Rosenberg (New York: Academic Press, 1987), p. 55.
57. Rosenberg and Barry, *The Transformed Cell,* pp. 85–86.
58. The white blood cells, or leukocytes, are traditionally classified according to their morphology. One of these morphological categories, the lymphocytes (so named because they are abundant in the lymphatic system and the lymph nodes), is involved in cellular immune reactions. It was assumed that IL-2 activated mainly the lymphocytes. For practical reasons, however (the separation of lymphocytes from other cat-

egories of white blood cells is labor-intensive), researchers sometimes incubated with interleukin the entire white blood cells, and not the lymphocytes alone.

59. S. Gillis and K. A. Smith, "Long-term culture of tumor-specific cytotoxic T-cells," *Nature,* 368 (1977), 154–155.

60. Michael T. Lotze et al., "*In vitro* growth of cytotoxic human lymphocytes: IV. Lysis of fresh and cultured autologous tumor by human lymphocytes cultured in T-cell growth factor (TCGF)," *Cancer Research,* 41 (1981), 4420–25.

61. E. A. Grimm et al., "Lymphokine-activated killer cell phenomenon: Lysis of natural killer-resistant fresh solid tumors by interleukin-2 activated autologous human peripheral lymphocytes," *Journal of Experimental Medicine,* 155 (1982), 1823–41; M. Rosenstein et al., "Lymphokine activated killer cells: Lysis of fresh syngeneic NK-resistant murine tumor cells by lymphocytes cultured in interleukin-2," *Cancer Research,* 44 (1984), 1946–53.

62. S. A. Rosenberg, "The adoptive immunotherapy of cancer: Accomplishments and prospects," *Cancer Therapy Reports,* 68 (1984), 244–255; J. C. Yang, J. J. Mule, and S. A. Rosenberg, "Characterisation of the murine lymphokine-activated killer precursor and effector cell," *Surgical Forum,* 36 (1985), 408–410.

63. The morphological and functional tests are not perceived as independent because it is assumed that surface markers play a role first in the recognition and then in the killing of target cells; L. L. Lanier and J. H. Phillips, "Effectors, repertoire and receptors involved in lymphocyte mediated MHC unrestricted cytotoxicity," *Annales de l'Institut Pasteur (Immunologie),* 139 (1988), 433–478.

64. Usually the targets are tumor cell lines maintained in the laboratory. Although cell lines are standardized, their susceptibility to lysis by cytotoxic lymphocytes may vary because of variability in cell-culture conditions. Target cell variability is even greater in tests that employ fresh, uncultured tumor cells.

65. E.g., T. Timonen et al., "Cultures of purified human natural killer cells: Growth in the presence of IL-2," *Cellular Immunology,* 72 (1982), 198; R. Suzuki et al., "Natural killer (NK) cells as responders to interleukin-2 (IL-2)," *Journal of Immunology,* 130 (1983), 981–987.

66. Michel Serres, *La traduction* (Paris: Editions de Minuit, 1974).

67. The different presentations of LAK cells probably reflected not a deliberate use of rhetorical devices aimed at convincing different audiences, but rather oscillations in the degree of certainty attributed to the existence of these cells by the scientists who studied them. On the transformation of "scientific facts" that circulate between esoteric and exoteric circles see Ludwik Fleck, *Genesis and Development of a Scientific Fact*

(1935), trans. Fred Bradley and Thaddeus J. Trenn (Chicago: University of Chicago Press, 1985), pp. 105–107. Fleck proposed that such transformation does not represent a distortion of a single truth (e.g., of specialists) in order to adapt it to a different public (e.g., general practitioners), but divergent and incommensurable truths.

68. Rosenberg, "Adoptive immunotherapy of cancer using lymphokine-activated killer cells and recombinant interleukin-2."

69. The aim of these IL-2 injections was to maintain a high biological activity of injected LAK cells and/or to generate new LAK cells in the body; A. Mazumdar and S. A. Rosenberg, "Successful immunotherapy of natural killer resistant established pulmonary melanoma metastases by the intravenous adoptive transfer of syngeneic lymphocytes activated *in vitro* by interleukin-2," *Journal of Experimental Medicine,* 159 (1984), 495; J. J. Mule et al., "Adoptive immunotherapy of established pulmonary metastases with LAK and recombinant interleukin-2," *Science,* 225 (1984), 1487–89; S. A. Rosenberg et al., "Regression of established pulmonary metastases and subcutaneous tumor mediated by systemic administration of high dose recombinant IL-2," *Cancer Research,* 45 (1985), 3735–41.

70. R. Lafranière and S. A. Rosenberg, "Successful immunotherapy of murine experimental hepatic metastases with lymphokine activated killer cells (LAK) and recombinant interleukin-2 (RIL-2) can mediate the regression of both immunogenic and non-immunogenic sarcomas and an adenocarcinoma," *Journal of Immunology,* 135 (1985), 4273–80.

71. S. E. Ettinghausen et al., "Systemic administration of recombinant interleukin-2 stimulates *in vivo* lymphoid cell stimulation in tissues," ibid., pp. 1488–97.

72. J. H. Donohue et al., "The systemic administration of purified interleukin-2 enhances the ability of sensitized murine lymphocyte lines to cure a disseminated syngeneic lymphoma," ibid., 132 (1984), 2123–28.

73. Rosenberg, "Adoptive immunotherapy of cancer using lymphokine-activated killer cells and recombinant interleukin-2"; idem, "The development of new immunotherapies for the treatment of cancer using interleukin-2," *Annals of Surgery,* 208 (1988), 121–135.

74. Elisabeth A. Grimm and S. A. Rosenberg, "The human lymphokine-activated killer cell phenomenon," in *Lymphokines,* ed. E. Pick and M. Candy (New York: Academic Press, 1983), vol. 9, pp. 279–311.

75. S. A. Rosenberg et al., "Biological activity of recombinant human interleukin-2 produced in *Echerichia coli,*" *Science,* 223 (1984), 1412.

76. Kenney, *Biotechnology,* p. 171.

77. In the early 1980s the production of recombinant IL-2 was an anticipated event, and one may assume that Rosenberg's attempts to cure cancer with high concentrations of the molecule were not unrelated to

his hopes of obtaining access to large quantities of it; Rosenberg and Barry, *The Transformed Cell.*

78. Michael T. Lotze et al., "*In vivo* administration of purified human interleukin-2: Half-life and immunologic effects of the Jurkat line derived interleukin-2," *Journal of Immunology,* 134 (1985), 157–166. Seven cancer and five AIDS patients participated in this trial.

79. M. T. Lotze et al., "*In vivo* administration of purified human interleukin-2: Half-life, immunological effects and the expansion of peripheral lymphoid cells *in vivo* with recombinant IL-2," ibid., 135 (1985), 2865–75. Twenty cancer patients participated in this trial.

80. Toxic effects were also observed in laboratory animals; Y. L. Matory et al., "Toxicity of recombinant human interleukin-2 in rats following intravenous infusion," *Journal of Biological Response Modifiers,* 4 (1985), 377.

81. Rosenberg explained that his earlier failures, together with the success of animal studies, convinced him that his duty was to try even harder; Rosenberg and Barry, *The Transformed Cell.*

82. Rosenberg's studies were not the first published attempt to apply IL-2-activated cells to cancer therapy in humans. A year earlier Israeli physicians had attempted to activate a patient's lymphocytes in the test tube with crude, cell-derived IL-2, then to inject the activated lymphocytes into subcutaneous tumor metastases; Aliza Adler et al., "Intralesion injection of interleukin-2 expanded autologous lymphocytes in melanoma and breast cancer patients: A pilot study," *Journal of Biological Response Modifiers,* 3 (1984), 491–500. Localized IL-2 therapy was, the authors of this study claimed, well tolerated by patients and in some cases led to regression of malignant nodules. Attempts at localized application of IL-2 were discontinued later, perhaps because partial regression of cancer nodules might have seemed a modest achievement when compared with the impressive results of systemic therapy with LAK/IL-2 reported by Rosenberg's group.

83. Teitelman, *Gene Dreams,* pp. 188–190.

84. S. A. Rosenberg et al., "Observations on the systemic administration of autologous lymphokine-activated killer cells and recombinant interleukin-2 to patients with metastatic cancer," *New England Journal of Medicine,* 313 (1985), 1485–92. Publications in prestigious medical journals increased the visibility of IL-2.

85. "Cancer patience," *Wall Street Journal,* December 16, 1985; de Vita quoted in "The search for a cure," *Newsweek,* December 16, 1985. On the media's enthusiastic reception of the announcement of the new therapy see James T. Patterson, *The Dread Disease: Cancer and Modern American Culture* (Cambridge, Mass.: Harvard University Press, 1987), pp. 295–296.

86. For cases of "responsive" malignant tumors, melanoma and kidney cancer (renal cell carcinoma), IL-2/LAK treatment looked even more impressive: four cases (out of seven) of malignant melanoma, and three cases (out of three) of kidney cancer responded to the new therapy.

87. John R. Durant, "Immunotherapy of cancer: The end of the beginning?" *New England Journal of Medicine,* 316 (1987), 939–940.

88. R. K. Oldham, "Patient funded cancer research," ibid., pp. 46–47.

89. According to the *Wall Street Journal,* individual therapeutic contracts at Biotherapeutic were priced at $19,400 per IL-2-treated patient; "Cancer patience."

90. Biotherapeutic's brochure, Contract Research Services, Franklin, Tenn., 1985.

91. William H. West et al., "Constant infusion of recombinant interleukin-2 in adoptive immunotherapy of advanced cancer," *New England Journal of Medicine,* 316 (1987), 898–905. The IL-2/LAK therapy was again found to be most efficient in melanoma and renal cell carcinoma.

92. M. T. Lotze et al., "High doses of recombinant interleukin-2 in the treatment of patients with disseminated cancer," *Journal of the American Medical Association,* 256 (1986), 3117–24. The therapeutic effects of IL-2 were attributed to the activation of LAK cells in the patient's body.

93. Charles G. Moertel, "On lymphokines, cytokines and breakthroughs," ibid., p. 3141.

94. A report to the conference "Biological Therapy of Cancer," organized by the Cetus Corporation at Chapel Hill, North Carolina, in September 1986, explained that to date, 4 of 30 renal cell carcinoma patients enlisted in extramural trials of IL-2/LAK therapy had responded to treatment (compared with 9 of 10 patients in Rosenberg's original trial). No complete remissions were seen in the extramural trials; Arthur Klausner, "Clinicians question adoptive immunotherapy," *Bio/Technology,* 4 (1986), 1044.

95. E.g., John C. L. Wang et al., "A phase II clinical trial of adoptive immunotherapy for advanced renal carcinoma using mitogen-activated autologous lymphocytes and continuous-infusion interleukin-2," *Journal of Clinical Oncology,* 7 (1989), 1885–91; Janice P. Dutcher et al., "A phase II study of interleukin-2 and lymphocyte activated killer cells in patients with metastatic malignant melanoma," ibid., pp. 477–485; Jeffrey W. Clark et al., "Interleukin-2 and lymphocyte activated killer cell therapy: Analysis of a bolus interleukin-2 and a continuous infusion interleukin-2 regimen," *Cancer Research,* 50 (1990), 7343–50. Opponents of the new method noted that melanoma and renal cell carcinoma are precisely those with the highest rates of spontaneous regressions. Moreover, the spontaneous regression of renal cell carcinoma was

linked with psychological factors; R. T. D. Oliver, "Surveillance as a possible option for management of metastatic renal cell carcinoma," *Seminars in Urology,* 7 (1989), 149–152. Oliver added, however, that IL-2-induced permanent regressions of tumors were more frequent than spontaneous regressions of malignant tumors.

96. S. A. Rosenberg et al., "Experience with the use of high-dose interleukin-2 in the treatment of 652 cancer patients," *Annals of Surgery,* 210 (1989), 474–485. Later, when Rosenberg's group refined its selection of patients and decided to treat all of them with very high doses of IL-2 (thus increasing the toxicity and the costs of therapy), they obtained 6.7 percent long-term regressions of melanoma and renal cell carcinoma; S. A. Rosenberg et al., "Treatment of 283 consecutive patients with metastatic melanoma or renal cell cancer using high-dose bolus interleukin-2," *Journal of the American Medical Association,* 271 (1994), 907–913.

97. Amy H. Kargel et al., "Myocarditis or acute myocardial infection associated with interleukin-2 therapy of cancer," *Cancer,* 66 (1990), 1513–16; Kargel et al., "Pathologic finding associated with interleukin-2 based immunotherapy for cancer: A post-mortem study of 19 patients," *Human Pathology,* 21 (1990), 493–502. Sepsis—not an obvious consequence of a treatment aimed at the stimulation of immune mechanisms—was the main cause of therapy-linked deaths. The article "Pathologic finding associated with interleukin-2 based immunotherapy for cancer" ended with an affirmation (expressed in litotes): "Not unlike other forms of therapy of cancer, IL-2-based immunotherapy does not appear to be without significant toxicity" (p. 501).

98. Kirk D. Denicoff et al., "The neuropsychiatric effects of treatment with interleukin-2 and lymphokine-activated cells," *Annals of Internal Medicine,* 107 (1987), 293–300; Bettie S. Jackson et al., "Long-term biopsychosocial effects of interleukin-2 therapy," *Oncology News Forum,* 18(4) (1991), 693–690. Jackson et al. hoped, on the basis of estimates of response levels and patients' survival extrapolated from Rosenberg's 1985 article, to be able to follow the long-term effects of IL-2 therapy, but the high mortality of IL-2-treated patients did not allow them to develop statistically valid estimates of long-term effects of that therapy (p. 689).

99. Durant, "Immunotherapy of cancer," pp. 939, 940.

100. E.g., N. Thatcher et al., "Recombinant interleukin-2 given intrasplenically and intravenously for advanced malignant melanoma," *British Journal of Cancer,* 60 (1989), 770–774; S. Negrier et al., "Interleukin-2 with or without LAK cells in metastatic renal cell carcinoma: A report of a European multicenter study," *European Journal of Clinical Oncology,* 25, supp. 3 (1989), s21–s28; David R. Parkinson et al., "Inter-

leukin-2 therapy in patients with metastatic malignant myeloma: A phase II study," *Journal of Clinical Oncology,* 8 (1990), 1650–56.

101. A. K. Ghosh et al., "Lack of correlation between peripheral blood lymphokine-activated killer (LAK) cell function and clinical response in patients with advanced malignant melanoma receiving recombinant interleukin-2," *International Journal of Cancer,* 43 (1989), 410–414; M. C. Favrot et al., "Functional and immunophenotypic modifications induced by interleukin-2 did not predict response to therapy in patients with renal cell carcinoma," *Journal of Biological Response Modifiers,* 9 (1990), 167–177.

102. Lewis L. Lanier et al., "Natural killer cells: Definition of cell type rather than a function," *Journal of Immunology,* 137 (1986), 2735–39; Arabella B. Tilde, Kyogo Itoh, and Charles M. Balch, "Human lymphokine-activated killer (LAK) cells: Identification of two types of effector cells," ibid., 138 (1987), 1068–73; Ronald B. Herberman, "Lymphokine-activated killer cell activity," *Immunology Today,* 8 (1987), 178–181.

103. Wolf H. Fridman, "New immunotherapeutic approaches: The use of cytokines to stimulate the immune system or to control the growth of malignant lymphoid cells," *European Journal of Clinical Oncology,* 25 (1989), 1525–28; Ernest C. Borden and Paul M. Sondel, "Lymphokines and cytokines as cancer treatment: Immunotherapy realized," *Cancer,* 65, supp. 1 (1990), 800–814; Florence C. Antoine, "1971–1991: Biological therapy moves form the bench to the bedside," *Journal of the National Cancer Institute,* 83 (1991), 530–532; Samuel Hellman, editorial, "Immunotherapy for metastatic cancer. Establishing a 'proof of principle,' " *Journal of the American Medical Association,* 271 (1994), 945–946.

104. Ken Marumo et al., "Immunologic study of human recombinant IL-2 low dose in patients with advanced renal cell carcinoma," *Urology,* 33 (1989), 219–225.

105. Ghosh et al., "Lack of correlation"; Favrot et al., "Functional and immunophenotypic modifications"; Jeff A. Sosman et al., "Prolonged interleukin-2 (IL-2) treatment can augment immune activation without enhancing antitumor activity in renal cell carcinoma," *Cancer Investigation,* 9 (1991), 35–48. The increased expression of MHC antigens, some investigators proposed, might facilitate the recognition and destruction of malignant cells by immune mechanisms.

106. Joshua T. Rubin et al., "Immunohistochemical correlates of response to recombinant interleukin-2 based immunotherapy in humans," *Cancer Research,* 49 (1988), 7086–92. The authors found that tumors of the majority of the patients who responded to IL-2 treatment showed high levels of MHC antigens. The increase in expression of MHC antigens on tumor cells by IL-2 became the basis of a new approach to cancer therapy developed by Rosenberg's group—the reinjection into patients

of their own cancer cells, modified by the insertion of the gene of IL-2. The cancer-modified cells, it was hoped, would express higher levels of MHC antigens and would therefore be more readily recognized as "foreign," then destroyed by the body's immune mechanisms; Rosenberg and Barry, *The Transformed Cell*. This approach—a variant of specific immunization with cancer cells—might be seen as an implicit acknowledgment of the difficulties of manipulating cytotoxic T cells and as a return to traditional, antigen-centered immunological methods.

107. In the words of Borden and Sondel, enthusiastic supporters of cancer immunotherapy, "we still do not understand which of the pleiotropic biological effects of interleukin-2 results in antitumor activity"; "Lymphokines and cytokines as cancer treatment," p. 809.

108. Kendall A. Smith, "Interleukin futures," *Bio/Technology*, 7 (1989), 664.

109. Robert Oldham, the founder of Biotherapeutic Inc., expressed what some considered an extreme view of the importance of the alliance between the laboratory and the clinic: such an alliance, he asserted, should be based on the direct transfer of research innovations from the test tube to the patient, not on extensive preclinical studies: "there are no good pre-clinical models, and in my opinion there are likely never going to be any very good ones. If you look at the clinics, you cannot even use your observations in one breast cancer patient to predict what is going to happen in the next. So, where humans predict so poorly for human activity I have a great deal of difficulty understanding how we're going to improve the situation with any pre-clinical model"; Oldham quoted in Arthur Klausner (coordinator), "The biotechnology forum on cancer biotherapy," *Bio/Technology*, 6 (1988), 136–140.

110. C. Da Fano, "A cytological analysis of the reaction in animals to implanted carcinomata," *Fifth Scientific Report of the Imperial Cancer Research Fund*, 5 (1912), 57–78.

111. I. Yron, P. J. Spiess, and S. A. Rosenberg, "*In vitro* growth of murine T cells: V. The isolation and growth of lymphoid cells infiltrating syngeneic solid tumors," *Journal of Immunology*, 125 (1980), 238–245.

112. Linda M. Muul et al., "Identification of specific cytolytic immune responses against autologous tumor in humans bearing malignant melanoma," ibid., 138 (1986), 989–995.

113. S. A. Rosenberg, P. J. Spiess, and R. Lafranière, "A new approach to the adoptive immunotherapy of cancer with tumor infiltrating lymphocytes," *Science*, 223 (1986), 1318–21.

114. In contrast, LAK cells were generated in short-term cultures (three to four days), so their preparation was less labor-intensive.

115. S. A. Rosenberg et al., "The use of tumor-infiltrating lymphocytes and interleukin-2 in the immunotherapy of patients with metastatic melanoma," *New England Journal of Medicine*, 319 (1988,) 1676–80.

116. R. K. Oldham et al., "Continuous infusion of interleukin-2 and tumor-

derived activated cells as treatment of advanced solid tumors: A National Biotherapy Study group trial," *Molecular Biotherapy,* 3 (1991), 68–73.

117. M. T. Lotze et al., "Mechanisms of immunologic antitumor therapy: Lessons from the laboratory and clinical applications," *Human Immunology,* 28 (1990), 198–207.

118. Rosenberg, "Adoptive immunotherapy of cancer."

119. S. A. Rosenberg et al., "Gene transfer into humans: Immunotherapy of patients with advanced melanoma using tumor-infiltrating lymphocytes modified by retroviral gene transduction," *New England Journal of Medicine,* 323 (1990), 570–578.

120. Ibid., p. 571; Denis Cournoyer and C. Thomas Caskey, "Gene transfer into humans: A first step," ibid., pp. 601–603.

121. Rosenberg's attempts to cure cancer with TILs transfected with gene for tumor necrosis factor (TNF) were strongly criticized in 1992 by an NIH scientific oversight panel; Christopher Anderson, "Gene therapy researcher under fire over controversial cancer trials," *Nature,* 360 (1992), 399–400.

122. E.g., Malcolm S. Mitchell et al., "Low-dose cyclophospamide and low-dose interleukin-2 for malignant melanoma," *Bulletin of the New York Academy of Medicine,* 65 (1989), 128–144; K. Marumo et al., "Immunologic study of human recombinant interleukin-2 (low dose) in patients with advanced renal cell carcinoma," *Urology,* 33 (1989), 219–225. In some studies, low doses of interleukin were injected subcutaneously in cancer patients, and the authors of these studies affirmed that IL-2 administered in that way was clinically and immunologically active; J. Atzpodien et al., "Low-dose subcutaneous recombinant interleukin-2 in advanced human malignancy: A phase II outpatient study," *Molecular Biotherapy,* 2 (1990), 18; R. C. Stein et al., "The clinical effects of prolonged treatment of patients with advanced cancer with low-dose subcutaneous interleukin-2," *British Journal of Cancer,* 63 (1991), 275.

Some authors affirmed that "high doses" (5 to 10×10^6 Cetus units/M^2/day) of interleukin-2 could also be administered in an outpatient setting; Ronald M. Bukowski et al., "Phase II trial of high-dose intermittent interleukin-2 in metastatic renal cell carcinoma: A Southwest Oncology Group study," *Journal of the National Cancer Institute,* 82 (1990), 143–146; Robert L. Krigel et al., "Renal cell carcinoma: Treatment with recombinant interleukin-2 plus β interferon," *Journal of Clinical Oncology,* 8 (1990), 460–467.

123. The concepts of "low" and "high" doses were relative. IL-2 doses described as "low" might vary from as much as 3.6×10^6/U/M^2/day (e.g., Mitchell et al., "Low-dose cyclophosphamide and low-dose interleukin-

2 for malignant melanoma") to as little as 4×10^4/U/M^2 day (e.g., J. Wand et al., "Adoptive immunotherapy for stage IV renal cell carcinoma: A novel protocol utilizing periodate and interleukin-2 activated autologous lymphocytes and continuous infusion of low-dose interleukin-2," *American Journal of Medicine*, 83 [1987], 1016–23). A dose of 3×10^6/U/M^2/day was labeled "high" in one study; N. Javadapour and M. Lalehzarian, "A phase I–II study of high-dose recombinant human interleukin-2 in disseminated renal cell carcinoma," *Seminars in Surgical Oncology*, 4 (1988), 207–209.

124. S. A. Rosenberg, "The development of new immunotherapies for the treatment of cancer using interleukin-2," *Annals of Surgery*, 208 (1988), 121–135; "Interleukin-2: Sunrise for immunotherapy?" *Lancet*, 1989, p. 308.

125. E.g., E. Shiloni et al., "Sequential dacarbazine chemotherapy followed by recombinant interleukin-2 in metastatic myeloma," *European Journal of Cancer and Clinical Oncology*, 25, supp. 3 (1989), s45–s49; R. O. Dilman et al., "Recombinant interleukin-2 and adoptive immunotherapy alternated with dacarbazine therapy in melanoma: A National Biotherapy Study Group trial," *Journal of the National Cancer Institute*, 82 (1990), 1345–49; N. Thatcher et al., "Recombinant interleukin-2 with flavone acetic acid in advanced malignant melanoma: A phase II study," *British Journal of Cancer*, 61 (1990), 618–621.

Therapies akin to standard chemotherapies, combining one or more cytokines with other anticancer drugs, were used increasingly in the early 1990s; José Alexandre M. Barbuto and Evan M. Hersh, "Role of cytokines in cancer therapy," in *Human Cytokines: Their Role in Disease and Therapy*, ed. Brahat B. Aggraval and Raj K. Puri (Cambridge, Mass.: Blackwell Science, 1995), pp. 503–524; Anne Taylor and Martin Gore, "Principles of cytokine therapy," in *Oncology: A Multidisciplinary Textbook*, ed. Alan Horwich (London: Chapman & Hall Medical, 1995), pp. 161–177.

126. L. Bergmann, "Malignant melanoma: Prognosis and actual treatment: Strategies with chemotherapy and biological response modifiers," *European Journal of Cancer and Clinical Oncology*, 25, supp. 3 (1989), s31–s36; D. R. Parkinson et al., "Interleukin-2 alone and in combination with other cytokines in melanoma: The investigational approach at the University of Texas M. D. Anderson Cancer Center," *Cancer Treatment Reviews*, supp. A, 1989, pp. 39–48.

127. D. R. Parkinson, "Lessons from the clinical trials of interleukin-2," *Natural Immunity and Cell Growth Regulation*, 9 (1990), 242–252; Bergmann, "Malignant melanoma."

128. Teitelman, *Gene Dreams*.

129. T. Cicardelle and K. Smith, "Interleukin-2: Prototype for the new gen-

eration of immunoactive pharmaceuticals," *Trends in Pharmaceutical Sciences,* 19 (1989), 239–242; J. Hodgstone, "Data directed drug design," *Bio/Technology,* 9 (1991), 19–21; Robert Burns and Glenn Rifkin, "Companies targeting drug delivery," ibid., 8 (1990), 513–522.

130. Frances R. Balkwill, "Cytokine therapy of cancer: The importance of knowing the context," *European Cytokine Network,* 5(4) (1994), 379–385.

131. Eli Kedar and Eva Klein, "Cancer immunotherapy: Are the results discouraging? Can they be improved?" *Advances in Cancer Research,* 59 (1992), 245–322; quotations pp. 292, 293.

132. A. Klausner, "Unlocking IL-2's business potential," *Bio/Technology,* 4 (1986), 622–624; Kenney, *Biotechnology,* p. 171; Teitelman, *Gene Dreams,* p. 189.

133. Amgen had a patent dispute with Cetus that was settled in 1988 in a decision that was largely favorable to Cetus; Robert H. Benson, "Patent wars," *Bio/Technology,* 4 (1986), 1064–68.

134. Klausner, "Unlocking IL-2's business potential."

135. Cetus Corporation, *Proleukin-2: An Abbreviated Monograph* (Emeryville, Calif., 1989). Renal cell carcinoma is a rare cancer, and the profits that can be expected from the sale of a drug for this particular disease are limited. However, obtaining a marketing permit earmarked for a cure for a rare disease may open the way to other uses of the same molecule.

136. Betty Dodet, "Eurocetus à la conquête du marché européen," *Biofutur,* November 1989, pp. 84–85.

137. "Les petites firmes de biotechnologies financées par le capital-risque," ibid., December 1984, pp. 56–57; Pierre-Jean Raugel, "La création de sociétés indépendantes spécialisées en biotechnologies et en biologie en France," ibid., May 1990, pp. 95–104.

138. John Hodgson, "Proleukin slowing the CPMP merry-go-round," *Bio/Technology,* 8 (1990), 894–895.

139. Mark Ratner, "The Cetus experience: Troubles with clinical designs and data presentation," ibid., pp. 815–817.

140. "Pharmaceutical: The miracle is missing," *Time,* August 13, 1990, p. 57. In January 1992 the FDA accorded Cetus the right to market IL-2 for therapeutic use in renal cell carcinoma, but the granting of this restricted marketing permit came too late to prevent Cetus' financial troubles.

141. Hodgson, "Proleukin slowing the CPMP merry-go-round."

142. Filippo La Monica, "Cetus commentaries," *Bio/Technology,* 9 (1991), 197.

143. Isabelle Trocheris, "Chiron/Cetus. Les adieux de la baleine," *Biofutur,*

October 1991, pp. 54–56. Cetus Corporation became the Cetus Oncology Division of Chiron Corporation.

144. Fields quoted in Ann Gibson, "Chiron/Cetus," *Science,* 253 (1991), 503–504. In 1994 interleukin-2 was still not a commercial success, and its prospects were not encouraging; for example, its French producer, Russel-Uclaf, decided to abandon the development and commercialization of its IL-2; Dodet, "Cytokines in the clinics," p. 369.

145. Ratner, "The Cetus experience"; Teitelman, *Gene Dreams,* p. 189.

146. Cetus, *Annual Report,* 1988, p. 1. On p. 2 there is a different statement of Cetus' mission: "This is the year we are making it happen . . . In the key areas of our business, we have taken the crucial steps—steps that point us in a direction of success and profitability." On the possible influence of psychological factors on spontaneous remissions of kidney cancer see Oliver, "Surveillance as a possible option."

147. Rosenberg presented another variant of this belief when he asserted that the migration of TILs to the tumor site demonstrated that tumors possess specific antigens and can therefore be cured by immunotherapy. This claim equates the possibility of an immune reaction against a tumor with the possibility of efficient cure of cancer induced by immune mechanisms; Rosenberg and Barry, *The Transformed Cell.*

148. Jacques C. Norderman, "A message from the president," Cancer Research Institute, *Annual Report,* 1991, p. 3. Emily Martin discusses popular representations of immunology in *Flexible Bodies: Tracking Immunity in American Culture from the Days of Polio to the Age of AIDS* (Boston: Beacon Press, 1994).

149. Unruly behavior is often described as a "cancer" that the "social body" needs to get rid of; Susan Sontag, *Illness as Metaphor* (New York: Random House, 1977); Patterson, *The Dread Disease.*

150. Rosenberg, "Adoptive immunotherapy of cancer," p. 41.

151. Fabien Gruhier, "Cancer, la grande découverte," *Le Nouvel Observateur,* February 1, 1989, pp. 84–86.

152. Yves Christen and Jean-Claude Revy, "Un exploit photographique! Le merveilleux voyage de l'interleukine. Le cancer combattu par l'autodéfense," *Le Figaro Magazine,* May 5, 1991, pp. 87–94. The article presented a series of electronmicroscope photographs of killer cells surrounding a malignant cell.

153. Timothy E. Cook and David C. Colby, "The mass-mediated epidemic: The politics of AIDS on the nightly network news," in *AIDS: The Making of Chronic Disease,* ed. Elisabeth Fee and Daniel M. Fox (Berkeley: University of California Press, 1992), p. 85.

154. Panem, *The Interferon Crusade,* p. 99.

155. Critically oriented doctors are sometimes willing to admit that the profession has a pronounced tendency to make exaggerated therapeutic

claims (see, e.g., Collin Dollery, *The End of an Age of Optimism* [Nuffield: Nuffield Provincial Hospitals Trust, 1972], pp. 21, 32), but this tendency is attributed to ignorance, lack of critical spirit, and insufficient training in the scientific method in medicine.

156. On popular representations of science and "miracle making," see John C. Burnham, *How Superstition Won and Science Lost: Popularizing Science and Health in the United States* (New Brunswick, N.J.: Rutgers University Press, 1987).

157. One article was a study by Burton A. Waisbren, "Observations on the combined systemic administration of mixed bacterial vaccine, Bacillus Calmette-Guerin, transfer factor and lymphoblastoid lymphocytes to patients with cancer 1974–1985," *Journal of Biological Response Modifiers*, 6 (1987), 1–19. The author treated 139 patients with a combination of several "old" immunotherapies: mixed bacterial vaccine (Coley's toxins), BCG, "transfer factor" (a factor secreted by activated lymphocytes), and lymphocytes stimulated in the test tube. The treatment was well tolerated by patients and induced significant prolongation of life in comparison with historical controls. In several cases it also led to the complete disappearance of symptoms. The other article was by Robert J. Krane et al., "Treatment of metastatic renal cell carcinoma with autolymphocyte therapy: Low toxicity outpatient approach to adoptive immunotherapy without use of *in vivo* interleukin-2," *Urology*, 35 (1990), 417–422. The authors treated patients suffering from advanced renal cell carcinoma with an infusion of autologous lymphocytes (2×10^9) depleted of suppressor T cells and activated in the test tube by a mixture of autologous lymphokines. That treatment too was well tolerated by patients, and the authors of the study affirmed that 33 percent (12 of 36) experienced either stabilization or regression of their tumor(s). At the time the article was published, 9 of the long-term survivors (25 percent) had survived for two years or more (in historical controls, survival at two years was estimated at 10 percent or less).

158. Krane et al., "Treatment of metastatic renal cell carcinoma," p. 421.

159. Waisbren, "Observations of combined systemic administrations," pp. 11, 12.

160. Rosenberg et al., "Observations on the systemic administration of autologous lymphokine-activated killer cells and recombinant interleukin-2 to patients with metastatic cancer," p. 1492. See also Rosenberg et al., "Experience with the use of high-dose interleukin-2 in the treatment of 652 cancer patients," p. 483; Negrier et al., "Interleukin-2 with or without LAK cells in metastatic renal cell carcinoma," p. 21; Sewa S. Legha, "Current therapy for malignant melanoma," *Seminars in Oncology*, 16(1) (1989), 34; Borden and Sondel, "Lymphokines and cytokines as cancer treatment," p. 800.

161. See also Evelleen Richards' comparison of a "low-tech" cancer therapy—vitamin C—and a "high-tech" cancer therapy—interferon; *Vitamin C and Cancer: Medicine or Politics?* (London: Macmillan, 1991).

162. The organization of Waisbren's paper closely recalls that of Nauts's papers on Coley's toxins: it contains long tables enumerating the diagnosis of each patient, the therapy that patient received, and the clinical results. The work by Krane et al. is more "modern" in style, but there too the accent is on increased length of survival, not on "biological tests" or carefully documented ("before" and "after" photographs, tomography measures) regression of tumor(s).

163. Niels K. Jerne, "Summary: Waiting for the End," *Cold Spring Harbour Symposia on Quantitative Biology,* 32 (1967), 591–603.

164. Michael B. Shimkin, *Contrary to Nature,* NIH Publication no. 76-720 (Bethesda, Md.: National Institutes of Health, 1976); John D. Durant, "Immunotherapy of cancer," pp. 939–941.

165. Derek de Solla Price, *Science since Babylon* (New Haven: Yale University Press, 1975).

166. Dorothy Windhorst, "International registry of tumor immunotherapy: The contribution of an information service of a new specialty," in Terry and Windhorst, *Immunotherapy of Cancer.*

167. Gordon Duff, "Clinical evaluation of cytokines," in *Cytokine Interactions and Their Control,* ed. A. Baxter and R. Ross (New York: John Wiley and Sons, 1991), p. 200.

168. Barbuto and Hersh, "Role of cytokines in cancer therapy"; Taylor and Gore, "Principles of cytokine therapy." The possibility of integrating cytokine treatment with routine chemotherapies also contributed to its acceptance by oncologists.

169. E. Richard Brown, *Rockefeller Medicine Men: Medicine and Capitalism in America* (Berkeley: University of California Press, 1973); Anne-Marie Moulin and Ilana Löwy, "La double nature de l'immunologie. L'histoire de la transplantation rénale," *Fundamenta Scientiae,* 4 (1983), 201–208; Stuart Blume, *Insight and Industry* (Cambridge, Mass.: MIT Press, 1992); Kenney, *Biotechnology.* This symbiotic relationship is often reflected in a single individual's performance of several professional roles (scientific researcher, industrial researcher, administrator, science policymaker) during his or her career.

170. On the career pattern of scientist-managers in the physical sciences, see, e.g., Peter Galison and Bruce Hevly, eds., *Big Science: The Growth of Large-Scale Research* (Stanford: Stanford University Press, 1992); in biology, Lily Kay, "Selling pure science in wartime: The biochemical genetics of G. W. Beadle," *Journal of the History of Biology,* 22(1) (1989), 73–101; and in medicine, Renée C. Fox and Judith Swazey, *Spare Parts* (Oxford and New York: Oxford University Press, 1992).

171. Robert Bud, *The Uses of Life* (Cambridge: Cambridge University Press,

1993). The career of Paul Ehrlich, one of the founders of immunology, is an example of such a link. See, e.g., Jonathan Liebnau, "Paul Ehrlich as a commercial scientist and research administrator," *Medical History,* 34 (1990), 65–78.

172. Important exceptions existed, however, especially in the drug industry, where a few leading firms grasped in the 1930s the importance of links with academic science. See, e.g., John P. Swann, *Academic Scientists and the Pharmaceutical Industry: Cooperative Research in Twentieth-Century America* (Baltimore: Johns Hopkins University Press, 1988); Daniel Bovet, *Une chimie qui guérit. Histoire de la découverte des sulphamides* (Paris: Payot, 1988).

173. The rapidity of this process, unlike, e.g., the gradual development of close collaboration between academic and industrial chemistry in the nineteenth century, probably contributed to the difficulty of establishing desirable norms and practices.

174. Paul Rabinow, "Serving the ties: Fragmentation and dignity in late modernity," *Knowledge and Society: The Anthropology of Science and Technology,* 9 (1992), 176.

4. The IL-2 Trial at the Cancer Foundation

1. Spatial separation between sites in which one manipulates animal products and those in which one manipulates human cells reduces the risk of contamination of human cells with animal viruses or mycoplasma. Limiting the risks of contamination was particularly important during the IL-2 trial because the cultured cells were to be injected into patients.

2. INSERM is roughly the French equivalent of the NIH. However, whereas the majority of NIH laboratories are concentrated at a single site, in Bethesda, Maryland, INSERM has no main center, and INSERM laboratories are located at numerous French teaching hospitals, university campuses, and medical schools.

3. Cancer Foundation employees had a high level of social protection, and it was difficult (both administratively and because of possible effects on the morale of other employees) to fire a worker who had spent more than 30 years on the job.

4. For example, I noticed that graduate students who worked in an immunology laboratory in an important American cancer treatment center complained that a research institute shared elevators with a pediatric oncology department. It was emotionally difficult, they explained, to start a day with the sight of bald, ghastly-looking small children.

5. See, e.g., Haroun Jamous, *La réforme des études médicales et des structures hospitalières* (Paris: CNRS, Centre des Etudes Sociologiques, 1967); Pierre Bourdieu, *Homo Academicus* (Paris: Editions de Minuit, 1989).

6. Ilana Löwy, "The impact of medical practice on biomedical research: The case of human leukocyte antigen studies," *Minerva,* 25 (1987), 171–200.

7. François was an M.D. who had not followed the usual pathway to promotion—from *interne* through *chef de clinique* to *professeur agrégé*—obligatory within the rigid structure of the French public hospital system, but instead had turned to a laboratory research career.

8. The medical division of the Cancer Foundation was at first exclusively dedicated to radiation therapy. Later the biology division developed research in experimental oncology, biochemistry, immunology, and virology, but the medical division remained for a long time dominated by radiation therapists.

9. Immunology did not enter the cancer clinics at that time and was not associated with the main wave of chemotherapy.

10. The French *internat* in medicine is a practical training of future doctors in teaching hospitals. French *internes,* that is, students who have passed a special exam, the *concours d'internat des hôpitaux,* are not burdened, however, by a very heavy workload. They often can choose the hospital wards in which they want to work, then negotiate their tasks. They can also temporarily interrupt their *internat* and switch to a different occupation such as training in a research laboratory.

11. Later I learned that in fact the French pharmaceutical firm manufacturing IL-2 had negotiated simultaneously with other French cancer treatment centers as well.

12. In the mid-1980s the arguments that LAK cells were a new subpopulation of cytotoxic lymphocytes and that IL-2/LAK therapy demonstrated the efficacy of immunological mechanisms in fighting human malignancies mutually reinforced each other. For a discussion of the mechanisms of mutual reinforcement of clinical and experimental studies see S. Leigh Star, "Triangulating clinical and basic research: British localizationists, 1870–1906," *History of Science,* 34 (1986), 29–48.

13. The group of physicians and scientists participating in the preparation of the IL-2 trial in 1987 should be distinguished from the official IL-2 group, a formal collaborative structure organized two years later to facilitate exchanges between clinicians and immunologists during clinical trials of IL-2 in adults.

14. The French IL-2 was reduced, while the IL-2 secreted by white blood cells was nonreduced. The chemical modification of the molecule was necessary because an American biotechnology firm held the patent for the cloned native molecule (that is, a molecule with the same structure as IL-2 found in the body).

15. "Nude" mice are mutant, hairless mice (hence their name) that, among other things, lack T cells and do not reject grafts (including tumor grafts) from genetically different donors.

16. These rumors were officially confirmed in 1987 during the annual meeting of the American Society of Clinical Oncology.

17. In 1981 four patients enrolled in a French clinical trial of interferon died suddenly and inexplicably from heart failure. The trial was immediately halted by the French Ministry of Health; "Interferon: Situation des essais cliniques en France," *Biofutur,* March 1983, p. 14.

18. During the early stages of IL-2/LAK study both Dominique and Chantal were rapidly propelled into the professional role of research technicians and mastered a whole range of new skills such as culture of white blood cells and work with radioactive compounds. Later, when the clinical trials of IL-2 became partly standardized, they were assigned to semi-routine tasks, while research-oriented tasks were performed by newly recruited, trained research technicians.

19. "Miracle yard" is an allusion to a beggars' gathering place described in Victor Hugo's *Notre Dame de Paris*.

20. Daniel knew that I would be working with him only part-time, but he hoped that my hours would fit neatly into the gaps in his timetable. Unfortunately, often just the opposite was true: the times when Daniel and I were occupied elsewhere frequently overlapped.

21. The aim of these studies was to repeat with the French IL-2 the results obtained by Rosenberg and his collaborators and to serve as a dry run for clinical experiments. No surprising results were expected, and none were found.

22. My guess is that Madeleine denied Pierre access to the cell sorter because she feared that as a more experienced laboratory researcher, he would otherwise take over control of the sole domain of the trial in which she could legitimately claim expertise.

23. See Arthur Klausner, "Clinicians question adoptive immunotherapy," *Bio/Technology,* 4 (1986), 1044.

24. As far as I know, the Cancer Foundation specialists did not discuss the possibility that the introduction of IL-2/LAK therapy should be delayed until it had been approved—or not approved—in the United States.

25. G. M. Brodeur et al., "Amplification of N-myc in untreated neuroblastoma correlates with advanced disease stage," *Science,* 224 (1984), 1121–24. For a different view, see Susan L. Cohn et al., "Lack of correlation of N-myc gene amplification with prognosis in localized neuroblastoma," *Cancer Research,* 55 (1995), 721–726.

26. Phase I trials test the toxicity and the tolerated dose of a tested drug; phase II trials, its effects in a given pathology.

27. The fact that a given clinical experiment was a part of multicenter trial was probably seen as an additional guarantee of its seriousness. Such a view, however, does not take into account that protocols of multicenter clinical trials do not necessarily reflect a negotiated agreement among

numerous specialists, but rather may represent the opinion of a single industrial sponsor and of a restricted organizing committee.

28. The philosopher was not my personal friend, and we did not have close professional relationships: Pierre just assumed automatic links between all the persons interested in "humanities in medicine."

29. Cytaphereses are usually conducted in blood donors, thus in adults. The process is long and uncomfortable but, the experts claim, not painful. The only information I was able to gather on the cytaphereses made in children during the IL-2 trial was that they "went all right."

30. TILs were expanded in culture in the presence of IL-2, then injected into patients.

31. Granulocyte colony stimulating factor (G-CSF) and macrophage-granulocyte colony stimulating factor (MG-CSF) stimulates the multiplication of white blood cells, while erythropoietin stimulate the proliferation of red blood cells. Oncologists use these cytokines, among other things, to hasten patients' recovery after intensive chemotherapy, which destroys the precursors of blood cells in the bone marrow.

32. This link was never proved, and it remained one possible hypothesis among many.

33. The IL-2 doses seemed to me ridiculously low. Later I learned that some American oncologists also used such low doses.

34. Similar rates of success in "responsive" tumors (melanoma and renal cell carcinoma) were reported by researchers who employed very different protocols of IL-2 or IL-2/LAK therapy.

35. The protocol, though nominally elaborated jointly by representatives of the industry and of the participating centers, was defined mainly by the IL-2 producer.

36. The initial lack of physiological response was explained later. The Foundation's researchers found that French IL-2 units were not the same as American units. One American IL-2 unit corresponded to approximately three French units, and when patients were given what was supposed to be a maximal tolerated dose, they in fact received only a third of the standard therapeutic dose of American IL-2.

37. A paper published later attributed the death from respiratory failure to the injection of too large a quantity of activated cells. After the publication of that paper, there was an additional case of treatment-related death (cardiac arrest after administration of IL-2) in a child treated by IL-2 and LAK at the second participating center. That case put an end to hints that the problems with the IL-2/LAK therapy were strictly center-related. Later publications discussed the possibility of higher toxicity of IL-2/LAK therapy in children.

38. At that point the Cancer Foundation's IL-2 project was financed by the two principal French cancer charities and by the French producer of

IL-2. The American producer of that molecule did not directly fund clinical trials, but supplied free interleukin and coordinated multicenter clinical experiments.

39. Indeed, after the publication of the article François was asked more often to talk on new developments in cancer therapy. He spoke mostly to semiprofessional groups (doctors, nurses) and lay audiences (fundraising meetings, the media).

40. IL-2 receptors are proteins on the cell surface that specifically bind IL-2. Cells devoid of the IL-2 receptor cannot be stimulated by this molecule.

41. Cells that adhered to plastic contained mainly monocytes, a specific class of white blood cells. Although the terms "adherent cells" and "monocytes" do not entirely overlap—the first is a functional definition of a subset of white blood cells, and the second a morphological category—they were often used interchangeably in the debates of the IL-2 group.

42. The Foundation's blood bank specialists finally agreed, though reluctantly, to perform cytaphereses for the preparation of LAK cells.

43. This problem was overcome later by the fact that TILs used in cancer therapy had to be cultivated from tumor fragments of the patient who was a candidate for TIL treatment.

44. Good biological response was usually defined as a strong increase in the total number of lymphocytes in the blood, an increase in LAK activity, and an increase in the proportion of subpopulations of T cells (NK, cytotoxic T cells) credited with antitumor activity in the total white blood cell population.

45. Partial response (PR) was defined as a 50 percent or greater decrease in the sum of products of all the diameters of measured lesions, without the appearance of new lesions. Stable disease (SD) was defined as a reduction of tumor volume smaller than that in partial response, or as an increase of less than 25 percent in the size of any measurable lesion without the appearance of new lesions or worsening of the symptoms. The large margins of each definition reflect the difficulty of measuring with precision the volume of tumors.

46. In the melanoma cases, nearly all observed regressions occurred in soft tissue sites (usually subcutaneous tumors), and the duration of response was often short (several weeks).

47. Physicians and scientists involved in high-risk, "heroic" therapies (e.g., S. A. Rosenberg and John M. Barry, *The Transformed Cell* [New York: Routledge, 1992]; Thomas E. Starzl, *The Puzzle People* [Pittsburgh: University of Pittsburgh Press, 1992], pp. 334–339) may repeatedly enumerate the "miracles" of a given therapy in order to convince their audience (and themselves) that risky therapeutic approaches are justified. In their book *Spare Parts* (New York and Oxford: Oxford Uni-

versity Press, 1992), Renée Fox and Judith Swazey quote a hospital chaplain's comment on this practice: "I have often seen transplant surgeons confronted with a clinical dilemma begin to invoke a litany of names, like a litany of Roman Catholic saints: 'it may be a really long shot,' they say, 'but remember Vernie and remember Tony and remember Carl and remember . . . and remember . . . and remember . . .' " (p. 199).

48. Clinical tests of substances that had obtained the marketing permit in France (*authorisation du mise sur le marché,* or AMM) were not financed by the special "biotherapy" funds of the French Health Ministry.

49. The clinical biology division was scheduled to include the previous immunology laboratory (renamed immunology unit), hematology unit, clinical immunology unit, blood bank unit, bacteriology unit, and biochemistry unit. It was defined as part of the "medico-technical services" of the hospital, which also include the pathology department, radiodiagnostic services, nuclear medicine services, and the hospital's pharmacy.

50. The Cancer Foundation Direction decided to develop in parallel a distinct service dedicated exclusively to the transfer of advanced biological technologies to the diagnosis and therapy of cancer. The new "transfer service," inaugurated in the spring of 1993, was headed by a newly recruited scientist and staffed by people from both the medical and the biological divisions of the Cancer Foundation. François become one of the two copresidents of its scientific council. Thus in 1993 François occupied an important role in linking the laboratory and the clinics in the Cancer Foundation, but he was not the sole director.

51. On the contribution of the translation of medical questions into fundamental biological ones to the solution of biological (rather than medical) problems see Olga Amsterdamska, "Between medicine and science: The research career of Oswald T. Avery," in *Medicine and Change: Historical and Sociological Studies of Medical Innovation,* ed. Ilana Löwy (London and Paris: John Libbey, 1993), pp. 181–212.

52. The planned integration of several research laboratories (clinical and preclinical research, industry-oriented research) into a clinical biology division closely associated with a cancer hospital could be viewed as a bold move at the Cancer Foundation. Such arrangements, however, are already quite common in leading cancer treatment centers in Israel and the United States.

5. Making the IL-2 Trial Work

1. Rosenberg's articles defined the application of IL-2 to the therapy of human cancer as "adoptive immunotherapy." See, e.g., S. A. Rosenberg, "The development of new immunotherapies for the treatment of cancer

using interleukin-2," *Annals of Surgery,* 208 (1988), 121–135; idem, "Clinical immunotherapy studies in the Surgery Branch of the U.S. National Cancer Institute," *Cancer Treatment Reviews,* 16, supp. A (1989), 115–121; idem, "Adoptive immunotherapy for cancer," *Scientific American,* May 1990, pp. 34–41. Rosenberg also used the term "adoptive immunotherapy" in a public hearing during which he presented his new treatment; Hearing of the National Cancer Institute Revisory Board, May 13, 1985.

2. The quotation is from a 1989 consent form (no. IRB-88-890). Earlier consent forms for clinical trials of IL-2 and LAK cells (e.g., those proposed by Rosenberg in 1986 and the one proposed in a 1986 extramural multicenter trial of IL-2 and LAK cells in melanoma) contained the sentence: "Interleukin-2 is a biological substance normally produced by the body in small amounts."

3. In the United States, clinical trials of interleukins were conducted by researchers from various professional backgrounds. Dr. Steven Rosenberg was trained as a surgeon (S. A. Rosenberg and John M. Barry, *The Transformed Cell* [New York: G. C. Putnam's Sons, 1992]); Dr. Robert Oldham was trained as an immunologist; and other IL-2 trials (especially those using IL-2 alone or in combination with other molecules) were initiated by medical oncologists with no particular interest in immunology.

4. Jean-Paul Gaudillière, "Biologie moléculaire et biologistes. La naissance d'une discipline" (Ph.D. diss., University of Paris 7, 1991).

5. Jean Dausset was awarded the Nobel Prize in Medicine for his contribution first to the discovery of human leukocyte groups (the HLA system) and then to the introduction of HLA typing to kidney transplantation, while Georges Mathé was among the first to introduce BCG into the therapy of human cancer.

6. Gaudillière, "Biologie moléculaire et biologistes." For example, an immunologist was chosen in the mid-1980s to head the most important French research institution, the Centre National de la Recherche Scientifique; another immunologist was elected as the first director of the influential governmental agency that centralizes French research on AIDS, the Agence Nationale de Recherche sur le Sida (ANRS).

7. Ilana Löwy, "The impact of medical practice on biomedical research: The case of human leukocyte antigen studies," *Minerva,* 25 (1987), 171–200.

8. The juxtaposition of preclinical studies describing IL-2 as a molecule that regulated immune responses with clinical studies on anticancer effects of that molecule implicitly reinforced the conclusion that the antitumor activity of IL-2 was mediated by immune mechanisms.

9. Some of the non-French-speakers, however, described IL-2 treatment

less precisely as "biotherapy" or as an undifferentiated "anticancer treatment."

10. This statement may be compared with the one by the pioneer of immunology, Paul Ehrlich: "Unfortunately, this differs in no way from all other scientific problems, since it just becomes more and more complicated"; quoted in Ludwik Fleck, *Genesis and Development of a Scientific Fact* (1935), trans. Fred Bradley and Thaddeus J. Trenn (Chicago: University of Chicago Press, 1979), p. 29.

11. The French government started to finance tests of "biotherapy of cancer" in 1991.

12. Another French clinical trial of IL-2 preceded the Cancer Foundation trial. It was conducted in collaboration with the American producer of interleukin.

13. Relations with the American biotechnology firm were always different. In February 1989 François mentioned that he never had the slightest idea how many hospitals in France were testing the American IL-2: "the Americans keep the secret to themselves." The American biotechnology in France claimed in the spring of 1990 that at that time there were nearly 50 clinical trials of IL-2 in France. This number, however, included all clinical trials of IL-2, not only attempts to apply the molecule to cancer therapy.

14. Quincke's edema or angioedema is an allergic syndrome expressed as rapid edema of the face and neck.

15. The clinicians' decision did not violate the formal criteria for inclusion of patients in that IL-2 trial. The list of conditions disqualifying a patient from enrollment in the American IL-2 trial did not include previous therapy with IL-2.

16. T. Philip et al., "High-dose chemotherapy with bone marrow transplantation as a consolidation treatment in neuroblastoma: An unselected group of stage IV patients over one year of age," *Journal of Clinical Oncology,* 5 (1987), 266–271.

17. One of the main dangers of bone marrow grafts is the patient's great susceptibility to infections during the postgraft period until the bone marrow is fully reconstituted. IL-2 therapy, some experts hoped, would accelerate the multiplication of bone marrow cells and thus shorten the dangerous postgraft period.

18. The authors' supposition that NK cells played an important role in the elimination of residual neuroblastoma cells was, as far as I know, based solely on indirect evidence and on theoretical considerations.

19. J. Casper et al., "The successful use of unrelated donors for twenty-three pediatric bone marrow transplants," *Blood,* 75(5), supp. 5 (1988), 382–383.

20. The introduction of the FACS technique into immunology has been

studied by Alberto Cambrosio and Peter Keating, "A matter of FACS: Constructing novel entities in immunology," *Medical Anthropology Quarterly,* 6 (1992), 362–384.

21. On the importance of reputation and trust in scientific work see Bruno Latour and Steve Woolgar, *Laboratory Life* (Beverly Hills: Sage, 1979); Steven Shapin, *The Social History of Truth* (Chicago: University of Chicago Press, 1994).

22. Annette decided to prepare a *diplôme d'études approfondies* (DEA), a degree that requires graduate students to follow a specific teaching curriculum and to conduct a small-scale research project. Obtaining a DEA is a precondition to starting a doctoral thesis, but a DEA may also be viewed as an independent degree. Thus medical students may prepare a DEA as an initiation to laboratory research.

23. This was by no means a peculiarity of the Cancer Foundation's IL-2 trial. See, e.g., Gerda Lerner's description of the proposal to enter her husband as an "out of protocol" patient in a clinical trial of chemotherapy for brain tumors; *A Death of One's Own* (New York: Simon and Schuster, 1978), p. 169.

24. On the importance of direct contacts between scientists and the media see Michel Callon, "La science par conférence de presse," *La Recherche,* 21 (1990), 1184–90.

25. In the United States scientists and physicians are occasionally asked to give public accounts of their projects, and such public hearings may be seen as a part of scientists' efforts to popularize their activity. There are no parallel "routine" public hearings of scientists in France. Political bodies or public committees invite scientists to their debates only when politicians consider important changes in science (or health) policies, or when things go wrong, as when the French parliament organized a hearing about the contamination of the nation's blood supply by the HIV virus.

26. On such risks in France, see, e.g., Axel Kahn, "Publier à tout prix," *La Recherche,* 21 (1990), 1190–91.

27. Her good-humored but effective resistance to some of the attempts to change the direction of her work perhaps point to the second possibility.

28. Being a woman was perhaps an additional difficulty. Nearly half of the Cancer Foundation doctors and scientists were women, but very few held positions of power in the Foundation.

29. A classic explanation of the incommensurability of different approaches to medicine was proposed by Ludwik Fleck, "Some specific features of the medical way of thinking" (1927), in *Cognition and Fact: Materials on Ludwik Fleck,* ed. Robert S. Cohen and Thomas Schelle (Dordrecht: Reidel, 1986), pp. 39–46; idem, *Genesis and Development of a Scientific Fact.* Thomas S. Kuhn's notion of incommensurability in *The Struc-*

ture of Scientific Revolutions (Chicago: University of Chicago Press, 1961) is probably indebted to Fleck's ideas.

30. The possibility that a given person may belong to more than one "social world" (or "thought collective") was proposed by sociologists of science; see, e.g., Susan Leigh Star, "Power, technologies and the phenomenology of standards: On being allergic to onions," in *The Sociology of Monsters: Power, Technology and the Modern World,* ed. John Law (London: Routledge, 1993). However, as Fleck had already pointed out in 1935, some combinations of allegiances to different thought collectives are more difficult to sustain than others; Fleck, *Genesis and Development of a Scientific Fact,* pp. 110–111.

31. On "trading zones" see Ilana Löwy, "The strength of loose concepts—boundary concepts, federative experimental strategies, and disciplinary growth: The case of immunology," *History of Science,* 30 (1992), 371–395.

32. Susan Leigh Star and James R. Griesemer, "Institutional ecology, 'translations,' and boundary objects: Amateurs and professionals in Berkeley's Museum of Vertebrate Zoology," *Social Studies of Science,* 19 (1988), 387–420.

33. One may distinguish among several types of such intermediary areas of interaction: the loosely structured "trading zone," which allows local coordination of the activities of members of distinct professional cultures that continue to disagree on the global meaning of terms; the more stabilized "pidgin zone," in which there is partial agreement on the meaning of shared terms and practices; and finally, a "creole zone," which is gradually transformed into an autonomous professional subculture; Peter Galison, "The trading zone: Coordinating action and belief in modern physics," Paper presented at a conference at the Institut Henry Poincaré, Paris, December 13, 1991; Löwy, "The strength of loose concepts."

34. For a more detailed discussion of this point see Löwy, "The strength of loose concepts."

35. It was less clear, however, if the distinction between different subpopulations of cytotoxic cells referred to structural differences (such as differences in specific proteins found on the surface of cytotoxic lymphocytes—the cluster of differentiation, or CD, markers), to functional differences (such as differences in the ability of cytotoxic lymphocytes to kill different targets), or to both; Lewis L. Lanneir et al., "Natural killer cells: Definition of cell type rather than function," *Journal of Immunology,* 137 (1986), 2735–39; T. Hercend and R. E. Schmidt, "Characteristics and uses of natural killer cells," *Immunology Today,* 9 (1988), 291–296; J. M. Michon and W. H. Fridman, eds., "23rd Forum in Immunology: Non-specific lymphoid effectors: Characterization and

activation mechanism," *Annales de l'Institut Pasteur—Immunologie,* 139 (1988), 433–478.

36. Giorgio Trincheri and Bice Perusia, "Human natural killer cells: Biologic and pathologic aspects," *Laboratory Investigation,* no. 350 (1984), 489–513.

37. Such "science-oriented" clinical trials should be distinguished from, e.g., "me-too" trials—trials in which a pharmaceutical company proposes to test a drug similar to a substance produced by their competitors—and from "improvement" trials, which test a molecule closely related to an existing drug but which, its producers claim, is more efficient or less toxic.

38. Subpopulations of lymphocytes were usually defined by their surface markers. Thus NK cells were defined as CD3(−) NKH1/(CD56)(+) cells; T-cytotoxic lymphocytes as CD3(+) NKH/CD56(−) cells; and IL-2 receptor-positive cells as CD25(+) cells. Morphological properties of lymphocytes were assessed through reaction with standard anti-CD monoclonal antibodies (cf. Cambrosio and Keating, "A matter of FACS"), while functional studies investigated the destruction of cells of established tumoral cell lines such as Daudi, Raji, or K-562 in the test tube.

39. A description of a positive correlation between, e.g., the increase in the proportion of cytotoxic T cells that carry on their surface the receptor to IL-2 and the reduction of tumor mass would not automatically establish an identity between the immunologist's concept of a "CD3(+) CD56(−) CD25(+) cell" and the oncologist's notion of a "killer lymphocyte": it would, however, facilitate their cooperation.

40. Samuel Hellman, Editorial, "Immunotherapy for metastatic cancer: Establishing a 'proof of principle,' " *Journal of the American Medical Association,* 271 (1994), 945–946.

41. Dominique Maraninchi, "Commentaire: Immunotherapie," *Journal of the American Medical Association,* French ed., 53 (May 1994), 5. Other investigators proposed, in contrast, that numerous physiological mechanisms, not only immunological ones, might account for the antitumor activity of IL-2; Eli Kedar and Eva Klein, "Cancer immunotherapy: Are the results discouraging? Can they be improved?" *Advances in Cancer Research,* 59 (1992), 245–322.

42. Editorial, "Traitement du mélanome malin ou du cancer rénal métastasés par de fortes doses d'IL-2," *Journal of the American Medical Association,* French ed., 53 (May 1994), 3–4.

43. The distinction between material, discursive (or literary), and social techniques employed by scientists was proposed by Steven Shapin, "Pump and circumstance: Robert Boyle's literary technology," *Social Studies of Science,* 14 (1984), 481–520.

44. LAK activity was mainly associated with non-MHC (major histocompatibility complex) restained NK cells, while TILs were viewed as MHC-restricted cytotoxic T lymphocytes.

45. Such aligning of efforts of distinct social groups was named "heterogeneous engineering" by sociologists of science; John Law, "On the method of long-distance control: Vessels, navigation, and the Portuguese road to India," in *Power, Action and Belief: A New Sociology of Knowledge,* ed. John Law (London: Routledge and Kegan Paul, 1986).

46. This claim remained controversial. Renal cell carcinoma is a rare cancer, so clinical trials of IL-2/LAK therapy usually involved only a small number of patients, making statistical evaluations difficult.

47. An article published by Hoang proposed that prostaglandin E-2 (PGE-2) and beta transforming growth factor (beta TGF) might play a role in the inhibition of LAK by adherent cells.

48. Such patterns were expected to reflect a combination of several "biological results." The data usually taken into consideration were the size of lymphocytic "rebound," levels of cytotoxic activity against established tumor lines (Raji, Daudi, K-562), the percentage of cytotoxic T cells—CD3($+$), CD56($-$) cells—and NK cells—CD3($-$), CD16($+$), CD56($+$) cells—and levels of soluble IL-2 receptor in the serum.

49. On the specificity of "conjectural knowledge" (e.g., clinical semiotic, clinical inference) as a distinct kind of cognitive activity see Carlo Ginzbourg, "Clues: Morelli, Freud, and Sherlock Holmes," in *The Sign of Three: Dupin, Holmes, Pierce,* ed. Umberto Eco and Thomas A. Sebeok (Bloomington: Indiana University Press, 1983), pp. 81–118.

50. See Warwick Anderson, "The reasoning of the strongest: The polemics of skill and science in medical diagnosis," *Social Studies of Science,* 22 (1992), 653–684. On 19th century debates on differences between "medical science" and the "art of healing" see Ilana Löwy, *The Polish School of Philosophy of Medicine: From Tytus Chalubinski (1820–1889) to Ludwik Fleck (1896–1961)* (Dordrecht: Kluwer, 1990).

51. Scientists (and philosophers of science) assume that the use of two independent methods to describe a given object (say, the identification of a bacterium by an immunological and a biochemical method) increases the robustness of that object. Such triangulation depends, however, on the assumptions (1) that the methods are truly independent (a problematic assumption, because methods of investigation are often a part of the same continuum); and (2) that the two methods indeed study the same object (also a problematic assumption, because the identification of a given object may depend on a method of investigation). Such "imperfect triangulation" is frequent in biomedical research. The supposition that phenomena studied in the laboratory are relevant to a clinical situation and vice versa may help to stabilize both clinical observations

and laboratory findings; Susan Leigh Star, "Triangulating clinical and basic research: British localizationists, 1870–1906," *History of Science,* 24 (1986), 29–48.

52. The idea that the persistence of "biological response," rather than its absolute levels, is important for an efficient destruction of malignant cells is as reasonable as the opposite proposal, namely that in order to eliminate disseminated tumor cells it may be above all important to induce high levels of cell-killing responses. Moreover, in the 1980s and 1990s oncologists developed cancer therapies (such as ABMT) based on the principle of short-term, very intensive chemotherapy, which aims at the elimination of all the malignant cells.

53. Alternatively, it is possible that Annette, like other participants, was aware of the trial's internal contradictions but, unlike her colleagues, transgressed the unwritten rules of the group by displaying them in public, an attitude that might have been judged immature or tactless.

54. The term "objective response" was introduced by Cancer Foundation researchers (in an article describing phase II of the IL-2 trial) to indicate the perceptible effects of IL-2 that did not fit the rigid definition of partial response (PR) (40 percent reduction of tumor volume).

55. The assertion that a given observation was valid for "most cases" when the number of responding patients was 6 is reminiscent of Woglom's 1929 criticism of cancer researchers that "80 percent of positive results may seem imposing at first glance, but it may, and all too frequently does, mean 4 out of 5"; William H. Woglom, "Immunity to transplantable tumors," *Cancer Review,* 4 (1929), 131. To be fair, however, one should add that Woglom was discussing experiments conducted with laboratory animals, not clinical studies.

56. Efforts to find correlations between the activation of specific subgroups of lymphocytes and clinical response were abandoned in 1991.

57. LAK therapy was discontinued at the Cancer Foundation around 1991. The attempts to treat with TILs melanoma patients who had failed to respond to IL-2 therapy also failed, and the Foundation's researchers published a note on this subject indicating that their results contradicted Rosenberg's claims.

58. In the United States the term "biotherapy" was at one point opposed (e.g., by representatives of the biotechnology industry) to the term "immunotherapy," but, as far as I know, such an opposition did not exist in France.

59. The superiority of the "nude mouse" model may be debatable. Such a model allows a direct observation of tumors that arise spontaneously in humans, not the standard tumors of laboratory mice. On the other hand, when a human tumor is transferred to a "nude mouse," the animal may be viewed merely as a passive recipient that allows the survival of the tumor.

60. The term "activated lymphoid killer cells" may refer to Rosenberg's studies. Rosenberg, however, employed the more precise expression "lymphokine activated killer cells."

61. NK cells were always viewed by immunologists as distinct from cytotoxic T cells. At the time the protocol was proposed (fall 1988) specialists usually agreed that LAK cells were a subpopulation of NK cells. The meaning of the term "cytotoxic lymphocytes" was not specified.

62. Graham A. Currie, "Immunotherapy of human cancer: Prospect and retrospect," in *Cancer and the Immune Response* (Baltimore: Williams and Wilkins, 1974), p. 81.

63. In semiotics, a "connoted system" is present when the "sign" becomes the "expression plane" or a "signifier" of a second system, e.g., when the style of a sentence transmits a separate message; Roland Barthes, *Le degré zéro de l'écriture* (Paris: Gonthier), pp. 163–168. On the multiple meanings of science in medicine see, e.g., Christopher Lawrence, "Incommunicable science: Science technology and the clinical art in Britain, 1850–1914," *Journal of Contemporary History*, 20 (1985), 503–520; John Harley Warner, *The Therapeutic Perspective: Medical Practice, Knowledge, and Identity in America* (Cambridge, Mass.: Harvard University Press, 1986); Stuart S. Blume, *Insight and Industry: On the Dynamics of Technological Change in Medicine* (Cambridge, Mass.: MIT Press, 1992).

64. On techniques of routine exclusion of "messiness" from science see Susan Leigh Star, "Craft vs. commodity, mess vs. transcendence: How the right tool became the wrong one in the case of taxidermy and natural history," in *The Right Tools for the Job,* ed. Adele Clarke and Joan Fujimura (Princeton: Princeton University Press, 1992), pp. 257–286.

65. One of the rules in the unwritten etiquette of the IL-2 trial was precisely not to ask (certainly not in public) detailed questions about patients' fate once their treatment ended. Thus I incidentally learned that some of the patients presented as successful cases of IL-2 therapies later died, but I had the strong feeling that seeking information as to why, when, and how they died would be viewed as a faux pas.

66. The desire to exclude physicians from a clinical experiment illustrates the limits of "informed consent." For clinicians, informed consent may mean that patients understand and assimilate all the information their doctors wish to give them. However, a "truly informed" patient, such as another specialist in the same area, may be seen as a highly problematic case.

67. Kirk D. Denicoff et al., "The neuropsychiatric effects of treatment with interleukin-2 and lymphokine-activated killer cells," *Annals of Internal Medicine,* 107 (1987), 293–301.

    As far as I know, all the patients who suffered from neurological disturbances during IL-2 therapy at the Cancer Foundation recovered completely after the interruption of interleukin treatment.

68. The term "habitus" was used by the French sociologist Pierre Bourdieu to define the portions of the social environment that are seen as "natural" and are not questioned by individuals who share that environment. The conviction that one's habitus is "natural" is acquired through a long process of socialization. Pierre Bourdieu, *Esquisse d'une théorie de la pratique* (Geneva and Paris: Droz, 1972); idem, "The specificity of the scientific field and the social conditions of the progress of reason," *Social Sciences Information*, 14(6) (1975), 19–47.

69. Cancer Foundation researchers did not discuss "unusual" effects of IL-2 therapy in a paper describing the phase II trial. Another group of French researchers who also described a phase II trial of IL-2 included in the "symptoms" table a column titled "unusual effects of IL-2/LAK therapy," but they did not comment upon these "unusual effects" in the text.

70. Cases of hypothyroidism following IL-2 therapy were reported by M. B. Atkins et al., "Hypothyroidism after treatment with interleukin-2 and lymphocyte activated killer cells," *New England Journal of Medicine*, 318 (1988), 1557–63; and P. A. van Liessum et al., "Hypothyroidism and goitre during interleukin-2 therapy without LAK cells," *Lancet*, 1989, p. 224.

71. On affixing a price to a theoretically priceless item—human life—see Theodore Porter, "Objectivity as standardization: The rhetoric of impersonality in measurement, statistics and cost-benefit analysis," *Annals of Scholarship*, 1992, pp. 19–59. The choices imposed upon health care professionals by cost-containment policies are discussed by Henry J. Aaron and William B. Schwartz, *The Painful Prescription: Rationing Hospital Care* (Washington, D.C.: Brookings Institution, 1984).

72. François also argued that TIL therapy was less expensive than the average bone marrow graft (he evaluated the costs of TIL therapy at 50,000 francs per patient and of heterologous bone marrow graft at 200,000 francs per patient).

73. Patients who did not complete at least two of the three cycles of IL-2 therapy were not included in publications. In contrast, patients who received only part of the total IL-2 dose (usually, more than 75 percent) were included.

74. On the role of black humor in helping the physician to cope with uncertainty and failure see Renée C. Fox, *Experiment Perilous: Physicians and Scientists Facing the Unknown* (Philadelphia: University of Pennsylvania Press, 1974), pp. 76–82.

75. The ironic attitude did not, however, prevent François from becoming very angry when he found himself during the radio program facing a colleague who was openly skeptical about the efficacy of interleukin therapy.

76. Such multifunctional scientific activities permit the construction of a given segment of knowledge and, at the same time, advance the social interests of actors; Steven Shapin, "History of science and its sociological reconstructions," *History of Science,* 20 (1982), 157–211; Gad Freudenthal and I. Löwy, "Ludwik Fleck's roles in society," *Social Studies of Science,* 18 (1988), 625–651.

77. A parallel may be drawn between the perception of some of the consequences of a new therapy as "secondary" or "side" effects, and the perception of some of the aspects of a clinical trial as "nonessential" or "marginal."

6. *A Science-Laden Pathology between Bench and Bedside*

1. Evelleen Richards, *Vitamin C and Cancer: Medicine or Politics?* (London: Macmillan, 1991); Stuart Blume, *Insight and Industry: On the Dynamics of Technological Change in Medicine* (Cambridge, Mass.: MIT Press, 1992).

2. Annemarie Mol, "What is new? Doppler and its others," in *Medicine and Change: Historical and Sociological Studies of Medical Innovation,* ed. Ilana Löwy (Paris and London: John Libbey, 1993), pp. 107–127.

3. Peter Medawar, *New York Review of Books,* March 28, 1968, quoted in Gunther Stent, *The Paradoxes of Progress* (San Francisco: W. H. Freeman, 1978); Kettering quoted in Kenneth T. Jackson, *Crabgrass Frontier: The Suburbanization of the United States* (New York and Oxford: Oxford University Press, 1985), p. 304.

4. Thomas P. Hughes, "The evolution of large technological systems," in *The Social Construction of Technological Systems,* ed. Wiebe E. Bijker, Thomas P. Hughes, and Trevor J. Pinch (Cambridge, Mass.: MIT Press, 1987), pp. 51–82.

5. Mark Berg, "The construction of medical disposals: Medical sociology and medical problem solving in medical practice," *Sociology of Health and Illness,* 14 (1992), 151–180.

6. For a different view, which allows for the coexistence of different types of medical practices, see John Pickstone, "Ways of knowing: Towards a historical sociology of science, technology and medicine," *British Journal of the History of Science,* 26 (1993), 433–458.

7. "Knowledge about diseases" and therapy, the Polish philosopher of medicine Edmund Biernacki explained in the late nineteenth century, have evolved separately, and usually only loose links exist between these two aspects of medical activity; Ilana Löwy, *The Polish School of Philosophy of Medicine: From Tytus Chalubinski (1820–1889) to Ludwik Fleck (1896–1961)* (Dordrecht: Kluwer, 1990), pp. 37–68. Similarly, the historian of technology Derek de Solla Price proposed that the practice

of medicine, like every technology, usually maintains only loose relationships with science; *Science since Babylon,* 2nd ed. (New Haven: Yale
University Press, 1975), p. 132.

8. Isabelle Baszanger, "From pain to person," in Löwy, *Medicine and
   Change,* pp. 155–170.

9. The trajectory of nearly every pathology can be negatively correlated
   with "life-style" elements. The question is not, however, if a severely
   undernourished AIDS patient will deteriorate more rapidly than one
   who is adequately fed, but if the progress of AIDS can be reversed or
   arrested by an appropriate diet.

10. Steven A. Rosenberg and John M. Barry, *The Transformed Cell: Un-
    locking the Mysteries of Cancer* (New York: G. P. Putnam's Sons, 1992),
    p. 34.

11. Ronald J. Glaser's book popularizing the role of the immune system in
    fighting diseases (including cancer) was called *The Body Is the Hero*
    (New York: Random House, 1976).

12. Charles E. Rosenberg, "Catechisms of health: The body in the prebel-
    lum classroom," *Bulletin of the History of Medicine,* 69 (1995), 197.

13. Anne Hunsaker Hawkins, *Reconstructing Illness: Studies in Pathogra-
    phy* (West Lafayette, Ind.: Purdue University Press, 1993), pp. 11–30.
    The search for meaning and control may explain why some cancer pa-
    tients supplement their "orthodox" therapy (and a few replace it) with
    "parallel therapies" conducted by practitioners who believe that every
    pathology can be arrested by appropriate "life-style" changes such as
    diet, exercise, or meditation; ibid., pp. 142–147.

14. Karen Osney Browstein, *Brainstorm* (New York: Avon Books, 1980).

15. Ibid., p. 189.

16. On medicine as the practice of "management of living" and changing
    the patient's behavior and expectations, see William Ray Arnay and
    Bernard J. Bergen, *Medicine and the Management of Living: Taming
    the Last Great Beast* (Chicago: University of Chicago Press, 1984).

17. Gerda Lerner, *A Death of One's Own* (New York: Simon and Schuster,
    1978).

18. Ted Rosenthal, *How Could I Not Be among You* (New York: Avon
    Press, 1979), p. 73, quoted in Arnay and Bergen, *Medicine and the
    Management of Living,* pp. 138–139.

19. Some unorthodox therapies of cancer attempt to stimulate the defense
    mechanisms of the body not through chemical manipulation of cells,
    but through the activation of psychic forces ("visualization technique").
    Patients are asked to imagine daily their "good" (immune) cells fighting
    and destroying the "bad" (malignant) ones; Barrie R. Cassileth et al.,
    "Survival and quality of life among patients receiving an unproven as

compared with conventional therapy," *New England Journal of Medicine,* 324 (1991), 1180–85.

20. Mark Granovetter, "The strength of weak ties," *American Journal of Sociology,* 78 (1973), 1360–80.

21. E.g., Bruno Latour, *Science in Action: How to Follow Scientists and Engineers through Society* (Cambridge, Mass.: Harvard University Press, 1987).

22. This expression is borrowed from Nelly Oudshoorn, *Beyond the Natural Body: Archeology of Sex Hormones* (New York and London: Routledge, 1994), p. 138.

23. Daniel S. Greenberg, "A sober anniversary of the 'war on cancer,' " *Lancet,* 1991, pp. 1582–83; Tim Beardsley, "A war not won," *Scientific American,* January 1994, pp. 131–138.

Acknowledgments

My most important debt is to the doctors, researchers, and technicians of the "Cancer Foundation," who for three years shared with me the ups and downs of a clinical experiment. They were wonderfully open-minded and hospitable, and I hope that my description of them in the book not only makes manifest the difficulties with which they struggled and the dilemmas they faced, but also shows their dedication, skill, and hard work. My second debt is to my home institution, the Institut National de la Santé et de la Recherche Medicale (INSERM), which offers me the (rare) opportunity to devote most of my time to research. And then there are all the colleagues and friends who contributed in numerous ways to this study. I wish to thank them, not in order to conform to the official rites of "university correctness," but to stress the importance of the collective aspects of my research. In an interview with the biologist-turned-science-policy-analyst Sandra Panem, the sociologist Jonathan Cole suggested to her that she had moved from a virology laboratory to science policy studies in order to be in the top 2 percent of her professional field. From my point of view such a perspective—to consider 98 percent of the colleagues in one's field as worse than oneself—would be a chilling one indeed. During my own, not always very smooth, transition from a laboratory researcher to a student of science, the discovery that the new area gave me a vast opportunity to meet interesting people and to learn from them encouraged me to persist in my reorientation. And contacts with colleagues continue to make my work both fruitful and enjoyable. It is a pleasure rather than a duty to acknowledge some of my debts.

My research for this book greatly benefited from discussions with Olga Amsterdamska, Isabelle Baszanger, Alberto Cambrosio, Renée Fox, Gad Freudenthal, Peter Keating, Sylvia Klingberg, Anne-Marie Moulin, and Fred Tauber. Patrice Pinell generously shared with me his knowledge of the history of cancer treatment in France, while Stuart Blume made available to me his (then unpublished) study of medical technology, which helped me to develop my view of experimentation in the clinics. Jean-Paul Gaudillière actively participated in the early stages of my research and continued to discuss it with me over the years. Many of the ideas in the book grew out of our dialogue. Aaron Cicourel helped me to overcome my "white page complex," to organize my thoughts and to start writing. His encouragement was crucial at a crucial moment. Isabelle Baszanger, Nicolas Dodier, Jean-Paul Gaudillière, Harry Marks, Dominique Pestre, and John Pickstone read the entire manuscript, made detailed comments, and helped me to improve it in many significant ways. If the end result does not always correspond to their high standards, the fault is exclusively mine.

The book was long in the making, and the historical research that accompanied it took even longer. In the meantime, some elements of the historical studies that appear in this volume were included in articles published elsewhere: in the *Bulletin of the History of Medicine* (1989), *Journal of the History of Biology* (1994), and *Science in Context* (1995).

Marie Bézard helped to produce the manuscript with her usual skill and kindness, while Dominique Villebrun and Annick Guénel helped with documentation. I am very lucky to have been able to work with Harvard University Press. Michael Fisher has been an understanding, efficient, and highly supportive editor. Ann Downer-Hazell has taken excellent care of technical aspects of the production of the book, and Ann Hawthorne has translated with a rare sensitivity my approximate English into the standard idiom.

Woody Sayre often helped me to clarify my thoughts and always boosted my morale. He also took on more than a fair share of housekeeping and childcare. Thanks to him, the potentially complicated exercise of balancing two academic careers and family life is not a burden but a joy. My children, Tamara, Daniel, Naomi, and Rachel, performed the salutary task of frequently and forcibly reminding me that there is life outside academia, and prevented me from losing my sense of proportion and my sense of humor.

Index

Abbot, Andrew, 53
Acute Leukemia Task Force, 46, 57–60, 62, 64
Adoptive immunotherapy of cancer, 84, 135, 142, 143, 265
AIDS, 12, 135; activists, 11, 36
Alsop, Stewart, 77
American Cancer Society (ACS), 37, 44, 46, 106, 122, 124, 126
American Society for the Control of Cancer, 38
Amsterdamska, Olga, 349n51
Anderson, Warwick, 294n39
Animal models of cancer, 28, 47, 59, 100, 114, 158, 345n15, 356n59; using grafted tumors, 84, 85, 90–96; importance of genetic homogeneity, 96–99, 113; critique of, 114–116; in IL-2 research, 134, 143, 176, 177, 207, 264
Atomic Energy Commission (U.S.), 46

Bacillus Calmette-Guérin (BCG), 107–109, 114, 126, 130, 220, 329n44
Bacterial products in cancer therapy, 29, 100, 123, 157, 158. *See also* Bacillus Calmette-Guérin; Coley's toxins, *Serratia marcescens*
Baszanger, Isabelle, 294n39, 360n8
Baumann, Zygmunt, 313n183
Benacerraff, Baruj, 107
Ben-David, Joseph, 292n22

Berg, Mark, 294n39
Bergonié, Jean, 37
Bernard, Jean, 67, 68
Biological Response Modifiers (BRM) Program of NCI, 122–124, 128, 201
Biotechnology industry, 31, 32, 117, 151, 158, 161–162; and interferon production, 124, 125; and IL-2 production, 142, 144. *See also* Cetus
Biotherapeutics, Inc., 137, 201. *See also* Oldham, Robert
Black humor, 276, 277
Blume, Stuart, 292n29
Bone marrow graft, 78, 194, 214, 351n17. *See also* Neuroblastoma
Bordet, Jules, 101
Bosk, Charles, 296n57
"Boundary objects," 248, 251, 258, 259, 262, 265, 287
Bourdieu, Pierre, 344n5, 358n68
British Medical Council, 112
Browstein, Karen Osney, 283–284, 285

Cancer Act of 1971, 64, 116, 120
Cancer charities, 10, 31, 39, 224
Cancer Chemotherapy Committee (CCC), 45, 46
Cancer Chemotherapy National Service Center (CCNSC), 43, 46–48, 54–60, 64
Cancer patients, 10, 26, 69; quality of life, 62–63, 68, 76, 289n5, 360n19;

Cancer patients (*cont.*)
and truth-telling, 70–71; and thera-peutic choices, 71, 74–76, 80–81; and visibility in clinical experiments, 213–214, 269–272
Cancer Research Institute (previously New York Cancer Research Institute), 110, 152
Canguilhem, Georges, 291n21
Cantell, Kari, 121
Cantor, David, 297n1
Carrel, Alexis, 94
Carter, Stephen K., 126
Case, J. T., 38
Cassileth, Barrie R., 306n107
CAT scan, 62, 258, 280, 283
Cellular immunology, 83, 106
Centre National de la Recherche Scienti-fique (CNRS), 171
Centres de Lutte Contre le Cancer (CLCC), 66, 67, 73, 216
Cetus, 135–137, 147–152, 155; Euro-cetus, 149, 150
Chester Beatty Research Institute (U.K.), 41
Choriocarcinoma, 57, 58
Cicourel, Aaron, 294n44
Clarke, Donald, 107
Clemmenson, Johannes, 97
Clinical trials, 51–54; randomization in, 48, 50, 53; debates on validity of, 49–50, 53
Clinical trials of anticancer therapies, 64–68; nonrandomized, 59, 60, 269; randomized, 123, 215, 216; multicen-ter, 187, 228–230, 346n27
Coca, Arthur, 159
Coleman, William, 302n62
Coley, William, 102–103
Coley-Nauts, Helen, 110, 111, 299n22, 318n64, 320n77
Coley's toxins, 41, 102–103, 104, 110–111, 322n107
Collins, Harry M., 21, 22, 295n47
Coltman, Charles, 152
"Connotation," 267, 357n63
Coolidge, William D., 38
Cooperative Clinical Group for the In-vestigation of Syphilis Treatment, 51, 52
Currie, Graham, 115, 117, 266

Cynicism, 277, 278
Cytapheresis, 178, 191, 202, 235, 236, 254, 347n29
Cytotoxic antisera, 101
Cytotoxic lymphocytes, 3, 86, 108, 120, 130, 133, 211, 248, 249, 251, 265. *See also* Killer T cells; Lymphokine-activated killer (LAK) cells; Natural killer (NK) cells; Tumor-infiltrating lymphocytes (TILs)

Da Fano, C., 89, 142
Damon Runyon Memorial Fund, 46
Dausset, Jean, 220, 350n5
De Kruif, Paul, 17
Délégation Générale de la Récherche, de la Science et de la Technologie (DGRST), 172
De Vita, Vincent, 75, 137
Dran, Henri, 39
Duclaux, Emile, 88
Durant, J. R., 140

Ehrlich, Paul, 87, 92
Endicott, Kenneth, 46, 55, 56, 58. *See also* Cancer Chemotherapy National Service Center
Erythropoietin, 193
European Organization for Research on the Treatment of Cancer, 67
Experimentation on humans, 68–69, 75, 104–105, 129, 320n82, 348n47

Fagot-Largeault, Anne, 50
Farber, Sidney, 42, 44
Feenberg, Andrew, 75, 302n61, 312n165
Feinstein, Alvin, 50
Fields, Robert, 150
Fleck, Ludwik, 22, 23, 290n15, 352n29
Flexner, Simon, 90
Fluorescein activated cell sorter (FACS), 132, 186, 233–234, 244, 246, 351n20
Food and Drug Adminstration (FDA), 11, 46, 60
Fox, Renée, 19, 293nn35,36, 343n170
Fox-Chase Cancer Center (Philadelphia), 219

Freireich, Emil, 75
French Association for Clinical Oncology, 221, 228, 241
French Ministry of Health, 171, 216, 241, 263
French Pediatric Oncology Group, 228, 229, 230, 241
Freudenthal, Gad, 359n76
Friedson, Eliot, 18, 293n33, 309n133

Gaudillière, Jean-Paul, 307n122
Geertz, Clifford, 23, 290n10
Geison, Gerald, 292n26
General Motors, 42, 136, 279
Gilman, Alfred, 40
Goodfield, June, 112
Goodman, Louis S., 40
Gresser, Ion, 120
Gutterman, Jordan, 110

Haddow, Alexander, 41
Hammer, Armand, 137
Hauschka, Theodore, 99
Hericourt, J., 102
Hevitt, Harold B., 116
"High-tech" medicine, 15, 151, 280
Holland, James, 75
Hunsaker-Hawkins, Anne, 283, 313n172
Hunter, Kathryn M., 291n18
Huxley, T. H., 112

IBM, 58, 59
Imperial Cancer Research Fund (London), 89, 92, 93
Institute of Laboratory Animal Resources, 47
Institut Gustave Roussy (Villejuif), 67
Institutional isomorphism, 72
Institut National de la Santé et de la Recherche Médicale (INSERM), 42, 51, 165, 172, 185, 241, 263, 344n2
Interferon, 4, 6, 76, 77, 85, 140, 141, 212; history as anticancer drug, 120–122, 179, 329n37; production of recombinant, 124–127, 329n41; hype, 154, 155, 201; interaction with LAK activity, 183–185, 188, 260

"Intermediary zone," 242–247, 248, 261, 278, 287
Isaacs, Alick, 120

Jackson Memorial Laboratories (Bar Harbor, Maine), 47, 97, 98, 318n56
James, John, 12
Jasmin, Claude, 68
Jerne, Niels, 159

Kay, Lily, 343n170
Kenney, Martin, 328n32
Kettering, Charles, 42, 279, 280
Kidney cancer (renal cell carcinoma): IL-2 in therapy, 3, 4, 8, 9, 149, 209, 212, 215, 216, 334n95; interferon in therapy, 125, 127, 212, 215
Kidney transplantation, 20, 85, 106, 202
Killer T cells, 119, 140, 142, 222, 233, 250, 257, 258
Knorr-Cetina, Karen, 21, 294n45
Kohler, Robert, 11, 290n9, 300n45, 315n12
Krim, Mathilde, 121

La Monica, Filippo, 150
Lasker, Mary, 44
Latour, Bruno, 21, 23, 291n20, 294n45, 361n21
Lawrence, Christopher, 292n27
Lerner, Carl, 78–79, 285
Lerner, Gerda, 78–79, 284, 285, 313n177
Leukemia: chemotherapy, 40, 44, 45, 57–60; acute lymphoblastic leukemia (ALL), 57, 58, 227, 229; animal models, 59, 111; BCG in therapy, 108–109; interferon in therapy, 125, 127, 328n36
Lewis, Jack, 78
"Life-style" considerations in disease, 280, 281, 287
Ligue Franco-Américaine Contre le Cancer, 38
Lindenmann, Jean, 120
Little, Clarence C., 97
Louis, Pierre, 16
Lymphokine-activated killer (LAK) cells, 29, 131–134, 137, 140, 143, 157; in

Lymphokine-activated killer (LAK) cells (*cont.*)
    therapy of renal cell carcinoma, 139, 149, 208–209, 216, 255; preparation, 165, 179, 180, 196, 232, 237, 244, 245; inhibition, 184–185, 188, 206–208, 244, 246, 254; in therapy of neuroblastoma, 189–194, 199, 200, 232; as "boundary objects," 250, 251, 256–258, 259
Lymphoma, 40, 125, 127; Hodgkin's, 59, 60
Lynch, Michael, 21

Major histocompatibility complex (MHC), 131, 141, 336n106
Marketing permits for anticancer drugs, 60, 149, 150, 340n135
Marks, Harry M., 51, 52, 53, 301n47, 303nn66, 67, 73, 304n75
Mathé, Georges, 107–108, 109, 110–111, 112, 113, 220
Measuring response to anticancer therapies, 275–276; "objective response," 61–62, 261; "measurable disease," 62, 276, 348n45
Medawar, Peter, 279, 280
Media images of cancer therapies, 12, 37, 171; of interferon, 122, 154; of IL-2, 136, 137, 151–156, 203–204, 240, 268, 348n39
Medical oncologists, 70, 109, 117, 146, 173, 268, 269, 273
Medical oncology, 28, 63–68, 73, 107
Medical Research Council (U.K.), 42, 51
Melanoma, 57, 266; IL-2 in therapy, 5, 8, 9, 138, 212, 215, 216, 239; BCG in therapy, 110, 113; interferon in therapy, 125, 127; TILs in therapy, 145, 209–210, 217
Memorial Hospital (New York), 42, 102, 103
Merton, Robert, 21
Metchnikoff, Elie, 87
Mortel, Charles, 138
Morton, D. L., 110
Morton, John J., 90
Moulin, Anne-Marie, 314n8, 321n92, 343n169

Murphy, James Baumgardner, 40, 89–92, 98, 108

National Cancer Institute (NCI), 39, 58, 65, 73, 110, 116, 120, 160, 287; screening programs, 42–44, 60; and cancer chemotherapy, 45, 61, 64, 75, 104; NCI/FDA Joint Task Force on anticancer drugs, 61, 69; and BRM Program, 122, 124; and IL-2 therapy, 136, 139
National Chemotherapy Program, 60, 64, 122
National Institutes of Health (NIH), 77, 129, 135
Natural killer (NK) cells, 6, 118, 119, 222, 250, 260; induction by interferon, 121, 128, 131, 133; induction by IL-2, 141, 227
NCI/FDA Joint Task Force on anticancer drugs, 61, 69
Neuroblastoma, 188; IL-2/LAK in therapy, 189–194, 199, 200, 247, 265; and bone marrow graft, 194, 226–230, 270, 274
Nicolle, Maurice, 88
Noriega, Johnny, 151, 152
Norris Cancer Hospital (Los Angeles), 37, 286
Nossal, Gustav, 85

Office of Scientific Research and Development (OSRD), 40, 42, 51
Old, Lloyd, 107
Oldham, Robert, 123, 127, 137, 201, 327n23, 337n109. *See also* Biological Response Modifiers (BRM) Program; Biotherapeutics, Inc.
Ordre des Médecins, 66
Organizational efficiency, 53, 54, 61
Oudshoorn, Nelly, 361n22
"Out of protocol" patients, 238–240, 271, 352n23

Panem, Sandra, 128, 154, 326n11
Park, Robert, 22
Parke-Davis Company, 103
Pasteur, Louis, 88, 328n35

Pathograpies, 70–79, 283–286, 313n173

Patient-derived biological materials, 9, 31, 235–236, 238, 246, 253, 261, 270

Philadelphia Institute for Cancer Research, 42, 54

Pickering, Andrew, 21

Pickstone, John, 293n32, 359n6

Pieters, Toine, 302n60, 326n11

Pinch, Trevor, 21, 294n45, 295n47

Pinell, Patrice, 297n6, 298nn13,15

Placebo effect, 48, 75

Polymerase chain reaction (PCR), 147, 150

Porter, Theodore M., 52, 302n62, 303n72

Public Health Service (U.S.), 51; Office for Cancer Investigations, 41, 103

Rabinow, Paul, 162

Radiation therapists, 38, 63, 109, 110, 174, 177

Radiation therapy for cancer, 37–38, 39, 54, 63, 66, 67, 82, 83

Raucher, Frank, 122

Renal cell carcinoma. *See* Kidney cancer

"Resistance" to transplanted tumors, 92–95, 97–98

Restivo, Sal, 21

Révy, Jean Claude, 153, 154

Rhoads, Cornelius, 42, 44

Richards, Evelleen, 76, 302n60

Richet, C., 102

Robinson, Ian, 50

Rockefeller Institute (New York), 40, 89, 90

Rokitanski, Karl, 16

Rosenberg, Charles, 283, 292n23, 306n108

Rosenberg, Steven, 29, 129–131, 133–137, 142–145, 152, 175, 200, 201, 209, 219, 223, 282

Rosenthal, Ted, 285

Rous, Peyton, 89, 94

Royal Cancer Hospital (U.K.), 41

Saint Louis Hospital (Paris), 67

"Science-laden" medical interventions, 280, 281, 287

"Scientific medicine," 15–18, 67, 80, 82, 280

Screening for anticancer substances, 42–44, 46, 47, 55, 82, 103, 122. *See also* Biological Response Modifiers (BRM) Program; Cancer Chemotherapy National Service Center

"Secondary effects" of Il-2 therapy, 2, 136, 139, 211, 230, 335n97; capillary leak syndrome, 207, 272; atypical, 208, 269, 274–275; psychiatric disorders, 213, 270, 272, 334n95

Serotherapy of cancer (specific), 84, 100, 101, 102, 104, 107

Serratia marcescens, 41, 102; *Serratia* polysaccharide, 41, 103

Serres, Michel, 133

Shapin, Steven, 296n62, 354n43, 359n76

Shapiro, Kenneth, 77

Shear, Murray, 41, 42

Silverstein, Arthur M., 314n8, 315n15, 321n92

Skoda, Joseph, 16

Sloan, Alfred, P., 42

Sloan-Kettering Institute (New York), 42, 43, 44, 54, 104, 121, 279

Smalley, Richard, 127

Smith, Kendall, 142

Snell, George, 97

Southam, Chester, 99, 104–105, 117, 320n82

Spencer, R. R., 99

Star, Susan Leigh, 21, 294n45, 345n12, 353nn30,32, 357n64

Stereotyped images of biomedical research, 12–13, 277, 278

Strander, Hans, 121

Sturdy, Steve, 300n34

Surgeons, 109, 110, 173, 217, 238, 253

Surgical treatment of cancer, 37, 39, 82, 83

Swann, John P., 344n172

Swazey, Judith, 19, 293n35, 343n170

Tanigushi, Tadatsugu, 124, 129

Technical efficiency, 53, 54, 61

Teitelman, Robert, 327n18

Terry, William, 113

Therapeutic protocols, 226–230, 231, 265, 273–274
"Thick description," 11, 32, 163
Thompson, E. P., 34, 35
Tribondeau, Louis, 37
Tumor immunology, 28, 92, 98, 99–100, 111, 118
Tumor-infiltrating lymphocytes (TILs), 142–145, 196, 257, 258; preparation, 165, 192, 199, 209, 245, 246, 255–256; in melanoma therapy, 209–210, 253
Tumor necrotic factor (TNF), 144, 172, 219, 260
Tumor-specific antigens, 98, 99, 114

U.S. Congress, 44, 45, 46, 75

Vaccination against cancer (specific), 84, 100, 101, 102, 104, 107, 109

Veterans Administration (U.S.), 46, 48, 51, 55

Warner, John Harley, 292n26
Weiss, David, 115
Weiss, Geoffrey, 152
Weissman, Charles, 124
Weisz, George, 301n49
Woglom, William, 84, 94, 95–96, 97
Woolgar, Steve, 21, 23, 294n45

X rays: in cancer therapy, 37, 38, 59, 90, 91; in cancer diagnosis and monitoring, 62, 258, 277; in cancer research, 90, 315n23

Zenzen, Michael, 21
Zubrod, Gordon, 46, 58, 60. *See also* Cancer Chemotherapy National Service Center

RETURN